GENETIC RISK, RISK PERCEPTION, AND DECISION MAKING

RECENT TITLES PUBLISHED BY ALAN R. LISS, INC. FOR MARCH OF DIMES BIRTH DEFECTS FOUNDATION

Birth Defects Compendium, Second Edition, Daniel Bergsma, *Editor*

BIRTH DEFECTS: ORIGINAL ARTICLE SERIES

1982 — Volume 18

No. 1 **Craniofacial Anomalies: New Perspectives,** Carlos F. Salinas, *Editor*
No. 3A **Annual Review of Birth Defects, 1981, Prenatal Diagnosis and Mechanisms of Teratogenesis,** William L. Nyhan and Kenneth Lyons Jones, *Editors*
No. 3B **Annual Review of Birth Defects, 1981, Dysmorphology,** William L. Nyhan and Kenneth Lyons Jones, *Editors*
No. 4 **Children With Sex Chromosome Aneuploidy: Follow-Up Studies,** Donald A. Stewart, *Editor*
No. 5 **Cumulative Index: Birth Defects: Original Article Series Volumes I (1965)–XVI (1980),** Natalie W. Paul, *Editor*
No. 6 **Genetic Eye Diseases: Retinitis Pigmentosa and Other Inherited Eye Disorders,** Edward Cotlier, Irene H. Maumenee, and Elaine R. Berman, *Editors*
No. 7 **Thalassemia: Recent Advances in Detection and Treatment,** Antonio Cao, Ugo Carcassi, and Peter T. Rowley, *Editors*

1983 — Volume 19

No. 1 **Dentition: Genetic Effects,** Ronald J. Jorgenson, *Editor*
No. 3 **Primary Immunodeficiency Diseases,** Ralph J. Wedgwood, Fred S. Rosen, and Natalie W. Paul, *Editors*
No. 4 **Nervous System Regeneration,** Bernard Haber, J. Regino Perez-Polo, George A. Hashim, and Anna Maria Giuffrida Stella, *Editors*
No. 5 **Annual Review of Birth Defects, 1982, Birth Defects: Clinical and Ethical Considerations,** Sara C. Finley, Wayne H. Finley, and Charles E. Flowers, Jr., *Editors*

1984 — Volume 20

No. 1 **CMV: Pathogenesis and Prevention of Human Infection,** Stanley A. Plotkin, Susan Michelson, Joseph S. Pagano, and Fred Rapp, *Editors*
No. 3 **Craniofacial Mesenchyme in Morphogenesis and Malformation,** Kenneth S. Brown and Carlos F. Salinas, *Editors*

1985 — Volume 21

No. 2 **Diagnostic Accuracy: Effect on Treatment Planning,** Robert J. Shprintzen and Natalie W. Paul, *Editors*
No. 5 **The Patient Within the Patient: Problems in Perinatal Medicine,** Bruce K. Young, *Editor*

1986 — Volume 22

No. 1 **Bone Marrow Transplantation for Treatment of Lysosomal Storage Diseases,** William Krivit and Natalie W. Paul, *Editors*
No. 3 **Prospective Studies on Children With Sex Chromosome Aneuploidy,** Shirley G. Ratcliffe and Natalie W. Paul, *Editors*

1987 — Volume 23

No. 1 **Genetic Aspects of Developmental Pathology,** Enid F. Gilbert and John M. Opitz, *Editors*

Please contact the publisher for information about previous titles in this series published by Alan R. Liss, Inc.

March of Dimes Birth Defects Foundation
Birth Defects: Original Article Series, Volume 23, Number 2, 1987

GENETIC RISK, RISK PERCEPTION, AND DECISION MAKING

Proceedings of a Conference Held
July 28–29, 1986, Leuven, Belgium

Editors

Gerry Evers-Kiebooms, PhD
Center for Human Genetics
University of Leuven
Leuven, Belgium

Jean-Jacques Cassiman, MD
Center for Human Genetics
University of Leuven
Leuven, Belgium

Herman Van den Berghe, MD
Center for Human Genetics
University of Leuven
Leuven, Belgium

Géry d'Ydewalle, PhD
Laboratory of Experimental Psychology
University of Leuven
Leuven, Belgium

ALAN R. LISS, INC., NEW YORK

To enhance medical communication in the birth defects field, the March of Dimes Birth Defects Foundation publishes the *Birth Defects Compendium (2nd Edition)*, an *Original Article Series*, a *Reprint Series*, *Nursing Staff Development Modules*, *Genetics in Practice* (a quarterly newsletter), and provides a series of films and related brochures.

Further information can be obtained from:

Professional Education Department
March of Dimes Birth Defects Foundation
1275 Mamaroneck Avenue
White Plains, New York 10605

Published by:
Alan R. Liss, Inc.
41 East 11th Street
New York, New York 10003

Views expressed in articles published are the authors', and are not to be attributed to the March of Dimes Birth Defects Foundation or its editors unless expressly so stated.

Library of Congress Cataloging-in-Publication Data

Genetic risk, risk perception, and decision making.

(Birth defects, original article series ; v. 23, no. 2)
Includes index.
1. Medical genetics—Congresses. 2. Genetic counseling—Decision making—Congresses. 3. Prenatal diagnosis—Decision making—Congresses. 4. Health risk assessment—Congresses. I. Evers-Kiebooms, G. II. Series.
RG626.B63 vol. 23, no. 2 616'.042 s 86-34264
[RB155] [616'.042]
ISBN 0-8451-1064-0

The March of Dimes Birth Defects Foundation is dedicated to the goals of preventing birth defects and ameliorating their consequences for patients, families, and society.

As part of our efforts to achieve these goals, we sponsor, or participate in, a variety of scientific meetings where all questions relating to birth defects are freely discussed. Through our professional education program we speed the dissemination of information by publishing the proceedings of these and other meetings. From time to time, we also reprint pertinent journal articles to help achieve our goals. Now and then, in the course of these articles or discussions, individual viewpoints may be expressed which go beyond the purely scientific and into controversial matters. It should be noted, therefore, that personal viewpoints about such matters will not be censored but this does not constitute an endorsement of them by the **March of Dimes Birth Defects Foundation**.

CONTENTS

LIST OF SPEAKERS

Howard CANN, Centre d'Etude du Polymorphisme Humain, 3, rue d'Ulm, 75006 PARIS, FRANCE

Jean-Jacques CASSIMAN, K.U. Leuven, Centrum voor Menselijke Erfelijkheid, Campus Gasthuisberg, Herestraat, B-3000 LEUVEN, BELGIUM

Gerry EVERS-KIEBOOMS, K.U. Leuven, Centrum voor Menselijke Erfelijkheid, Campus Gasthuisberg, Herestraat, B-3000 LEUVEN, BELGIUM

Jean-Pierre FRYNS, K.U. Leuven, Centrum voor Menselijke Erfelijkheid, Campus Gasthuisberg, Herestraat, B-3000 LEUVEN, BELGIUM

Patrick HUMPHREYS and Dina BERKELEY, The London School of Economics and Political Science, Houghton Street, LONDON WC2A 2AE, U.K.

Stephen G. PAUKER, Tufts University School of Medicine, New England Medical Center, 171 Harrison Avenue, BOSTON MA 02111, U.S.A.

Susan PERLMUTTER-PAUKER, Boston Center, Department of Genetics, Harvard Community Health Plan, 147 Milk Street, BOSTON MA 02 109, U.S.A.

Gordon F. PITZ, University at Carbondale, Department of Psychology, CARBONDALE, ILLINOIS 62901, U.S.A.

Anne SWERTS, K.U. Leuven, Centrum voor Menselijke Erfelijkheid, Campus Gasthuisberg, Herestraat, B-3000 LEUVEN, BELGIUM

Audrey TYLER, Medical Genetics, Heath Park, CARDIFF CF4 4XW, U.K.

Herman VAN DEN BERGHE, K.U. Leuven, Centrum voor Menselijke Erfelijkheid, Campus Gasthuisberg, Herestraat, B-3000 LEUVEN, BELGIUM

Charles A.J.VLEK, Vakgroep Sociale Psychologie, Rijksuniversiteit Groningen, Kraneweg 2, 9718 JP GRONINGEN, NEDERLAND

Robert VLIETINCK, K.U. Leuven, Centrum voor Menselijke Erfelijkheid, Campus Gasthuisberg, Herestraat, B-3000 LEUVEN, BELGIUM

Géry d'YDEWALLE, K. U. Leuven, Departement Psychologie, Afdeling Algemene en Experimentele Psychologie, Tiensestraat 102, B-3000 LEUVEN, BELGIE

PREFACE

The technology available to human geneticists for the diagnosis of an ever increasing number of heritable diseases and traits has evolved over the last twenty years to an arsenal of sophisticated, be it routine, tests. While the contribution of gross chromosomal anomalies, such as trisomies, to genetic pathology has been long recognized, small structural chromosome defects are now being detected, by high resolution banding techniques, in syndromes previously considered to be due to single gene defects. The recent application of recombinant DNA technology to human genetics has, once more revolutionized this discipline. Specific DNA-probes visualize various structural changes in genomic DNA, or polymorphic sites in DNA sequences closely linked to a particular gene. The diagnosis and carrier detection of many a disease, even poorly understood in its pathogenesis, is becoming a reality. Indeed, more genetic information is available on more and more people.

All this contrasts sharply with the knowledge, awareness and understanding of the general public, the actual consumers of these matters. The need for appropriate information, and for support in the decision making about genetic problems has reached a critical stage. Genetic counseling, which aims at the prevention of handicaps by giving appropriate information to those concerned, places people before complex and/or painful decisions for which they are poorly prepared but which nevertheless require responsible decision making.

In the field of risk perception a large body of research has been devoted to judgmental heuristics. These were studied in the laboratory as well as in real life situations. Concepts and theories concerning "perceived risk" and "acceptable risk" have been developed during the last decade. The evaluation of technological risks (e.g., safety of the implantation of LPG

terminals or nuclear reactors) was the most important application field for risk analysis and risk perception.
The boundary between risk perception and decision making is not always clear. Attempts were made to establish a compendium of the cognitive mechanisms and processes involved in judgement and decision making tasks. Based on this understanding, procedures were developed for helping people make important decisions. These decision aids were applied to a broad range of problems, e.g., program evaluation, managerial planning. Applications in the field of personal decisions however were very limited.

Over the years, several members of the Center for Human Genetics of the Unversity of Leuven in Belgium, realized that the genetic counseling situation has many elements in common with other situations dealing with risk perception and decision making under uncertainty. A symposium would provide the opportunity to exchange information between the two fields in a mutual concern to explore if, and to what extent, concepts, theories and models from the field of risk perception and decision making could be helpful in providing information on genetic problems and in supporting the decision making process. The enthusiast response of many researchers, working in the field of risk perception and decision making, made the organization of the present symposium on July 28 and 29th a reality.

After a general introduction on the "Impact of genetics on society", the first day of the symposium was dedicated to presentations concerning the state of the art in the field of genetics. New developments in cytogenetics, classical genetics and in the diagnosis by linkage at the DNA-level were reviewed. Recent studies by the Center for Human Genetics of the University of Leuven evaluating the impact of genetic counseling and prenatal diagnosis were presented during this first session. During the second day of the symposium experts in the field of risk perception and decision making discussed their theoretical models and decision aiding technologies in general or applied to the field of genetic risk perception and to decision-making involving 'genetic risks'. Experimental approaches to some aspects of genetic risk perception and decision making were also briefly presented during this meeting.
The gap existing between the two fields and the possible use of "decision support programs" in genetic counseling was critically and thoroughly discussed at the end of the symposium. The main points of this discussion are included here and an effort was made to reproduce the interventions of the different discussants as faithfully as possible.
The conference provided an excellent platform for geneticists, psychologists and social scientists to explain their respective disciplines to each other. The possible contribution of research work on risk perception and decision making to the quality of the genetic counseling, aimed at

helping people with genetic problems, was explored.
The problems are complex and this conference could not possibly discuss all aspects of the subject. Nevertheless, the basis was laid for further fruitful exchanges and cross-fertilization of the different fields in the future and as such this symposium can be considered to be a unique event.

Acknowledgments

The editors are extremely grateful for the organizational and editorial assistance of Ms M. De Dobbeleer. Together with Ms E. Vander Heyden she can also take full credit for the quality of the layout and the typing of these proceedings. Mrs D. Manet and Mrs A. Swerts are acknowledged for revising some of the manuscripts and Mrs C. Verjauw for technical assistance. Mr K. Rondou skillfully prepared all the photographic work.

The financial support from the University of Leuven, from the National Science Foundation Belguim, and from the March of Dimes Birth Defects Foundation is gratefully acknowledged.

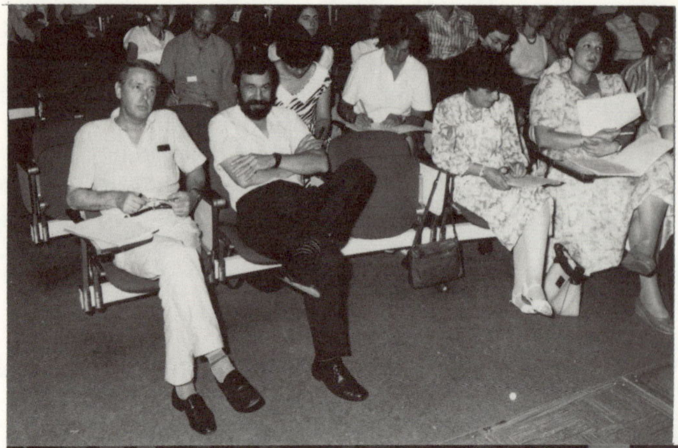

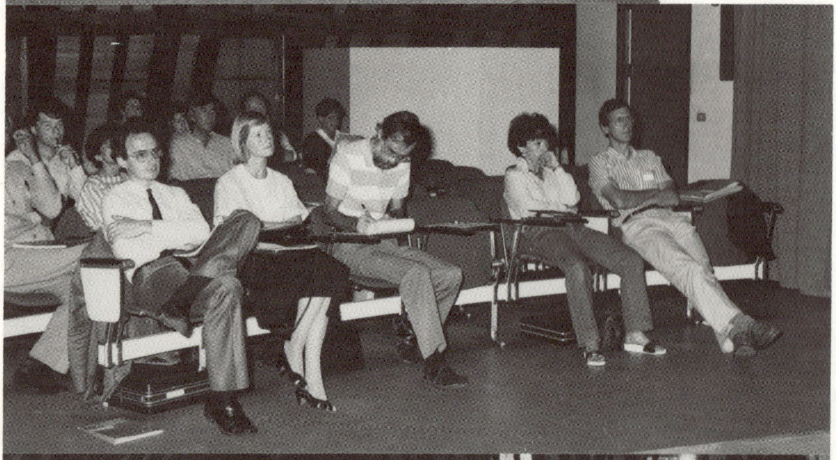

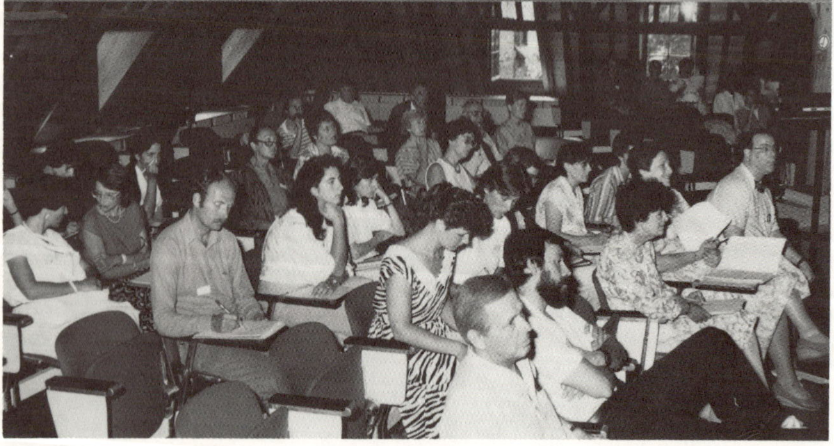

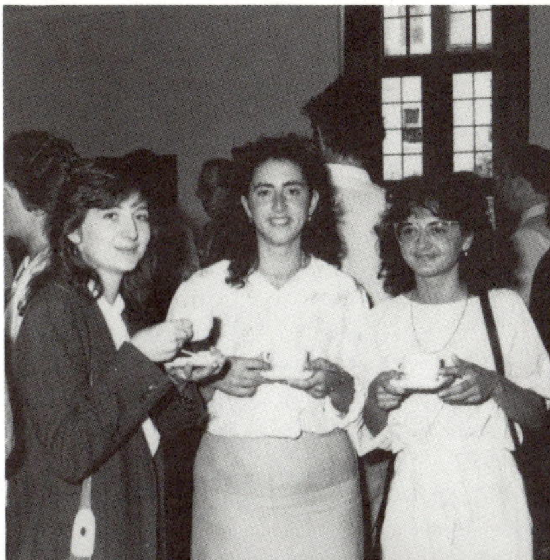
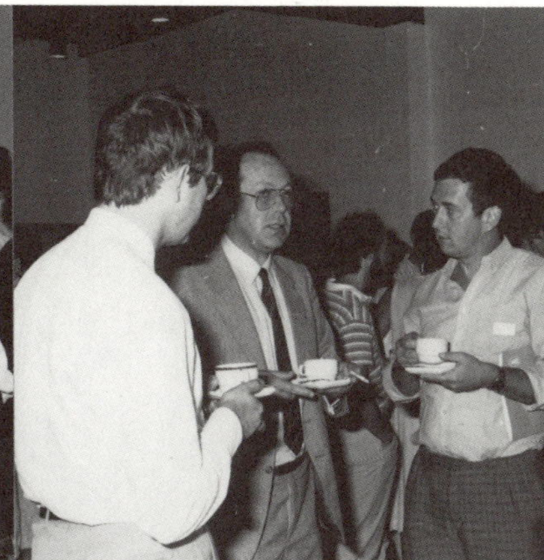
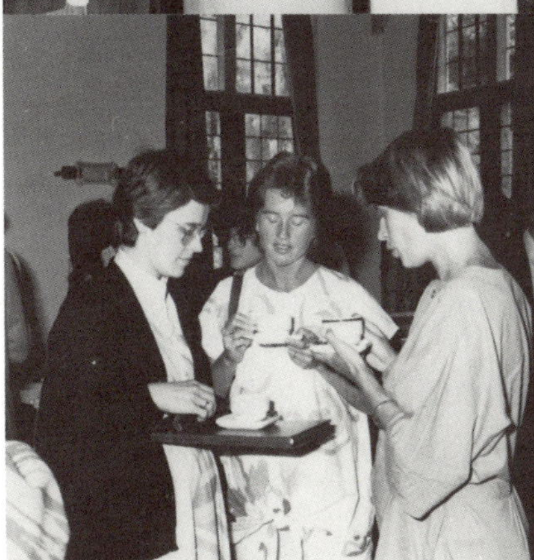
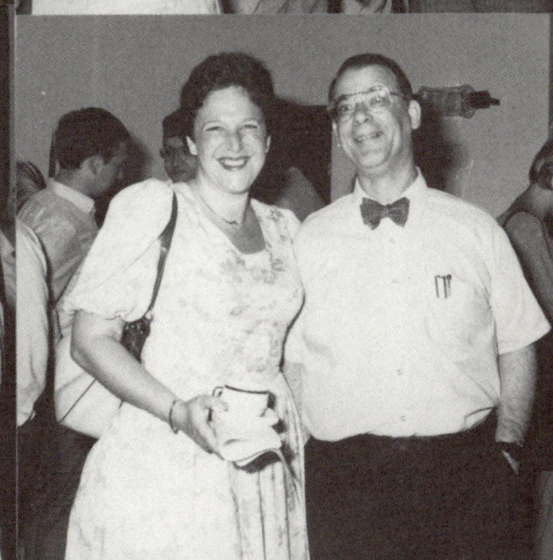
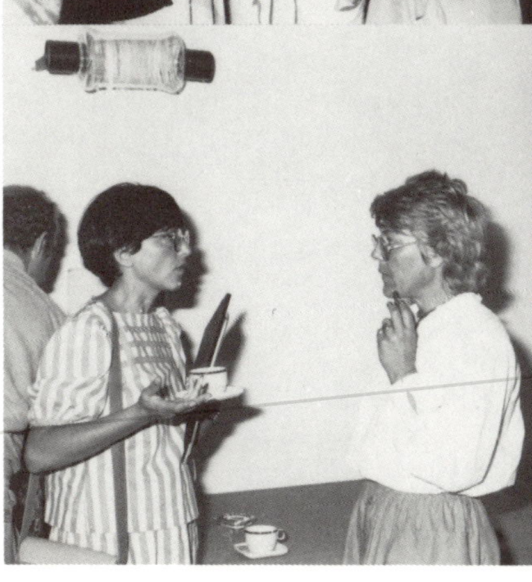
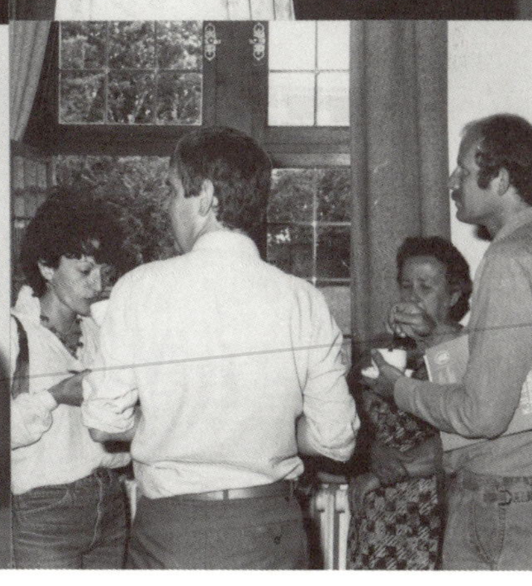

IMPACT OF GENETICS ON SOCIETY

Herman VAN DEN BERGHE

Center for Human Genetics, K.U.Leuven
Campus Gasthuisberg, Herestraat, B-3000, Leuven, Belgium

Modern genetics, especially human genetics, although it has many of its roots in the 19th and in the first half of the 20th century, is largely a science of the past 30 years.

Evidence that DNA is a genetic molecule capable of changing the heredity of bacteria was reported in 1949; the double helix leading to the explanation of how the molecules of life replicate and how they code for the vital substances we need was established in 1953. Human chromosomes and those of other mammals were not clearly visualized until 1956. Reverse transcriptase and restriction enzymes which opened the way for recombinant DNA were discovered in 1970, and the first recombinant DNA molecules, derived from two different parental molecules, using simple test tube procedures were produced in 1973.
Today, barely 13 years later, recombinant DNA techniques are used in all scientific and economic areas of modern biology.

In agriculture more and larger crops can be harvested, plants are made resistant to parasites, they are being modified to produce their own fertilizers, and new recombinant plants are being designed. Biotechnology based on recombinant DNA techniques now produces industrial quantities of naturally substances such as insulin and other hormones that previously had to be extracted with tremendous efforts and at exorbitant costs from animals or deceased human individuals, thus creating totally new possibilities for euphenic treatment of genetic and other diseases.

The first human gene was sequenced only 9 years ago. Since then, more than 500 human structural genes have been sequenced, plus a whole series of anonymous DNA-sequences. For some genetic disorders, gene therapy is already appearing on the horizon, in the first place by bone marrow transplantation, but correction by other methods is likely to break

Birth Defects: Original Article Series, Volume 23, Number 2, pages 1–5

through in the near future. From what has already been achieved in the field, one may also predict that perhaps within the next five to ten years, and almost certainly before the end of this century, the majority of frequent genetic diseases, be they dominant, recessive or X-linked, will be detectable early in embryonic life and at any moment thereafter. It can hardly be predicted what other developments may be expected during the same period. Perhaps they will include the first steps of molecular behavioral genetics, thus entering an area which at present is still a box of Pandora. In any case, modern genetics will make tomorrow's society totally different from what it was until now. For the first time man will shape himself the things to come, including his own genetic heritage. From now on Shakespeare's words "...there is a divinity that shapes our ends, rough hew-them how you will" (Hamlet V, ii, 10) will no longer be valid. More than ever before, will there be a need for normative descriptions of what human society should be like. We have had some of such predictions and normative descriptions in the past : Plato's Republic and Laws, Thomas More's Utopia written here in Leuven, Huxley's Brave New World, Well's The Shape of Things to Come, and George Orwell's 1984. Those efforts were the work of individuals, and they were not always projecting an ideal world. Today, large groups of natural scientists, technologists, social engineers working in universities, industry and government bodies, subsidized by government as well as private funds are investigating what advances are likely to be made, time tables for their achievement, and the effects they will have on war and peace, on social structure and virtually all other aspects of human existence. Planning in our society of today and tomorrow is no longer a simple matter of looking ahead five years, and explorations of the future are pursued with great vigor. With regard to this future, one question dominates all others, namely whether there even will be a future, because of the continuous treat of nuclear war. If, however, we will be spared from such a nuclear holocaust, our future will see genetics involved to a very large extent in medicine and public health, law and politics, agriculture and industry, nuclear developments and space exploration, and last but not least, with religion and social relations.

Will this involvement be for the good or for the bad of mankind, of human evolution ? There is a feedback between biology and culture. Ethical beliefs have evolutionary consequences, just as ongoing human evolution creates ethical problems. I'll not try to make predictions of what the general impact of genetics on society will be, let alone make normative prescriptions. What I would like to do in these few minutes is on the basis of what we know today, to raise a few questions about the possible immediate impacts of the tremendous development in human genetics on individuals, families and society of today.

I'll not raise a question which has come up several times in the past, and which I am sure will be heard again when some of the possible impacts of genetics on society will be discussed : **Is all this research necessary;** it is clear that new knowledge creates new problems; why then always pushing things further and further. In other words, is freedom of research, as a supreme expression of man's natural curiosity one of the highest values we should cherish, or should society control the directions research is taking. History learns us at least two things in this respect. First : Science has never been entirely free. Centuries ago, scientists could be physically contained; think of Galilei. Now methods are more subtle : one may simply lose one's support. Second : Despite all possible difficulties, man, throughout history has always done and applied everything he could.

A following, more directly pertinent question is that of **Natural selection versus intervention.**

During the past 20 years man has gained considerable insight in where he comes from (evolution), how by chromosomal changes and mutations under selection pressure, this evolution took place, how the same mechanisms of chromosome changes and gene mutations now are a source of major problems that threaten life or impede its quality; what the intimate nature is of his genetic material, and how he can change it. Faced with these abnormalities and armed with those insights man no longer accepts this burden as such; man is no longer willing to submit himself to blind natural selection, especially when he observes what he considers to be deficiencies in the selection process; man wants to intervene, ideally by repairing the genetic errors he observes, but that goal is not yet within reach immediately. Therefore he wants to trace, to diagnose these errors as much as possible, and he tries to prevent them from being passed on to the next generation; in addition he wants to complete the "imperfect" prenatally occurring natural selection by diagnosing genetic errors in utero and terminating the pregnancy.

All this is to be seen in the context of a mutual influence of society on the scientist, the geneticist, and of the geneticist on society. One of the recent changes in western society is that reproduction has been quantitatively regulated even to the extent that there is no replacement at the present time, but also that there is a very big concern about the quality of the children that are born.
Here we observe that a centuries-long impact of christianity has been lost in recent years : **Man in this society of to-day can no longer find any sense in suffering, especially when it hits him, on a genetic basis, in his existential prolongation which is the child.**
Therefore, man, faced with genetically determined abnormalities and suffering tries, as much as possible, to diagnose the presence of abnormal genes and prevent their occurrence.

The way this is done is primarily through diagnostic genetic services, which also provide ample information to the individuals and families concerned, so that they can make decisions in responsible freedom about having children or to have more children. This whole procedure called genetic counseling will eventually have a considerable impact on society, as abnormal genes can be increasingly diagnosed, including the harmless carrier-status of recessive genes. The impact of this necessarily non-directive procedure will not be fast. Its effect on the gene-pool of the population will however be considerable with time.
The basic ethical question here is : what to tell, to whom, when and how ? Many problems arise here : it speaks for itself that the diagnosis made and the information given must be correct, that information should only be given to whom is asking for it, at the appropriate time and in a non-directive way. Besides diagnosis and counseling at the individual level, there is also diagnosis and information at the level of the population. So far genetic screening is done in industrialized countries, for some 8-10 inborn errors of metabolism, some of which can be phenotypically helped or corrected by medication starting immediately after birth. Tomorrow, however, recombinant DNA technology will allow for screening of e.g. carriers of cystic fibrosis and other frequent or less frequent genetic diseases. Shall we organize such a screening, what will be its impact on people ? or society ? Time is lacking to analyze all these problems in depth and I will only mention a few which come up immediately.

1. If considerable emphasis is put on prevention of genetic disease, is not there a danger that a child which despite prevention programs is born with a genetic disease will be considered as a "missed prevention" with all the possible consequences?
2. Will identification of a carrier-status not lead to discrimination of all sorts (jobs, schools etc..)?
3. Will any pressure be put on carriers not to marry, not to have children ? If nevertheless they do have children, possibly even abnormal ones, will they not be penalized?
4. What may be the impact of genetic diagnosis on social security, on health insurance? We now live in a paradigm that every person has the same chances to become sick. In the future, genetic diagnosis will show individual risks of having genetic diseases, cardiovascular morbidity, cancer. Shall society give up solidarity?

These are just a few important questions that illustrate how big the impact of genetics on society may possibly become.

A depressing observation is

1. that genetic knowledge is increasing at a tremendous rate, which by itself is all right
2. but that society is not prepared to receive this information, let alone to do something with this information that has a sound ethical basis.

> Every human being is involved in the ethical, social and political problems of his age of science, problems that are multiplying in geometrical progression in the wake of scientific and technological advances. Making the right decisions in individual cases may seem trivial, yet it requires a considerable amount of information that has to be acquired and integrated. The collective decision of what man wants to do with its species is not trivial at all, and the development of an effective and just machinery for collective ethical decision making should have a high priority on mankind's agenda. Only an informed society can accomplish this task. That is why an understanding of genetics, of the new biology and of the evolutionary outlook are indispensable ingredients in the cultural heritage of every person.

Here I would personally drop a pessimistic note : I do not see how we can provide enough information to a large enough proportion of society, within the shortest possible time which should be long enough to integrate this enormously growing body of information into sound human ethics which includes not only the moral ideal of goodness, but also the scientific ideal of perfect knowledge, the esthetic ideal of beauty, and the economic ideal of abundance understood as sufficient to give everybody all possible chances, including the less-valid, the handicapped individuals.
I am afraid that with technology and knowledge growing so fast, but with this knowledge being in the hands of scientists only, that by simply offering this technology to the population at large, we are now taking a very big responsibility, and that with only a handful of people we are very deeply influencing an unprepared society.

I want you to think about it.

CHROMOSOMAL ANOMALIES AND AUTOSOMAL SYNDROMES

Jean Pierre FRYNS

Center for Human Genetics, K.U. Leuven
Campus Gasthuisberg, Herestraat, B-3000 Leuven, Belgium

INTRODUCTION

The detailed study of human chromosome morphology began in 1956 when the correct number of human chromosomes was reported as 46. With the so-called conventionally stained chromosomes only numerical and relatively large structural abnormalities could be detected. Human cytogenetics was revolutionized by the discovery that quinacrine staining under ultraviolet light produces a unique banding pattern for each chromosome (Casperson et al., 1971). A band is defined as a region which can be distinguished from a neighboring region on the basis of its difference in staining intensity, and therefore permits a more detailed analysis of chromosomal rearrangements such as, among others, translocations, deletions and duplications. Since then, several other banding procedures have been developed. A G-banded karyotype is shown in figure 1.

Here we will first discuss different types of autosomal aberrations i.e., numerical aberrations, structural rearrangements (ring chromosomes, deletions and duplications) with special attention for a number of clinically recognizable syndromes which are associated with such specific chromosomal changes.

The advent of more detailed banding techniques combined with the availability of prometaphase chromosomes in the further delineation and classification of human malformation syndromes will be discussed in a paragraph on the new cytogenetics.

Finally, the contribution of cytogenetics in the diagnosis of mental retardation and of recurrent early fetal wastage will be illustrated and discussed.

Birth Defects: Original Article Series, Volume 23, Number 2, pages 7–32

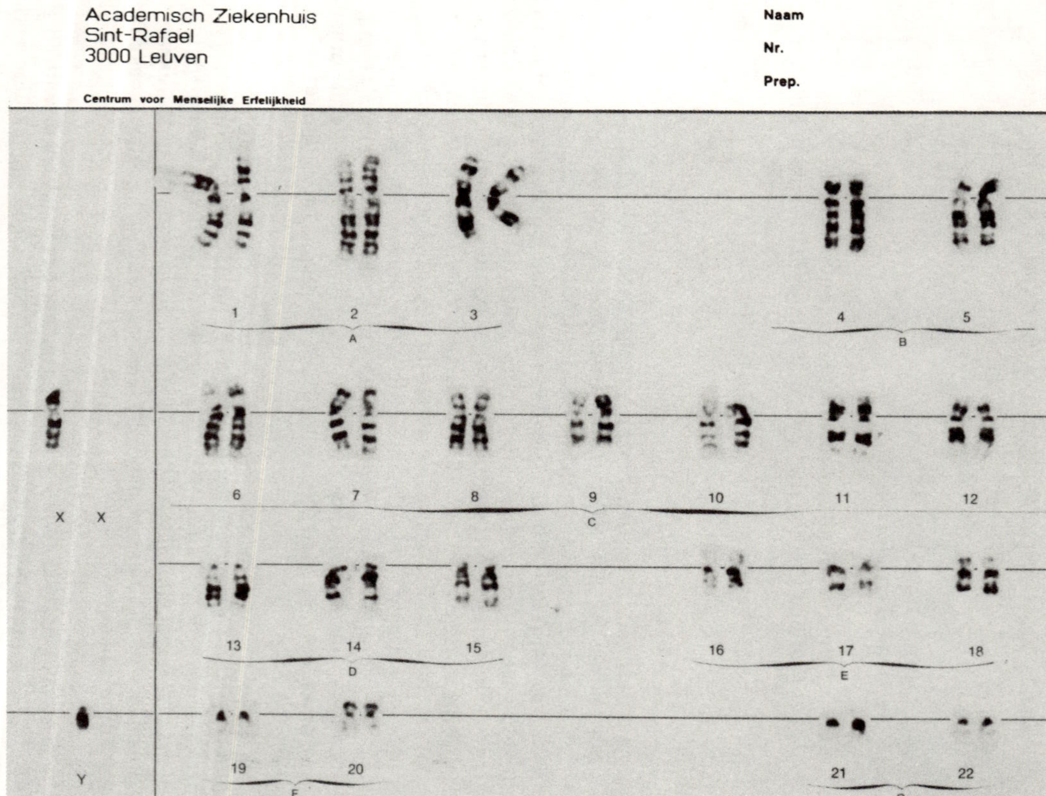

Figure 1 : G-banded karyotype : 46, XY normal male karyotype

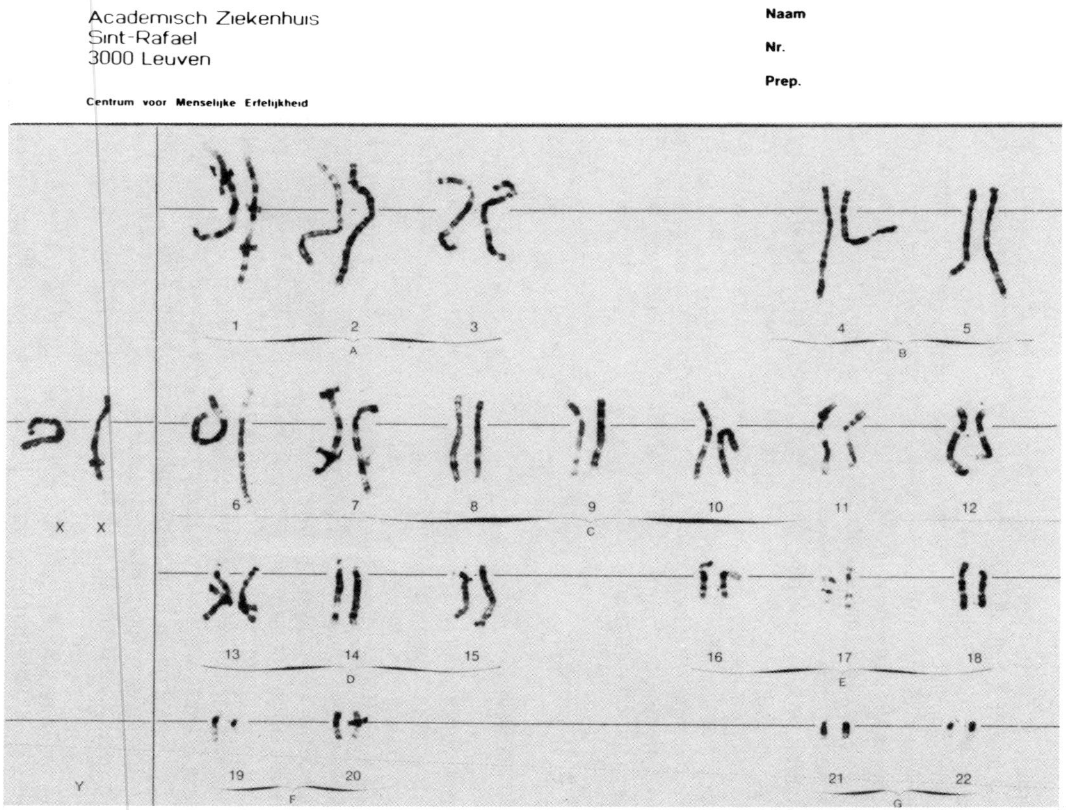

Figure 2 : Prometaphase chromosome banding

I. AUTOSOMAL ABNORMALITIES

1.1. Numerical aberrations

Numerical rearrangements consist essentially of trisomies which result from meiotic non-disjunction and are largely dependent on increasing maternal age. All possible trisomies are produced and seen in spontaneous abortions, but only a few are observed at birth. Monosomies are, as a rule, not compatible with birth, and they are even rarely found in products of early fetal wastage. Mosaicism is a postzygotic event and occurs at an early cell division after fertilization. It results in the birth of an individual with two or more cell lines having a different chromosome constitutions. With a few exceptions, numerical rearrangements occur de novo in patients born to parents having normal karyotypes. The best documented exception is a mosaic state in a parent without phenotypic expression, while it has also been suggested that certain specific chromosome rearrangements (i.e., translocations) may increase the risk of non-disjunction for any other chromosome (Lejeune et al., 1963) possibly due to interchromosomal effect.

1.1.1. Trisomy 21

General data

Down syndrome is the predominant single cause of mental retardation. Ten to twenty percent of inmates in institutions for the mentally retarded have Down syndrome. Down syndrome, Mongolism or trisomy 21, has been known as a clinical entity since Langdon Down described the clinical features in 1866. As early as 1932 the dutch ophthalmologist Waardenburg suggested that Down syndrome might be caused by a chromosomal aberration (Waardenburg, 1932). In 1959 Lejeune et al. (1959) described an extra chromosome called 21 or G21 in this syndrome. After the introduction of the Q-banding it became clear that the extra chromosome was a small acrocentric with a broad band of intense fluorescence and a distal pale band, very different from chromosome 22. It has also been shown that it was probably a triplication of the distal Q12 pale band which causes the clinical picture in trisomy 21.

The incidence of 21 trisomy is 1.45 per 1000, or about 1 for every 700 births. The maternal age is a well known etiological factor. Mean maternal age is 34.4 years as compared to 28.2 years in the general population. The biological basis of the maternal age effect is far from being understood. Many mechanisms have been suggested, such as delayed fertilization and ageing of the ovaries, but none has been convincingly proven.

Clinical diagnosis of 21 trisomy must be made at birth and rapidly confirmed by karyotype analysis to avoid giving erroneous information to the parents. Generalized muscular hypotonia and joint hyperlaxity are the most striking clinical features at birth, and are associated with a round, flat face with flat occiput, upslanting of palpebral fissures, epicanthal folds, and Brushfieds spots in the irides. The hands and feet are small, with characteristic incurvation of the 5th finger due to brachymesophalangy, and an increased space between the first two toes. Life expectancy is dependent on the presence of internal malformations of which cardiovascular anomalies (mainly atrioventricular defects) and gastroenterological malformations (duodenal obstruction) are the most frequent. The introduction of antibiotics and heart surgery has considerably improved the general life expectancy and life quality in the individual 21 trisomy patient.

Cytogenetics

In most cases 21 trisomy is due to a free trisomy (95 %), resulting from non-disjunction during meiosis in one of the parents, which correlates with advanced maternal age. The use of the different banding techniques, makes individual differences mainly in the short arms of chromosome 21 visible, and these heteromorphisms have been used to identify the supernumerary chromosome in Down syndrome as paternal or maternal. Non-disjunction in a maternal first meiotic division is the most common cause. About 60 % of the informative cases are of this type. Paternal non-disjunctions were observed on the average in 20 % of the cases (for review see Mikkelsen, 1985). The percentage of second division errors in maternal oogenesis is much lower than the percentage of first division errors. In paternal gametogenesis there are nearly equal 1st and 2nd division errors.
Mosaicism is observed in 2 % of 21 trisomies. In these individuals usually two cell lines, one with a free trisomy and one with a normal karyotype, are found. It is considered that mosaicism is a postzygotic event occurring after fertilization. A great phenotypic variability is observed in these individuals ranging from nearly normal to a classical 21 trisomy phenotype.

In some 5 % of the patients, 21 trisomy is due to a translocation. These translocations can either occur <u>de novo</u> or be transmitted by one of the parents. These translocations are usually centric fusion or Robertsonian type translocations involving most frequently a chromosome 14 (14/21 translocation) or a 21 or 22 (21/21 or 22/21 translocation) (see Table 1).

Recurrence risks

Most authors consider that for young mothers the recurrence risk is 1-2% in free trisomies, while for older mothers this risk is limited to that inherent to the maternal age. When a translocation is detected in the parents, the risk of recurrence depends on the type of translocation and on the sex of the carrier parent. For a t(21q21q) in the parent, all gametes are abnormal and produce only monosomic or trisomic zygotes. When the translocation occurs between a 21 and a D or a 22, the risk is different according to the sex of the parent carrier. If the mother is the carrier, the risk of recurrence is about 16 %, if it is the father the risk is lower than 5 %.

Table 1 : Different types of translocations in Down syndrome

1. t(21q Dq)	54 per 100 (55 % de novo)
	- t(21q/14q) : 58.5 %
	- t(21q/13q) : 22 %
	- t(219/15q) : 19.5 %
2. t(21q Gq)	41 per 100 (95 % de novo)
	t(21q21q) : 84 %
	t(21q22q) : 16%
3. others (tandem translocations)	5 per 100 (22 % de novo)

1.1.2. Trisomy 18

After the original description by Edwards et al. in 1960, trisomy 18 has been generally recognized as one of the most common multiple malformation syndromes. The incidence of this autosomal trisomy syndrome is approximately 1 in 3000 liveborns, with a 3 :1 preponderance of females versus males.

Clinical diagnosis at birth can be suspected on the basis of the presence of a typical malformative pattern.
Prenatal growth retardation with polyhydramnios and small placenta are generally present.
A general hypertonicity is seen in the neonatal period. Clenching of the hands is typical with the index finger overlapping the fourth and the fifth fingers. Craniofacial stigmata include short palpebral fissures, microstomia, micrognathia, small, poorly lobulated ears and prominent occiput. Abundant lanugo extends on the forehead, the cheeks and the neck. The thorax is short and the pelvis small. A low arch dermal ridge configuration is found on the fingertips. Short, dorsiflexed great toes, hypoplasia of the nails, and absence of the distal interphalangeal creases are constant limb anomalies. Subcutaneous adipose tissue and skeletal

muscles are poorly developed. Many other external and internal malformations may be present. Failure to thrive is pronounced and survival is limited. More than 50% of the affected individuals die within the first six weeks, and only 10 % live longer than six months.

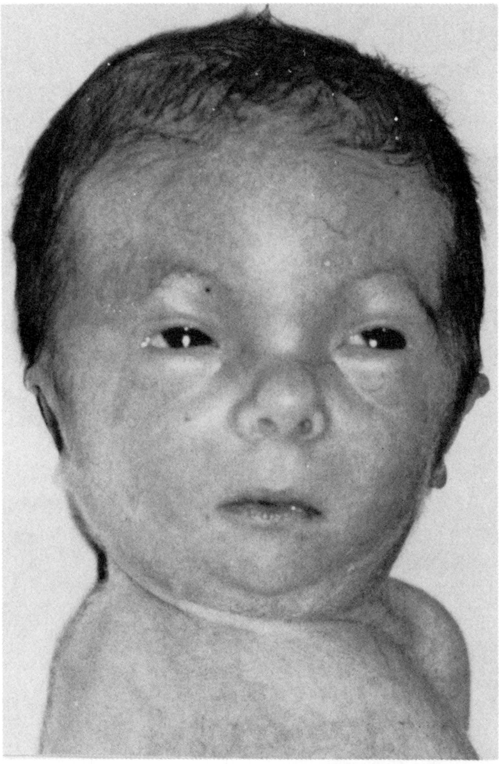

Figure 3 : The typical facial features in trisomy 18

In more than 90 % of the cases a complete trisomy 18 is found. Partial trisomies 18 may be the unbalanced product of a parental balanced autosomal translocation.
A limited number of partial trisomies 18 are reported in which clinical diagnosis of trisomy 18 was made at birth (Fryns et al., 1978a).
The bands of chromosome 18 which all patients with partial trisomy 18 and full trisomy 18 phenotype had in common were 18q11-q12. On the basis of these data Turleau and de Grouchy (1977) formulated the hypothesis that bands 18q11-18q12 might be responsible for most of the signs of trisomy 18, including failure to thrive and early death. Recently a

partial 18q12 trisomy, due to intrachromosomal duplication, was found in a deeply mentally retarded boy (Fryns et al., 1979a). The dysmorphism in this case demonstrates that trisomy of band 18q12 is not accompanied by a full or incomplete trisomy 18 phenotype, indicating that this phenotype may be due to the sole 18q11 band.

1.1.3. Trisomy 13

Trisomy 13 syndrome, first described in 1960 by Patau et al. (1960), constitutes a clinically recognizable malformative syndrome. The most salient clinical anomalies are craniofacial stigmata, deformities of the limbs and mid-line fusion defects. Microcephaly, sloping forehead, low-set poorly lobulated ears and a short neck are associated with one or several of the following features : midline scalp defects and midline haemangiomata, cleft lip and cleft palate. Eye anomalies vary from colobomata, microphthalmia to anophthalmia. Midface and forebrain defects are present in 75% of the patiens and include arrhinencephaly and holoprosencephaly of which proboscis and cyclopia are the most severe expressions.

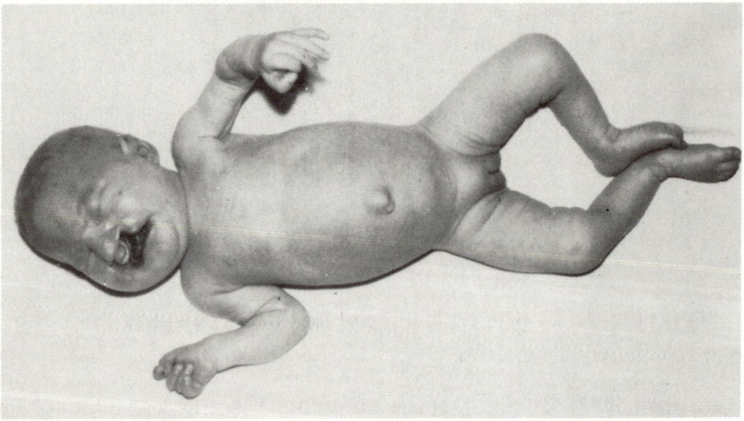

Figure 4 : A newborn with trisomy 13 syndrome

Postaxial polydactyly of the hands and, less frequently, of the feet, is one of the most distinct abnormalities of the limbs. As in 18 trisomy overriding of the fingers may be present with the second and fifth fingers overlapping the third and the fourth. The fingers frequently are in flexion contracture. The nails are small and hyperconvex.

Over 70% of the patients die within the first month of life. The limited survival is due to the pre- and postnatal growth failure, and to the associated internal anomalies of which congenital cardiovascular defects, polycystic kidneys and malrotation of the intestine are the most important. Of the three major autosomal trisomy syndromes, 13 trisomy seems to be the less common, occurring in approximately 1/7000 live births.

Cytogenetic findings

In the vast majority a classical free 13 trisomy is found (47, XX or XY, +13), due to a parental meiotic non-disjunction (de Grouchy and Turleau, 1978). Mosaic 13 trisomy, in which a normal karyotype is found in a variable percentage of the cells, may account for a less typical clinical syndrome and longer survival. Much less frequently, 13 trisomy syndrome is due to a translocation trisomy, either occurring de novo or being the result of a meiotic malsegregation in a parent, carrier of a 13/D Robertsonian translocation. Partial trisomies of different parts of chromosome 13 have been reported (Schutten et al., 1978). They exhibit more or less typical stigmata of the 13 trisomy syndrome. From these observations the conclusion can be made that the classical 13 trisomy syndrome, in contrast with 18 trisomy syndrome, is not due to a trisomy of a specific band or subband of chromosome 13.

1.1.4. Trisomy 8 mosaicism

Whereas complete 8 trisomy is incompatible with life due to the presence of severe internal malformations, mosaic trisomy 8 has been reported in an increasing number of individuals, even with normal IQ (Fryns et al., 1977d). They all present a characteristic clinical syndrome with quadrangular head, large everted ears, and relative micrognathia (Fig. 5). Differential diagnosis in the prepubertal male with Marker X-syndrome and Willams syndrome may be difficult on clinical grounds only. The most typical and diagnostic findings in trisomy 8 mosaicism, however, are the deep, furrowed palmar and plantar creases.

1.2. Ring chromosomes

1.2.1. Ring chromosome 15 syndrome

Ring chromosome 15 is the only autosomal ring chromosome anomaly which is accompanied by a clinical recognizable syndrome, and which in contrast with other ring chromosomes is not associated with severe developmental retardation.

Up to the present time less than 20 patients with ring chromosome 15 have been reported. We have observed four patients with this anomaly, and were able to further delineate the clinical characteristics of this chromosomal syndrome (Fryns et al., 1979b, 1981a). Pre- and postnatal growth retardation is pronounced in all patients. Five year follow-up of the oldest two patients, 12 and 6 years old at the present time, shows dwarfism in both with statures 15 cm below the third percentile for age. Psychomotor retardation is variable. In two patients mental retardation is limited (IQ's 65 and 70 respectively, at the ages of 12 and 4 years), but in the third patient psychomotor retardation is moderate (IQ 55 at the age of 6 years). No gross malformations are present, but the craniofacial appearance is typical with triangular face, microretrognathism, and tendency to have an oldish appearance. Hands and feet are generally small, with clinodactyly and brachymesophalangy of the fifth finger.

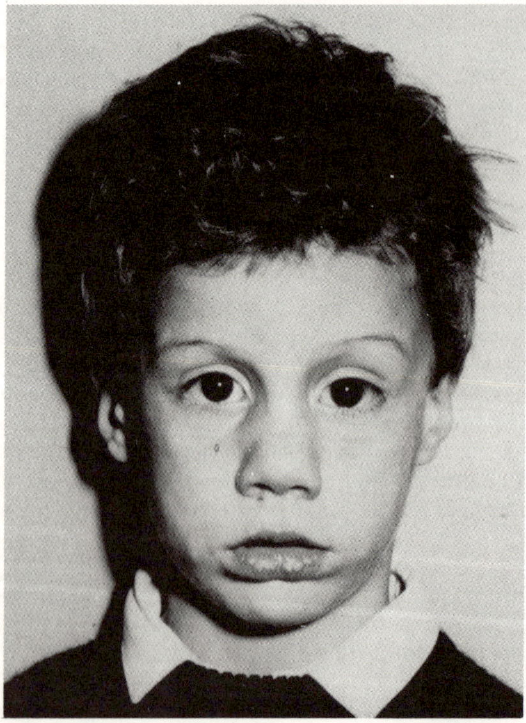

Figure 5 : Trisomy 8 in a 5-year-old boy

Before chromosomal analysis was performed, two of these patients were diagnosed as Silver syndrome, as they combined pre- and postnatal growth retardation with clinodactyly and brachymesophalangy V.

1.3. New chromosomal syndromes. Partial monosomies and trisomies

In the prebanding period, 1959-1970, an increasing number of numerical chromosomal abnormalities were reported.
Structural chromosomal rearrangements, more specifically smaller duplications and deletions remained undetectable with these techniques. After the advent of the different banding techniques more than 120 clinically recognizable syndromes associated with a small partial duplication or monosomy were delineated.

Within this period it became also evident that small structural autosomal changes are not associated with severe malformations and high lethality, but may result in minor somatic stigmata, good life expectancy and moderate to severe mental retardation.

Rather than giving an enumeration of the different "chromosomal syndromes", the typical phenotype associated with specific chromosomal changes will be illustrated by a few examples.

1.3.1. The short arm of chromosome 9. "Type and contretype" in partial 9p trisomy and 9p monosomy

After the original publication by Rethoré et al. (1970) trisomy for the short arm of chromosome number 9 became a clinically recognizable syndrome. Of all the stigmata craniofacial dysmorphism is the most specific (Fryns and Van den Berghe, 1980). The forehead is high and broad. In childhood there is a large fontanel and a broad metopic suture. Brachycephaly is most apparent in young children; the other stigmata become more evident after the first years of life : relative enophthalmos, antimongoloid slant of the palpebral fissures, mild hypertelorism, a globulous, large nose, short upper lip, large poorly lobulated ears, short neck and low hair-line. The extremities are slender with small hands and feet, hypoplasia of the phalanges, and dysplastic nails. Internal malformations occur rarely in this syndrome. All cases are mentally retarded.
In most cases of pure 9p trisomy, trisomy of the entire short arm of chromosome 9 is found, frequently as the unbalanced product of a familial translocation.

We reported one patient in whom intra-chromosomal duplication of 9p22→9p13 was accompanied by the full 9p syndrome (Fryns et al., 1979c). This observation indicates that the critical zone for the 9p trisomy pheno-

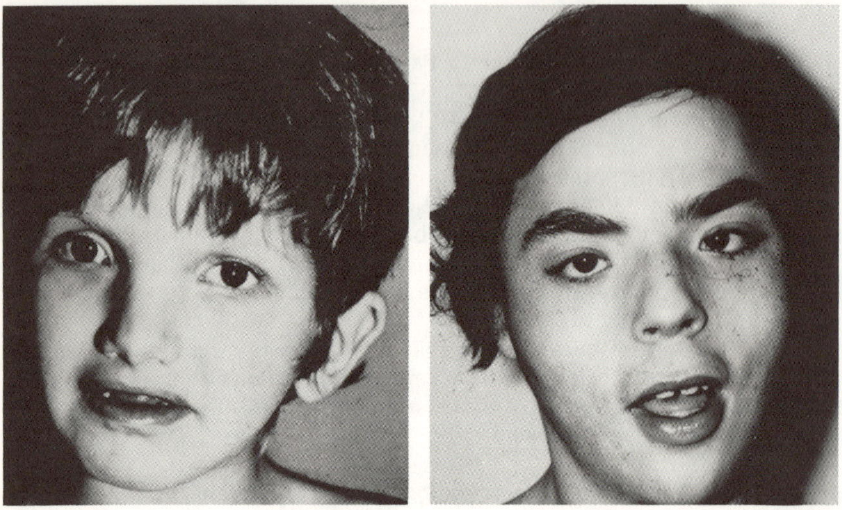

Figure 6 : The craniofacial stigmata in 9p trisomy (a) and 9p monosomy (b)

type is located within bands p22→p13, the segment for which the patient was trisomic. Addition of the 9q1 region to the 9p trisomy appears to have little effect on the phenotype. If, however, the partial trisomy also involves the regions 9q2 and 9q3, the malformative pattern becomes much more pronounced with severe failure to thrive and poor neurological condition. The craniofacial dysmorphism is less pronounced, but there are a large number of internal malformations (Fryns et al., 1978b). We observed two patients, who in addition to a 9p trisomy presented a 4q distal trisomy, and a distal 18pter monosomy, respectively (Fryns et al., 1981b, 1985). In both, the 9p phenotype dominated the expression of the concomitant chromosomal rearrangement.

We also discovered among our patients three cases with 9p deletion (Fryns, Unpublished observation), (Fryns et al., 1980; Deroover et al., 1978). The craniofacial findings in those were in "contretype" with the stigmata present in 9p trisomy : trigonocephaly, small palpebral fissures, mongoloid position of the eyes, mid-facial hypoplasia, thin upper lip with long philtrum, microstomia and retrognathia. An interesting observation was the change in craniofacial morphology in late childhood and adulthood (see Table 2). In all three patients a terminal 9p22 deletion was present, the result of a de novo germinal mutation. In two of the three, the

9p deletion was found to be of paternal origin, as evidenced by investigation of the 9qh C-polymorphism in both parents and in the patient.

Table 2 : Changes in craniofacial appearance of 9p deletion patients from the newborn period to adulthood

Newborn	Adulthood
trigonocephaly	disappears gradually
prominent metopic suture	less prominent
small palpebral fissures	present
mongoloid position of eyes	normal position
hairy eyebrows	present
hypertelorism	present
midfacial hypoplasia	less prominent to unchanged
small, upturned nose	small, beaklike nose
thin upper lip	present
long philtrum	present
high-arched palate	present
microstomia	present
retrognathia	disappears gradually

A remarkable observation was the finding of a nearly normal phenotype in a moderately mentally retarded boy with ring chromosome 9, despite the fact that 9p22 must have been deleted during the ring formation (Fryns et al., 1979d). This confirmed the unpredictable effect of ring chromosomes in general on the phenotype, which is probably related to the unstability of ring chromosomes, and the mosaic-state which is likely to exist in most patients.

1.3.2. Interstitial deletion of the long arm of chromosome 16 : a new clinically recognizable syndrome

In 1977 we reported a previously undescribed terminal deletion of the long arm of chromosome 16 in a newborn female (Fryns et al., 1977b). The child had a distinct craniofacial dysmorphism and other multiple congenital malformations. In the same year, Taysi et al. (1978) also reported a terminal 16q deletion in a male infant with features similar to those of our patient. Subsequently, we reported two other cases with strikingly similar clinical findings (Fryns et al., 1979e, 1981c). In one case, a 7-month-old male child had an apparently de novo reciprocal (5p; 16q) translocation. The breakpoint in the long arm of chromosome 16 was similar to one found in the previously reported patient (16q21) suggesting that certain parts of chromosomal material terminal to this band might be lost in the translocated chromosome (Fryns et al., 1979e). Our more recently reported case (Fryns et al., 1981c) was a 6 month-old girl with an interstitial deletion involving 16q13-22 region. Côté et al. (1980) described a male newborn with clinical findings similar to our three patients but with an apparently normal male karyotype. Finally, Lin et al. (1983) reported an infant with an interstitial deletion of the long arm of chromosome 16 (del(16)(q13q21)). The clinical findings were almost identical to those found by us (Fryns et al., 1977b). Although it is difficult to define the clinical variability of this new chromosomal syndrome, as it is based upon 6 patients only, the major clinical features suggestive of the diagnosis are as follows : all 6 patients presented severe problems of growth and development and malformations mainly confined to the head and the neck. Thus, the deletion involving the 16q21 band seems to be associated with a fairly specific clinical syndrome. The forehead is high, the anterior fontanel large and bulging with diastasis of the cranial sutures, and the metopic suture prominent. All 6 patients reported had a short neck, upward slanting palpebral fissures and low-set and/or dysmorphic ears. Two patients died in the neonatal period (Fryns et al., 1977b; Lin et al., 1983). Follow-up information on the four surviving patients is available. Whereas our second reported patient (Fryns et al., 1979e) is moderately mentally retarded and shows slight growth failure at the age of 6 years, the three other patients, including our third patient, are severely mentally retarded, with severe growth failure, recurrent respiratory infections and progressive renal insufficiency in one (Fryns et al., 1981c).

1.4. The new cytogenetics : specific chromosomal aberrations in human malformations syndromes

The introduction of high resolution banding techniques revealed the existence of small chromosomal changes (duplications or more frequently deletions) in an increasing number of human malformation syndromes.
The 8q deletion in Langer-Giedion syndrome is an example. In approximately half of the patients with Prader-Willi syndrome a variety of rearrangements involving chromosome 15 (15q11-13 deletion) have been described. Until now, the diagnosis of Prader-Willi syndrome was essentially based on the association of more or less typical clinical features : hypotonia and feeding difficulties, hypogonadism and cryptorchidism, mental retardation, obesity, hyperphagia and short stature. It is likely that with the help of better high resolution techniques small 15q11 deletions will be discovered in all patients with typical Prader-Willi syndrome, and that high resolution banding techniques will become a condition <u>sine qua non</u> for the final diagnosis of this syndrome. On the other hand, prometaphase chromosome studies have demonstrated that

Table 3 : Specific chromosomal anomalies in malformation syndromes

Malformation syndrome	Chromosomal finding
Prader-Willi syndrome	15q11deletion
Tricho-rhino-phalangeal syndrome type II (Langer-Giedion syndrome)	8q23-q24.1 deletion
Di George syndrome	22q11 deletion
Pierre-Robin syndrome	4qter deletion
Elfin face syndrome	15p deletion
Holt-Oram syndrome	14q interstitial deletion
Wiedemann-Beckwith syndrome	11p15 trisomy
Aniridia-mental retardation syndrome	11p13 monosomy

the Di George syndrome can be caused by at least two mechanisms : gene mutation or chromosome deletion. The Di George syndrome is a 3rd and 4th pharyngeal pouch syndrome, and includes aplasia of the thymus and parathyroids and congenital heart disease. De la Chapelle et al. (1981) reported partial 22q11 monosomy in a familial case, while in most other instances no chromosomal anomaly could be detected. In fact, Di George "syndrome" is not a real syndrome, but includes a number of associated anomalies which are the consequence of a single developmental defect which may be different from patient to patient. Also in the Pierre-Robin syndrome, with the classical triad of microretrognathia, glossoptosis and cleft palate, some patients with chromosomal abnormalities (4q deletion) have been reported (Fryns et al., 1981d). This confirms that, as is the case for the Di George "syndrome", Pierre-Robin "syndrome" covers a heterogeneous group of different entities with different etiology. These examples illustrate how high resolution banding techniques can help both in the further precise identification of a syndrome, or in the dissection of a seemingly unique syndrome into separate entities. It is very likely that a number of other multiple malformative syndromes, such as the Cornelia de Lange syndrome and the Rubinstein-Taybi syndrome, will ultimately be shown to have a chromosomal basis. In the Elfin-face syndrome we found a de novo reciprocal autosomal translocation involving the short arms of chromosome 15 in one patient (Fryns et al., 1982) but further confirmation in other patiens is necessary.

Finally, small deletions have been shown in some syndromes with multiple tumors, which presented as autosomal dominantly inherited conditions. They are not only important for the study of mental retardation, but also for the understanding of how the tumors may arise.

Table 4 : Collective data from surveys of mentally retarded patients

Reference	Total number of individuals investigated	Total number of chromosomal abnormalialities	Total number of patients with Down's syndrome	Other chromosomal abnormalities	Fragile X syndrome	Gonosomal abnormalities	Chromosomal variants
Singh et al. [1]	504	112 (22.2%)	89 (17.6%)	11 (2.2%)	-	12 (2.4%)	11 (2.2%)
Cassiman et al. [2]	857	132 (15.3%)	106 (12.4%)	23 (2.6%)	-	3 (0.3%)	No data
Mounoud et al. [3]	82	23 (28%)	18 (22%)	4 (4.8%)	-	1 (1.2%)	3 (3.6%)
Speed et al. [4]	2770	297 (10.7%)	250 (9%)	16 (0.6%)	-	31 (1.1%)	No data
Sutherland et al. [5]	588	90 (15.3%)	73 (12.4%)	12 (2%)	-	5 (0.9%)	No data
Bourgeois & Benezech [6]	600	54 (9%)	32 (4.2%)	18 (3%)	-	11 (1.8%)	19 (3.2%)
Hunter [7]	1811[a]	-	-	-	-	15 (0.8%)	No data
Tharapel & Summit [8]	200	5 (2.5%)	-	5 (2.5%)	-	-	1 (0.5%)
Jacobs et al. [9]	475	57 (12%)	40 (8.4%)	14 (2.9%)	-	3 (0.6%)	No data
Grace et al. [10]	512	57 (11.1%)	42 (8.2%)	10 (2.0%)	-	5 (0.9%)	23 (4.5%)
Faed et al. [11]	756	103 (13.6%)	91 (12%)	6 (0.8%)	-	6 (0.8%)	No data
Czeizel et al. [12]	246	76 (30.8%)	47 (19%)	8 (3.2%)	-	21 (8.5%)	No data
Gripenberg et al. [13]	1062	349 (32.8%)	305 (28.7%)	35 (3.2%)	-	10 (0.9%)	4 (0.4%)
Kondo et al. [14]	449	37 (8.1%)	33 (7.3%)	3 (0.6%)	-	1 (0.2%)	No data
Moghe et al. [15]	74	14 (18.9%)	-	7 (9.4%)	-	7 (9.4%)[b]	No data

Narahama [16]	74	11 (14.9%)		10 (13.5%)	-	1 (1.4%)	5 (6.8%)
Thoene et al. [17]	727	72 (9.9%)	23 (3.2%)	-	7 (0.9%)	No data	
Klein et al. [18]	183	39 (21.4%)	25 (13.7%)	12 (6.6%)	-	2 (1.1%)	11 (6%)
Nelson & Smart [19]	720	148 (20.5%)	127 (17.6%)	14 (2%)	-	7 (0.9%)	No data
Rasmussen et al. [20][c]	1905	354 (18.5%)	281 (14.7%)	40 (2.2%)	-	33 (1.7%)	10 (0.5%)
Venter and Op't Hof [21]	2533	523 (20.6%)	397 (15.7%)	84 (3.3%)	56 (2.2%)	20 (0.8%)	No data
Nielsen et al. [22][d]	476	76 (16%)	58 (12.2%)	13 (2.7%)	2 (0.4%)	5 (1%)	Yes, but no detailed data
Present study	1991	424 (21.3%)	295 (14.9%)	59 (2.9%)	12 (0.6%)	120 (6%)	
Pooled data	19 594	2953 (15.1%)	2351 (11.9%)	427 (2.1%)	116 in 5000 (2.3%)	218 (1.1%)	207 in 7112 (2.9%)

Taken from Fryns et al., 1984.

[a] Males investigated for supernumerary Y chromosomes

[b] A case of double trisomy 48,XXY,+21 is also included to the Down syndrome group

[c] In this study five loco typico inversions 9 considered as polymorphic variants were included in "balanced" structural abnormalities, the correction was made by the present authors to include them into chromosome polymorphic variants

[d] The frequency of fragile X syndrome is estimated on the basis of data from the two last references and the present study, i.e. for the 5 000 of mentally retardates.

II. CHROMOSOME STUDIES IN MENTAL RETARDATION

After the advent of the different cytogenetic banding techniques, an increased number of studies have been reported on the incidence of chromosomal abnormalities in the population of mentally retarded (Table 4).

During the past few years, we studied a population of 2160 moderately and severely mentally retarded, of which 1233 were males and 937 females. They were living in different institutes, and their age varied between 2 and 60 years, with 75 % of the patients being between 2 and 21 years old. In 1991 of the 2160 patients a cytogenetic study was performed. In 169 patients no karyotype was done, as they all presented mental retardation of acquired pre-, peri- and postnatal origin. Additionally, in 23 patients with clinical diagnosis of Down's syndrome (17 males and 6 females) no karyotype was obtained, but they are included in the Down syndrome group. In all karyotyped patients chromosomal investigation was performed with at least Giemsa-banding and Quinacrine fluorescence. Additional banding techniques, (R-, C-banding) and prometaphase banding were performed whenever further investigation of the chromosomal abnormality was required. A fragile X-screening using M199 culture medium was performed in 354 males, and was found to be positive in 57 males i.e., 16.1% of the screened population. Of the 30 females who were screened, a fragile X was detected in one patient only.

Table 5 summarizes the results of this study.

Table 5 : Cytogenetic findings in the populations under investigation

Total number of patients in 8 institutions under investigation	2160	(100%)
Total number of patients who were chromosomally investigated	1991	(92.2%)
Number of patients with chromosomal aberrations	424	(21.3%)
Patients with Down's syndrome[a]	295	(14.9%)
Patients with other chromosomal aberrations	71	(3.5%)
Patients with fragile X syndrome[b]	58	(2.9%)
Patients with chromosomal variants	120	(6%)

[a] Included 23 patients (17 males and 6 females with features of Down's syndrome who were not chromosomally investigated).

[b] 57 males and 1 female. Screening for fragile X in 354 males (16.1 % positive) and 30 females (3.3 % positive).

The chromosomal abnormalities (71 patients) different from 21 trisomy, can be subdivided in six groups (Table 6).

Table 6 : Chromosomal abnormalities (71 patients) different from 21 trisomy

	Number of patients
1) partial autosomal trisomies	14
2) partial autosomal monosomies and ring chromosomes	15
3) "balanced" reciprocal translocations	7
4) Robertsonian translocations	10
5) sex-chromosome abnormalities	10
6) varia :	
(1) small accessory chromosomes	12
(2) paracentric inversions	2
(3) mosaic triploidy	1

COMMENTS

1. As illustrated in Table 4 the percentage of Down syndrome patients is variable in the different studies, which is, in our opinion, probably due to differences in the selection criteria for admission of patients to these types of institutions in different countries. On the other hand the frequency of "other chromosomal aberrations" is remarkably stable : the postbanding chromosome technology contributed only 2 to 3% new cytogenetic diagnoses in the mentally retarded in all large scale surveys (Gripenberg et al., 1980; Rasmussen et al., 1982; Venter and Op't Hof, 1982) and this is confirmed in the present study. Although this percentage is low, the correct diagnosis in these patients led to the detection of high-risk families as illustrated in the present material, and made genetic counseling (and, eventually, prenatal diagnosis) in phenotypically normal carriers possible. In the present study, fibroblast cultures for chromosomal analysis were performed in 20 patients with gross dysmorphic stigmata but without a definite clinical syndrome and with a normal karyotype in the lymphocytes. In 2 of them the fibroblast culture showed an abnormal karyotype in 100 % of the cells : a tetrasomy 21 in one patient, and a triploidy in an adult patient with severe dysmorphism and frog like position of the toes. Although this experience is limited to 2 positive cases it seems necessary to perform karyotype analysis from different tissues, if possible, to properly diagnose certain, clinically well selected patients.

2. The present study demonstrates that fragile X screening in institutionalized populations of mental retardates is a complementary and

very important tool in the etiological diagnosis of the mentally handicapped. Up to the present time, fragile X screening has been performed in 354 males and 30 females, and was found to be positive in 58 patients (57 males (16.1 % positive) and 1 female (3.3 % positive)). The diagnostic contribution of fragile X screening is numerically just as important as the advanced chromosome banding techniques, and its contribution to the prevention of mental retardation is even greater, as the diagnosis of fragile X syndrome in one index male patient usually leads to the detection of several female relatives who might be carriers of this X-linked recessively inherited condition.

III. CHROMOSOME REARRANGEMENTS IN COUPLES WITH RECURRENT FETAL WASTAGE

A number of genetic centers have now accumulated sufficient data to document the high incidence of structural chromosomal rearrangements in couples with recurrent fetal wastage. We performed a cytogenetic study in 1555 couples with recurrent fetal wastage, i.e., at least two first trimester abortions. Besides orceine staining G- and R-banding were routinely applied in all patients.

Table 7 summarizes the number and respective incidence of the different structural rearrangements in this group and it shows the incidences of the same structural rearrangements in a total number of 52,179 patients chromosomally investigated in this center for various other indications.

In addition to reciprocal balanced autosomal translocations and Robertsonian D/D, D/G and G/G translocations, we also detected para- and pericentric inversions, small accessory chromosomes, Xp and Xq deletions and one patient with ring chromosome 21. Pericentric inv(9)(p11q13) was excluded on the basis that it was considered to be a normal variant only. These types of structural chromosomal rearrangements were thus detected (see Table 7) in 6.36 % of this population. This is almost seven-fold higher than the incidence of chromosomal abnormalities in a general population. More than 50 % of the chromosomal abnormalities were reciprocal balanced translocations, and almost 30 % were Robertsonian, mostly D/D translocations. Peri- and paracentric inversions accounted for 6 %, and 4 %, of all chromosomal abnormalities detected. There was no significant prevalance of female carriers of balanced reciprocal translocations, but in the Robertsonian translocation carriers the female/male ratio was 2.5 :1. Further data are needed to evaluate whether peri- and paracentric inversions, and other chromosomal rearrangements such as small accessory chromosomes, X deletion and autosomal rings, are more frequent in patients with recurrent fetal wastage.

Table 7 : Number and incidence of structural chromosomal anomalies

	A. in the total number of 52,179 chromosomally investigated patients		**B.** in 1,555 couples with recurrent fetal wastage
rcp translocations :	167 (3.2 per 1000)		56 (36 per 1000)
Rob translocations :			
D/D	76 (1.5 per 1000)	142	23 (15 per 1000)
D/G	39 (0.7 per 1000)		4 (2.5 per 1000)
G/G	27 (0.5 per 1000)		1 (0.6 per 1000)
Inversions			
Pericentric :	25 (0.5 per 1000)		6 (3.9 per 1000)
Paracentric :	19 (0.36 per 1000)		4 (2.5 per 1000)
Small accessory chromosomes :	32 (0.6 per 1000)		3 (1.9 per 1000)
Xp and Xq deletions :	13 (0.2 per 1000)		1 (0.6 per 1000)
r(21) :	1 (0.01 per 1000)		1 (0.6 per 1000)
Total :	399 (7.6 per 1000)		99 (63.6 per 1000)

GENERAL CONCLUSIONS

The development of human cytogenetics has largely contributed to the delineation of an increasing number of human malformation and/or mental retardation syndromes associated with specific chromosomal abnormalities. After the description of so-called numerical chromosome abnormalities in the prebanding period (1959-1970), the introduction of the different banding techniques resulted in the individualisation of more than 120 malformation syndromes associated with specific larger or smaller chromosomal rearrangements as duplications and deletions. Moreover, the development of prometaphase banding techniques revealed small, but consistent chromosomal changes in an increasing number of human malformation syndromes as, among others, Prader-Willi syndrome, tricho-rhino-phalangeal syndrome type I and II and the aniridia-Wilms tumor complex.

The highest incidence of chromosomal rearrangements has been found in the study of the severely mentally retarded (> 20 %) and in couples with recurrent first trimester fetal wastage (6-7 %). Particularly in these two fields the diagnostic contribution of cytogenetics was of extreme help in the genetic counseling of individuals and parents confronted with these problems.

REFERENCES

Caspersson, T., Gahrton, G., Lindsten, J. et al.
Automatic karyotyping of quinacrine mustard stained human chromosomes.
Exp. Cell Res. 67, 233-235, 1971.

Côté , G.B., Papadakou-Lagoyanni, S. and Kairis, M.
Fryns syndrome without deletion 16q.
Ann. Génét. 23, 171-172, 1980.

de Grouchy, J. and Turleau, C.
Atlas des Maladies Chromosomiques.
Expansion Scientifique Française, Paris, 1977.

de la Chapelle, A., Herva, R., Koivisto, M. and Aula, P.
A deletion in chromosome 22 can cause Di George syndrome.
Hum. Genet. 57, 253-256, 1981.

Deroover, J., Fryns, J.P., Parloir, C., Haegeman, J. and Van den Berghe, H.
Partial monosomy of the short arm of chromosome 9. A distinct clinical entity.
Hum. Genet. 44, 195-200, 1978.

Down, J.L.H.
Observations on an ethnic classification of idiots.
Clin. Lect. Rep. London Hosp. 3, 259, 1866.

Edwards, J.H., Harnden, D.G., Cameron, A.H., Crosse and V.W., Wolff, O.H.
A new trisomic syndrome.
Lancet i, 787, 1960.

Fryns, J.P., Bussuyt, C. and Van den Berghe, H.
8-Trisomy syndrome.
Acta Paediatr. Belg. 30, 55-58, 1977a.

Fryns, J.P., Melchior, S., Jaeken, J. and Van den Berghe, H.
Partial monosomy of the long arm of chromosome 16 in a malformed

newborn : karyotype 46,XX,del(16)(q21).
Hum. Genet. 38, 343-346, 1977b.

Fryns, J.P., Detavernier, F., Van Fleteren, A. and Van den Berghe, H.
Partial trisomy 18q in a newborn with typical 18 trisomy phenotype.
Hum. Genet. 44, 2, 201-207, 1978a.

Fryns, J.P., Smeets, E., Eggermont, E., Delire, C. and Van den Berghe, H.
Partial trisomy 9q- in a polymalformed newborn, karyotype : 47, XX, + del(9)(q33).
Acta Paediatr. Belg. 31, 237-240, 1978b.

Fryns, J.P., Vinken, L., Marien, J. and Van den Berghe, H.
Partial trisomy 18q12, due to intrachromosomal duplication, is not associated with typical 18 trisomy phenotype.
Hum. Genet. 46, 341-344, 1979a.

Fryns, J.P., Timmermans, J., D'Hondt, F., François, B., Emmery, L. and Van den Berghe, H.
Ring chromosome 15 syndrome.
Hum. Genet. 51, 43-48, 1979b.

Fryns, J.P., Casaer, P. and Van den Berghe, H.
Partial duplication of the short arm of chromosome 9 (p13→p22) in a child with typical 9p trisomy phenotype.
Hum. Genet. 46, 231-235, 1979c.

Fryns, J.P., Lambrechts, A., Jansseune, H. and Van den Berghe, H.
Moderate mental retardation and nonspecific dysmorphic syndrome associated with ring chromosome 9.
Hum. Genet. 50, 29-32, 1979d.

Fryns, J.P., Bande-Knops, J. and Van den Berghe, H.
Partial monosomy of the long arm of chromosome 16 : a distinct clinical entity ?
Hum. Genet. 46, 115-120, 1979e.

Fryns, J.P. and Van den Berghe, H.
Trisomy of the short arm of chromosome number 9 : a clinical entity.
Acta Paediatr. Belg. Suppl. XIII, 97-104, 1980.

Fryns, J.P., Pedersen, J.C., Duyck, H., Fabry, G. and Van den Berghe, H.
Deletion of the short arm of chromosome 9. A clinically recognizable entity.
Eur. J. Pediatr. 134, 201-204, 1980.

Fryns, J.P., Jaeken, J., Devliegher, H., Debucquoy, P., Eggermont, E. and Van den Berghe, H.
Ring chromosome 15 syndrome.
Acta Paediatr. Belg. 34, 47-50, 1981a.

Fryns, J.P., Aron, M., Devliegher, H., Eggermont, E. and Van den Berghe, H.
A malformed newborn with 9p and 4q trisomy.
Ann. Génét. 24, 48-50, 1981b.

Fryns, J.P., Proesmans, W., Van Hoey, G. and Van den Berghe, H.
Interstitial 16q deletion with typical dysmorphic syndrome.
Ann. Génét. 24, 124-125, 1981c.

Fryns, J.P., Timmermans, J., Hoedemaekers, J., Emmery, L. and Van den Berghe, H.
Pierre-Robin anomalad, moderate mental retardation and distal 4q deletion.
Ann. Génét. 24, 187-188, 1981d.

Fryns, J.P., Van der Hauwaert, L.G., Dumoulin, M. and Van den Berghe, H.
The Elfin face syndrome and the short arm of chromosome 15.
Ann. Génét. 23, 181-182, 1982.

Fryns, J.P., Kleczkowska, A., Kubien, E., and Van den Berghe, H.
Cytogenetic findings in moderate and severe mental retardation. A study of an institutionalized population of 1991 patients.
Acta Paed. Scand. Supplement 313, 1984.

Fryns, J.P., Haspeslagh, M., De Mûlenaere, A. and Van den Berghe, H.
9p trisomy/18p distal monosomy and multiple cutaneous leiomyomata. Another specific chromosomal site (18pter) in dominantly inherited tumors ?
Hum. Genet. 70, 284-286, 1985.

Gripenberg, U., Hongel, K., Knuutila, S., Kähkönen, M. and Leisti, J.
A chromosome survey of 1 062 mentally retarded patients. Evaluation of a long-term study at the Rinnekoti Institution, Finland.
Hereditas 92, 223-228, 1980.

Lejeune, J., Gouthier, M. and Turpin, R.
Les chromosomes humains en culture de tissus.
C. R. Acad. Sci. Paris 248, 602, 1959.

Lejeune, J., Lafourcade, J., Berger, R., Vialatte, J., Boeswillwald, M., Seringe, P. and Turpin, R.

Trois cas de délétion partielle du bras court d'un chromosome 5.
C.R. Acad. Sci (Paris) 257, 3098-3102, 1963.

Lin, C.C., Lowry, R.B. and Snyder, F.F.
Interstitial deletion for a region in the long arm of chromosome 16. Hum. Genet. 65, 134-138, 1983.

Mikkelsen, M.
Down anomaly : new research aspects of an old and well known syndrome.
In : Medical Genetics : Past, Present, Future. Alan R. Liss, Inc. pp. 293-307, 1985.

Patau, K., Smith, D.W., Therman, E,, Inhorn, S.L. and Wagner, H.P.
Multiple congenital anomaly caused by an extra autosome.
Lancet i, 790-793, 1960.

Rasmussen, K., Nielsen, J. and Dahl, G.
The prevalence of chromosome abnormalities among mentally retarded persons in a geographically delimited area of Denmark.
Clin. Genet. 22, 244-255, 1982.

Rethoré, M.O., Larget-Piet, L., Abonyi, D., Boeswillwald, M., Berger, P., Carpentier, S., Cruveiller, J., Dutrillaux, B., Lafourcade, J., Penneau, M. and Lejeune, J.
Sur quatre cas de trisomie pour le bras cour du chromosome 9. Individualisation d'une nouvelle entité morbide.
Ann. Génét. 13, 217-232, 1970.

Schutten, H.J., Schutten, B.T. and Mikkelsen, M.
Partial trisomy of chromosome 13. Case report and review of literature.
Hum. Genet. 21, 95-99, 1978.

Taysi, K., Fishman, M. and Sekhon, G.S.
A terminal long arm deletion of chromosome 16 in a dysmorphic infant : 46,XY,del(16)(q22).
Birth Defects : Original Article Series 14, 6C, 343-347, 1978.

Turleau, C. and de Grouchy, J.
Trisomy 18qter and trisomy mapping of chromosome 18.
Clin. Genet. 12, 361-371, 1977.

Venter, P.A. and Op't Hof, J.
Cytogenetic abnormalities including the marker X chromosome in patients with severe mental retardation.
S. A. Med. J. 62, 947-950, 1982.

Waardenburg, P.J.
Das menschliche Auge und seine Erbanlagen.
Haag : Martinus Nijhoff, p. 47, 1932.

DIAGNOSIS OF GENETIC DISEASE BY LINKAGE ANALYSIS

Howard M. CANN, Daniel COHEN and Jean DAUSSET

Centre d'Etude du Polymorphisme Humain (CEPH), Paris, France

Introduction

There is intense interest in mapping the human genome because of the contribution of a well defined map of all chromosomes to diagnosis and prediction of genetic disease. Even in the absence of a specific test for a particular genetic disease, it is possible to detect the deleterious gene by one or more closely linked genetic markers on the same chromosome. A very rough estimate of the number of genes in the human haploid genome is 50,000-100,000. Such an estimate, rough as it is, suggests the enormity of an undertaking to map the human genome. Clearly, strategies are required to achieve this goal.

The human genetic map is being constructed by the interplay of physical techniques, which assign genes and other genetic markers to chromosomes and regions and individual bands of chromosomes, and linkage analysis, which determines genetic distance between these markers and their order along the chromosomes (Human Gene Mapping, 1985). The strategy for constructing a useful human genetic map involves placing evenly spaced genetic markers on all the chromosomes (Botstein et al., 1980). The span of the human genome has been estimated to be approximately 3300 centimorgans. A human genetic map containing at least 150 evenly spaced genetic markers along all chromosomes may put all genes within readily detectable distance of one or two markers. Of course, many more genes and genetic markers will have to be mapped to achieve such a goal. The map will be constructed, primarily, by linkage analysis.

Genetic linkage and gene order

Linkage implies that genes at two or more loci on the same chromosome

Birth Defects: Original Article Series, Volume 23, Number 2, pages 33–60

tend to be inherited together. Linkage between two or more loci can be demonstrated by noting that the genes at each of these loci on the same chromosome are co-inherited or segregate together in families. The farther apart gene loci are located on the same chromosome, the less likely gene markers at these loci will be inherited together because of their separation by recombination, the exchange of genetic material between homologous chromosomes. The frequency of recombination, which can be determined from family studies, is a reasonable measure of genetic distance between two loci, especially at relatively small map distances. Distance between loci on a genetic map is expressed in units called Morgans (or centimorgans). A Morgan is defined as the distance over which, on average, one genetic exchange (or crossing over) occurs when a large number of meioses are studied. Given this definition, it can be recognized that the probability of more than one crossover even occurring over a very short map distance is so small as to be negligible in contributing to an estimate of length. This is why the frequency of recombination (resulting from crossing over) is a reasonable measure of genetic distance for short map intervals. As genetic distance between two loci increases, the probability of more than one crossing over event increases, the even numbered events, such as the double crossover, cannot be detected between two loci and the observed recombination frequency will underestimate the distance between them. A more reasonable estimate of distance between widely separated loci is based on the sum of the distances between intervening loci. A recombination frequency of 50%, directly measured between two loci, cannot distinguish between linkage and independent assortment of the loci.

For a family to be informative for linkage, at least one parent must be heterozygous at two or more loci. The chromosomal distribution of the alleles at each of the heterozygous (linked) loci is called the phase. For human families, the phase for a parent with double or multiple heterozygosity is generally not known (unless grandparental genotypes are available), which means that recombinant events cannot be directly identified in the offspring. The interpretation of the genotype of each offspring as arising from a recombinant or non recombinant gamete depends on the phase of the parent. If the phase is unknown, the probability of the observed pedigree is the sum of the probabilities of the genotype distribution among the offspring for each possible parental phase (Figure 1). Thus, recombination can only be inferred from two generation nuclear families, parents and offspring, and the likelihood that the frequency of recombination is θ is computed from the probabilities of one or more informative pedigrees for that value of θ. An important strategy for efficient data collection in large scale linkage studies involves the use of large, phase known, human families.

$$z = \log \frac{f(y;\theta)}{f(y;0.5)} = \log 2^{s-1} \left(\theta^{a} (1-\theta)^{b} + \theta^{b} (1-\theta)^{a}\right) \quad \text{phase unknown}$$

$$z = \log \frac{f(y;\theta)}{f(y;0.5)} = \log 2^{s} \left(\theta^{a} (1-\theta)^{b}\right) \quad \text{phase known}$$

Figure 1 : Equations for lod scores for phase unknown and phase known families of the same mating type.

The mating is a double backcross, with one parent heterozygous at each of two loci and the other parent homozygous at each locus. The following symbols are employed : θ, the recombination frequency between two loci; y, the probability of the observed pedigree for the value of θ; s, the sibship size; a, the number of offspring in the sibship who show evidence of recombination or no recombination for each of the parental phases between the loci in a phase unknown family and who are identified as recombinants in a phase known family; b, vice versa. Note, s =a+b.

The detection of linkage between a pair of loci involves comparing the hypothesis, for a given value of θ, that the loci are linked, with the hypothesis that these are not linked, i.e., θ = 0.5 (Figure 1). The comparison of the two alternative hypotheses can be assessed with an odds (or likelihood) ratio, which is the probability of the pedigree for a given value of θ divided by the probability computed at 0.5. The log (base 10) of this ratio, the log of the odds ratio, is known as the lod, and for a given value of θ a lod (z) can be assigned to each pedigree of a series of informative families. These lod scores can be summed over a series of families for each value of θ used in the assessment of linkage. The lod score is one method, widely used, for testing significance of a series of observations (the pedigrees) about linkage. A lod score of 3, generally accepted as the lower limit of significance for a series of observations of θ between two loci (Morton, 1955), indicates an odds ratio of 1000:1 for linkage, at that value of θ , as compared to no linkage. When two loci are known to reside on the same chromosome, the lower limit for detection of linkage can be reduced. The most likely value of θ is that with the maximum lod value among a series of values of θ computed for the group of informative pedigrees under study. Generally the method of maximum likelihood is used to estimate the most likely value of θ .

When three or more loci are known to be linked, multiple crossover events can be identified or inferred, depending on knowledge of the parental phase. The ordering on the chromosome of three or more linked loci involves comparing distances between all pairs for the ensemble. The flanking markers will generally be those with the largest distance, which will immediately resolve the order for three loci (Figure 2). In contrast to ordering three (or more) linked loci from pairwise data, computer based methods are now available for estimation of recombination frequencies from the observed joint segregation of the loci and inference of order of these loci (Lathrop et al., 1984; 1985). Estimation is based on the maximum likelihood estimates of probabilities for all possible combinations of recombination events in the intervals between the linked loci.

$$\theta_{AB} = 0.10$$

$$\theta_{BC} = 0.06$$

$$\theta_{AC} = 0.16$$

(0.16)

A-----------B------C

0.10 0.06

Figure 2 : Relative map distances between three pairs of loci, A, B and C. The order of these loci on the chromosome is shown below.

When considering the mapping of multiple loci, the phenomenon of interference must be mentioned. Interference refers to the reduction of recombination when another genetic exchange has occurred in the vicinity. This suggests that crossing over events tend to interfere with each other, which leads to a non random distribution of recombination events along the chromosome. The phenomenon was first noted in linkage experiments involving three loci in Drosophila (Muller, 1916) and has been repeatedly observed in most, but not all, laboratory animals and plants. The relevance here is the significance for human linkage mapping. If, indeed, recombinant events in adjacent segments are not independent, the effect of interference must be incorporated into procedures for estimation of the recombination frequencies. Lathrop et al. (1985) have shown that the bias introduced by estimating recombination frequencies under an assumption of no interference is well within the standard error of the estimates for sample sizes likely to be used for human linkage studies. These and other tests support the conclusion that interference will have minimal effect on estimation of recombination frequencies and ordering of multiple linked human loci. Interference may also occur in the human organism, but it can be neglected given the limitations on collecting human data.

Efficient construction of the human linkage map

The construction of a linkage map consisting of evenly spaced genetic markers on all the chromosomes will be greatly facilitated by the use of efficient genetic markers, efficient data collection and efficient analysis of the data.

Efficient genetic markers

A genetic marker is any characteristic or trait which can follow the inheritance of a segment of DNA in families. Classically, genetic markers have been phenotypes associated with loci of known genes, which include clinical characteristics, i.e., inherited diseases, and a variety of normal traits usually detected by laboratory tests of blood components. For a genetic marker to faithfully trace inheritance of a gene, it must distinguish between any two alleles at the same locus in a heterozygous individual, tracking each allele in a family. In practice, segregation is followed in the offspring of a heterozygous parent. As already noted, only families with one or both parents heterozygous at two or more loci are informative for linkage analysis. The frequencies of heterozygosity for the genetic markers involved in a linkage study determine the frequency of informative families. Polymorphic gene loci, those with two or more codominant alleles occurring with relatively high frequencies in the population, provide desirable genetic markers for linkage studies. Note that the highest heterozygote frequency achievable for a two allele polymorphism is 0.5, resulting from equal allele frequencies of 0.5. Higher heterozygote frequencies are achievable with polymorphisms with multiple alleles occurring at equal or near equal frequencies. The efficiency of a genetic marker increases with its heterozygote frequency.

One of the most efficient genetic markers available for linkage studies is the human major histocompatibility complex, the HLA (genetic) system (Histocompatibility Testing, 1984). This complex genetic region has been assigned to the short arm of chromosome 6 and localized to band 21 by analysis of interspecific somatic cell hybrids (Francke and Pellegrino, 1977) and to higher resolution bands 21.1 and 21.3 by in situ hybridization of human metaphase chromosomes (Morton et al., 1984). The region spans 2-3 centimorgans (cM), may consist of about 3000 kb of DNA and contains at least 9 well defined, polymorphic loci (Figure 3). The number of alleles at the HLA-A and B loci, 0.8 cM apart, is at least 20 and 37 alleles, respectively, and at the HLA-DR locus, about 1 cM from HLA-B, at least 12 alleles. Some of the alleles at each locus are infrequent, and some others occur relatively frequently and with approximately equal frequencies. This means that almost everyone is heterozygous at, especially, the HLA-A and B loci, and for many families one parent is likely to carry a heterozygous genotype completely different from that of the other parent.

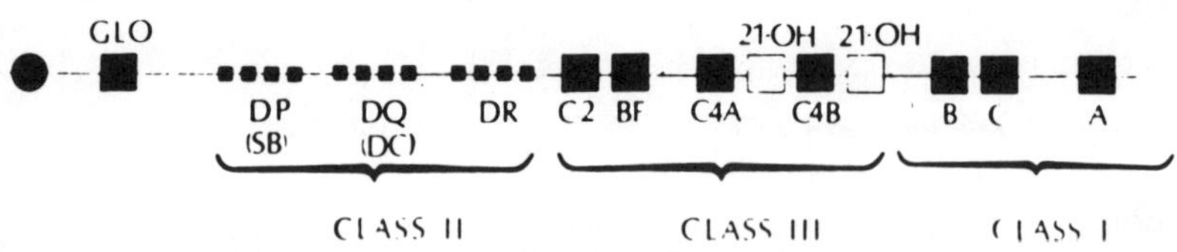

Figure 3 : Genetic map of the HLA region (White et al., 1984).

The centromere of chromosome 6 is at the extreme left of the map. Each square on the map represents a locus. GLO, the locus for the intracellular enzyme, glyoxalase I, is approximately 5 cM from the region. The names of the class I and class II loci are official names of the 1984 International Histocompatibility Testing Workshop. Class III loci, C2, Bf, C4A and C4B encode complement components. The loci, 21-OH are those of the genes for the P-450 enzyme, 21-hydroxylase. One of the 21-OH genes is inactive, perhaps a pseudogene, and is probably that next to C4A. Orientation of the class III loci to each other within the region is known. It is known that the 21-OH loci are very close to the C4 loci and 3' to them. The orientation of the class III region with respect to the flanking regions is unknown. The genetic distance from HLA-B to HLA-DR is 0.8-1.0 cM.

The phenotype encoded by these three polymorphic loci are cell surface proteins (peripheral blood lymphocytes are usually tested) which are detected by well characterized alloantiserums. The alleles at these loci are codominant, and ambiguity in tracking any of these alleles in families is infrequent. It should be noted that molecular genetic analysis of the HLA region has demonstrated additional loci for a total of at least 20 loci, not all polymorphic, and there is room for perhaps 100 genes. The polymorphism of the HLA region can even be extended by considering it as a complex locus. Instead of using the alleles at a single polymorphic locus as genetic markers, one can determine from family studies the haploid combinations of alleles from several (or all) linked polymorphic loci. Such combinations of alleles, residing on the same chromosome, are called haplotypes and can be used as genetic markers. The component alleles of an HLA haplotype will most of the time be inherited as a unit, with occasional exceptions because of genetic exchanges between chromosome 6 homologues, as predicted by a recombination frequency of 2-3% between the extremities of the region. One can expect fewer genetic exchanges by limiting the haplotypes to the more closely linked loci, HLA-A, B and C; the latter locus, between A and B, has at least 9 alleles. The number of allelic haplotypes expected in the population will be many times more than the number of the alleles at any one of the loci. The point to be made is that allelic haplotypes provide more efficient genetic markers than any of the single component loci.

Restriction fragment length polymorphisms provide a rich supply of genetic markers

The number of loci which could be used as markers for linkage analysis was rather limited until about seven years ago, when a new class of almost unlimited genetic markers became available, restriction fragment length polymorphisms (RFLPs) (Botstein et al., 1980). These polymorphisms of nucleotide sequences of genomic DNA can be detected with restriction endonucleases, a class of enzymes isolated from prokaryotic cells. Each of these enzymes cuts the DNA at a specific small sequence, usually of 4 or 6 nucleotide base pairs, but will not cut if one or more base pair in the restriction endonuclease site is changed (Figure 4). There are many specific sites for a single restriction endonuclease in genomic DNA (of the order of hundreds of thousands to millions of such sites), so that very many restriction fragments will be generated when the DNA is incubated under appropriate conditions with one of these enzymes. Polymorphism for a restriction site, can be inferred from comparing lengths of restriction fragments generated by the enzyme from that segment from various individuals. The many fragments of a restriction enzyme digest are ordered according to molecular size by electrophoresis,

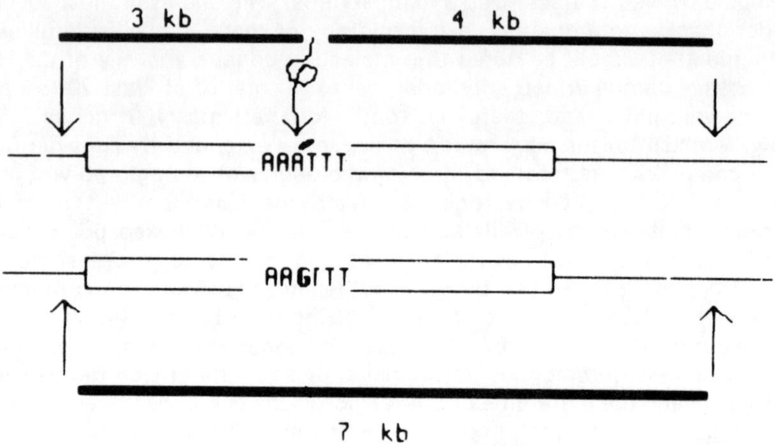

Figure 4 : Specificity of a restriction endonuclease site.
The enzyme recognizes the hexanucleotide sequence, AAATTT, and specifically cleaves the DNA at the site. Change of a single base in this site deletes the site. The restriction enzyme will no longer cut the DNA at this site.

and the fragments generated from a particular segment of genomic DNA can be recognized by hybridization with a radiolabelled cloned gene or sequence from the segment (Figure 5). RFLPs of specific DNA segments can also be created by insertion or deletion of a stretch of nucleotide base pairs. Individuals with the insertion will show a restriction fragment larger than that of someone who does not carry the insertion.

When a sequence cloned from a particular gene is used to probe the ordered restriction fragments, the RFLP detected will be located in or near one or more copies of the gene in the genome. When the origin of a cloned sequence is unknown, the RFLP it detects is called arbitrary or anonymous. All RFLPs, originating from genomic DNA, whether associated with known genes or arbitrary DNA segments, follow Mendelian laws of inheritance, and, thus, can be used as genetic markers. Each RFLP reflects a locus in a DNA segment, albeit an arbitrary locus in many instances, and the polymorphic fragments of that locus behave in populations and segregate in families as co-dominant alleles (Figure 6). Well over 100 restriction endonucleases are known, and it is almost always possible to find a RFLP in a specific DNA segment if one searches for polymorphism with many enzymes.

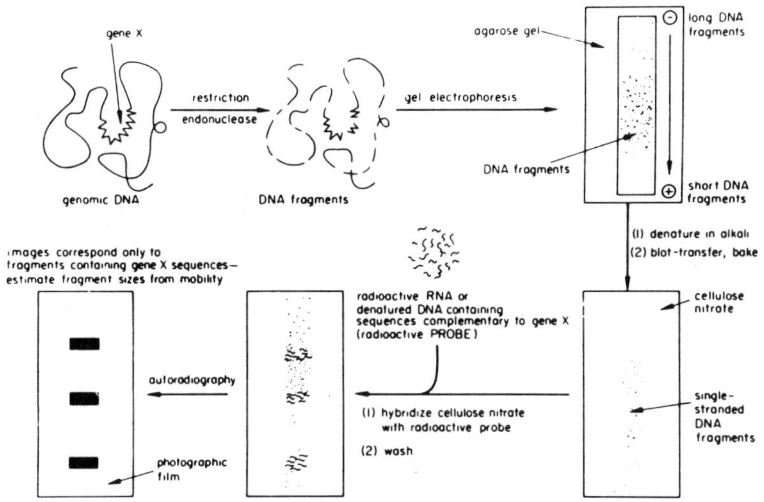

Figure 5 : Detection of restriction fragments (the Southern blot).
Cellular DNA is digested, under appropriate conditions, with a restriction endonuclease. The many restriction fragments are ordered, according to molecular size, by electrophoresis in agarose gel. The fragments are transferred to a hybridization membrane, maintaining the same order as in the gel. The fragments on the membrane are hybridized to a radiolabelled probe, which specifically hybridizes to complementary sequences. The fragments hybridized by the probe are visualized by autoradiography.

As already noted, the efficiency of linkage mapping increases if efficient genetic markers are used. RFLPs with high heterozygote frequencies have been found, especially when insertion of repeated sequences has been the basis for polymorphism (Bell et al., 1981; Jeffreys et al., 1985). Schumm et al. (1985) studied 160 RFLPs detected with a selected group of probes and found that 60% of these showed high heterozygote frequencies. DNA segments have been found with polymorphism of restriction sites of more than one enzyme, detected with the same probe (Barker et al., 1984). The sites for different restriction enzymes will generally not be identical, and polymorphism of different sites in the same segment is analogous to the multiple polymorphic loci of a complex genetic region, e.g., the HLA region. Thus, haplotypes consisting of combinations of allelic fragments from the different RFLPs of the same DNA segment can be defined, leading to a heterozygote frequency in excess of that for any one RFLP in such segments. The span of segments defined by cloned sequences is usually quite small in terms of genetic distance, and the frequency of recombination between arbitrary loci in a segment is likely to be low, certainly less than 1%. For practical purposes, the component allelic

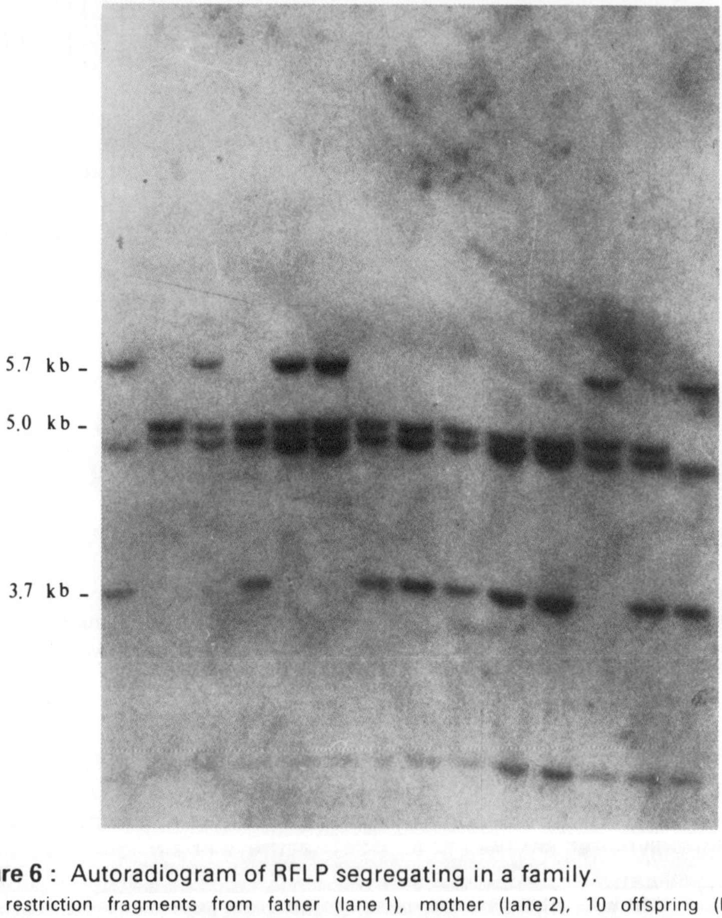

Figure 6 : Autoradiogram of RFLP segregating in a family.

TaqI restriction fragments from father (lane 1), mother (lane 2), 10 offspring (lanes 3 through 12), paternal grandfather (lane 13) and paternal grandmother (lane 14). The RFLP consists of 3 allelic fragments of molecular size 5.7, 5.0 and 3.7 kb, indicated in the figure. The father is heterozygous for the 5.7 and 3.7 kb fragments. The mother is homozygous for the 5.0 kb fragment. Thus, each offspring is heterozygous for the (maternal) 5.0 kb fragment and the 5.7 or 3.7 kb (paternal) fragment. The father of this family inherited the 5.7 kb fragment from his mother and the 3.7 kb fragment from his father. This RFLP is detected with a radiolabelled genomic cloned sequence located close to the HLA-B locus (Leach et al., 1986).

fragments will be inherited as a unit. It appears that numerous efficient markers can be found among RFLPs.

An important practical aspect of the use of RFLPs as genetic markers concerns the source of the genomic DNA. A peripheral blood sample provides the nucleated cells which are the source of the DNA. Lymphocytes from peripheral blood of an individual can also be used for the establishment of lymphoblastoid cell line, which serves as a permanent source of genomic DNA. Numerous samplings of the individual are avoided.

Over 300 fairly well characterized RFLPs have been reported (Human Gene Mapping 8, 1985). Many of these have been localized to chromosomes and chromosome bands by physical assignment techniques, and most are being used for linkage studies. The availability of RFLPs has indeed been a stimulus to large scale linkage mapping.

Efficient collection of data for linkage mapping : a reference panel of families with large sibships, both parents and all 4 grandparents

Families with large sibships, living parents and grandparents are especially informative for linkage mapping (Figure 7) (White et al., 1985). Each offspring affords the opportunity to assay for recombinant maternal and/or paternal chromosomes. It follows that the more offspring scored, the more secure will be the estimate of the recombination frequency, the basic unit of linkage mapping. The study of the grandparents of the sibship enables a determination of phase of the heterozygous parent(s), resulting in direct identification of offspring carrying recombinant or non recombinant chromosomes; only when both grandparents are themselves heterozygous for the same alleles at the loci under consideration will phase not be known. Lod scores for sibships arising from phase known parents are higher than for those where phase is unknown (see Figure 1), especially for smaller sibship sizes. It follows that linkage will be detected with fewer phase known than phase unknown families. Phase information can sometimes also be obtained from extended multigeneration families. The effort in collecting and sampling the often widely dispersed individuals of families with the latter structure must be considerably greater than working with two generation nuclear families plus grandparents. Furthermore, White et al. (1985) have provided data which indicate that collection of linkage data is more efficient with complete nuclear families plus grandparents than with extended families. The consideration of family structure is quite relevant to the design of large scale linkage mapping efforts.

The efficiency of data collection will be increased enormously with creation of a panel of test or reference families of optimal structure for development of the human linkage map. The idea is to accumulate data on segregation of a large number of genetic markers in the same group of families. Submitting the same group of chromosomes to many efficient markers should hasten detection of linkage among multiple loci and the estimation of gene/marker order. Parents of these families with one or both heterozygous parents will be studied for segregation. Eventually, parents in these families will be heterozygous at multiple loci, in the same and different linkage groups, thus facilitating the mapping of a new marker (Figure 7). The creation of such a reference panel of families implies a collaborative effort, not only for collecting numbers of families of the optimal structure, but also for accumulating the large number of RFLPs which will be tested in the panel. The collaboration, then involves many laboratories testing local probes on DNA from the same group of reference families. It becomes evident that for such a collaborative effort, an informative family is that with one or both parents heterozygous at a single locus; the linked locus (or loci) may be that of a marker in a collaborating laboratory. The support and coordination for the collaboration involves making DNA available from the test panel and collecting and analyzing the data from all participating laboratories.

```
 +---+              ---            +---+              ---
 |15 |--------------|16 |          |17 |--------------|18 |
 +---+        |     ---            +---+        |     ---
            +---+                              ---
            | 1 |------------------------------| 2 |
            +---+                |             ---
                                 |
  1 2       2 2       2 2        |       1 3    1 3 *   1 1
  2 2       2 2       2 2        |       1 2    1 2 *   2 2
  0 0       0 0       0 0        |       0 0    0 0     0 0
  4 4       1 4 *     1 4        |       1 4    4 4     4 4
  1 2       1 2 *     1 2        |       1 2    1 2 *   1 2
  3 3       1 3 *     1 3        |       1 3    3 3     3 3
                                 |
  ---------------------------------------------------------
  |    |    |    |    |    |    |    |    |    |    |    |
 --   --   --  +--+ +--+ +--+  --   --  +--+ +--+  --   --
| 3| | 4| | 5| | 6| | 7| | 8| | 9| |10| |11| |12| |13| |14|
 --   --   --  +--+ +--+ +--+  --   --  +--+ +--+  --   --


1 2  2 3  2 3  2 3  1 2  1 2  2 3  2 3  2 3  1 2  2 3  2 3
2 2  1 2  1 2  1 2  2 2  2 2  1 2  1 2  1 2  1 2  1 2  1 2
0 0  0 0  0 0  0 0  0 0  0 0  0 0  0 0  0 0  0 0  0 0  0 0
4 4  1 4  1 4  4 4  1 4  1 4  4 4  1 4  1 4  1 4  4 4  1 4
1 1  2 2  2 2  1 1  2 2  1 1  1 2  2 2  1 1  1 2  1 2  1 2
3 3  1 3  1 3  3 3  1 3  1 3  3 3  1 3  1 3  0 0  3 3  1 3
```

Figure 7 : Pedigree of a nuclear family and all 4 grandparents.

Genotypes/phenotypes of 5 marker loci are given beneath each individual. Closed squares represent males, and open squares females. A parent heterozygous at a locus is indicated by *.

Such a collaboration has been formed. The Centre d'Etude du Polymorphisme Human (CEPH) was organized in 1984 to hasten the mapping of the human genome by linkage analysis with DNA polymorphisms. The CEPH provides to collaborating investigators cellular DNA produced from cultured lymphoblastoid cell lines derived from each member of a reference panel of large families and a data base contributed to and shared by the investigators. Collaborating investigators use the DNA from the family panel to test informative families for RFLPs detected with their own probes. They contribute the results of these tests to the data base. As of July 1, 1986, 33 investigators in North America, Europe and Africa collaborate with the CEPH. It is estimated that approximately 500 probes are being used in the collaboration.

From 100 families available from various sources, almost all not selected for disease, a group of 40 families have been defined for the initial CEPH reference panel. The mean sibship size of these 40 families is 8.3, no family has less than 6 offspring and 23 families have 8 or more offspring. Cell lines are available for all four grandparents in each of 30 families of the reference panel. All of these families had been typed with various RFLPs and traditional genetic markers and been used for linkage assignments prior to entering the panel, enhancing their value as a reference population for linkage mapping. The CEPH has prepared and sent computer programs for data management and linkage analysis to collaborating investigators. CEPH manages the data base by computer and will monitor the growing genetic map continually with programs for detecting linkage and for determining order on a chromosome of multiple genetic markers.

The emphasis in creating the reference panel has been on the collection of normal families. The strategy for mapping the human genome involves placing evenly spaced genetic markers on all the chromosomes, primarily by linkage mapping, and there is no need to use generally poorly efficient disease loci for the task. It is likely that most of the evenly spaced markers on the human map will be RFLPs. Localization of disease loci will be made with linked markers which are also localized on the map. By emphasizing normal families, rather than those of patients with genetic disorders, for a reference panel, it is easier to find families with optimal structure for efficient collection of data for linkage analysis.

Efficient analysis of data

Traditionally, detection of linkage, the estimation of recombination frequencies and inference of order of linked genetic markers have depended on analysis of segregation of pairs of loci (so called 2 point tests). Recently, a series of papers have provided tests to support the contention that analysis of segregation of markers at three or more loci (multipoint tests) is more efficient (Lathrop et al., 1984; 1985). The interest in exploring the multilocus approach was raised, in part, in response to the realization that a large number of genetic markers were becoming available for linkage analysis and that linkage groups containing many markers could be envisioned. Furthermore, a test panel of families with optimal structure for collecting data for linkage, as just described, efficiently provides data for multilocus analysis, another impetus for evaluating this analytic approach.

Lathrop et al. (1985) have tested relative merits of two point and three point linkage analysis in estimating recombination frequencies. Tests were made by varying conditions pertaining to phase, mode of inheritance, number and frequencies of alleles for each locus, values of θ between adjacent loci and flanking loci and assumptions about interference. In general, under all conditions investigated, the efficiency of the estimates of recombination frequencies with three point analysis was the same as or greater than with 2 point tests. For three codominant loci, each with 2 alleles, the estimates of adjacent or flanking marker recombination frequencies were more efficient with three point analysis, especially with an assumption of no interference. Also, irrespective of the number of marker alleles, the estimate of θ for the two adjacent intervals was more efficient with three point analysis when the distance between flanking loci was held fixed. When the mode of inheritance for one marker was that of a rare autosomal dominant or a rate autosomal recessive trait, i.e., mimicking inheritance of a genetic disease, again increased efficiencies for estimates of θ were obtained with three point analysis, especially for the latter, linked to flanking markers, in phase known families. Efficiencies were also increased when each type of disease locus was a flanking marker. These results suggest that multilocus linkage analysis is the analytic technique of choice for construction of linkage maps, although formal proof of the advantage with more than three loci has not been demonstrated. These results also indicate the advantage of linking a disease locus to a linkage group, rather than to a single marker.

It is also possible to detect linkage by multilocus analysis (Lathrop et al., 1984). This involved determining the likelihood of the map location of a locus with respect to the members of a linkage group (Figure 8). The distances among loci in the group are held fixed, and the location of the locus under consideration, which could be previously untested, e.g., that of a disease, is varied in and outside the linkage group. For each value of map location, given as map distance from the same member of the linkage group, the likelihood of the location is computed from the probability of the joint segregation at all of these loci in the observed pedigree data as a function of location. This likelihood is divided by the likelihood for a location far removed from the linkage group, i.e., not linked, thus permitting the use of an odds ratio in detection linkage. Lathrop et al. (1984) have called the ratio of these Ln likelihoods of genetic location, "location scores".

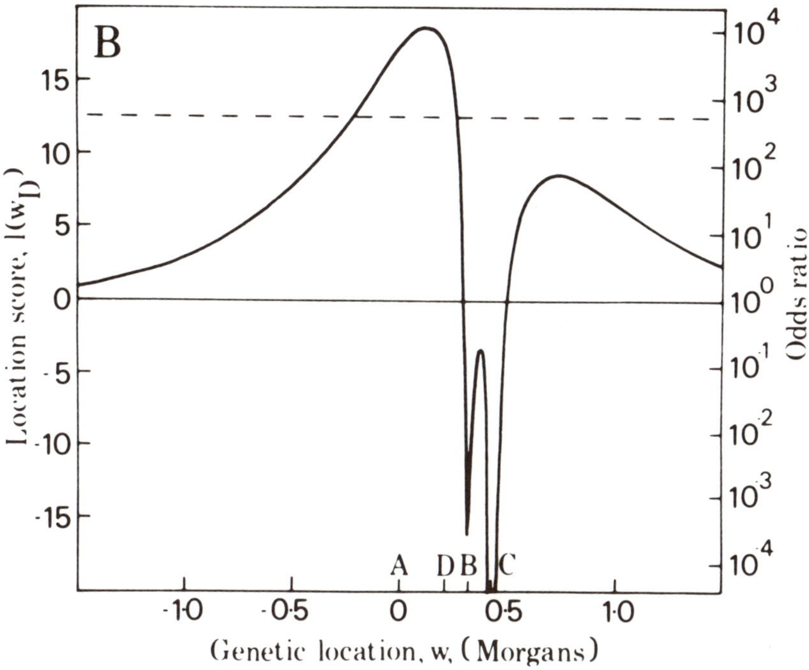

Figure 8 : Linkage and localization of a locus (D) to a linkage group, consisting of loci A, B and C, by location scores. Genetic distance, relative to locus A is on the abscissa. The ordinate shows the odds ratio for each location of D (right) and the corresponding location scores (-2 Ln Likelihood) (left).

If recombination frequencies can be more efficiently estimated with three point analysis, it follows that the precision of an estimate of order of three loci on the chromosome will be improved. For each possible order, the adjacent recombination frequencies can be estimated and a relative likelihood can be calculated. Each order, then, can be evaluated in relation to another order by ratios of the relative likelihoods (Figure 9).

The computer program package, LINKAGE (Lathrop et al., 1985), iterates maximum likelihood estimates of recombination frequencies for two or more loci and calculates the relative Ln likelihood for each iteration. For the analysis of more than three loci, no interference is assumed. The estimation of recombination frequencies for multiple loci can make use of data from families informative for subsets of loci. This attribute allows, for example, pooling of data from normal families and families of patients with a genetic disorder tested with one or more of the same markers. The package also provides lod score calculations for two loci and a graphic solution, with location scores, for likelihood calculations for assignment of linkage to multiple loci.

```
SPEEDY VERSION OF ILINK FOR CEPH PEDIGREES
CHROMOSOME ORDER OF LOCI :
  2  1  4  3
##############################################
THETAS:
 0.077 0.091 0.081
##############################################
-2 LN(LIKE) =  -4.46782192726951E+001
NUMBER OF ITERATIONS =       8
NUMBER OF FUNCTION EVALUATIONS =     42
PTG =  -5.43591072559617E-005
   3  2  1  4
##############################################
THETAS:
 0.173 0.070 0.075
##############################################
-2 LN(LIKE) =  -4.26983391185404E+001
NUMBER OF ITERATIONS =       7
NUMBER OF FUNCTION EVALUATIONS =     36
PTG =  -9.99494427979000E-005
EXIT CONDITIONS
Specified tolerance on normalized gradient
..............................................
```

Figure 9 : Joint estimation of adjacent recombination frequencies and the Ln relative likelihood for each of two orders of four loci.

Human linkage maps

Some human linkage maps have been constructed using estimation of recombination frequencies and inferring order on the chromosome by multilocus analysis. Drayna and White (1985) constructed a linkage map spanning the human X chromosome with 21 genetic markers assigned to various bands on the short and long arms; 20 of these markers are RFLPs. Figure 10 shows this map. The data for linkage analysis were generated from families with large sibship size and parents and all 4 grandparents studied. Individual markers and groups of markers are roughly evenly spaced along the X chromosome at intervals ranging from 10-40 cM. The order of some markers along the chromosome was inferred from band location and for a number of others from multilocus analysis of all possible orders of overlapping sets of four loci. The total length of the map is 185 cM. Other markers localized to the X chromosome can be efficiently and relatively quickly mapped by typing the same families used for constructing the map.

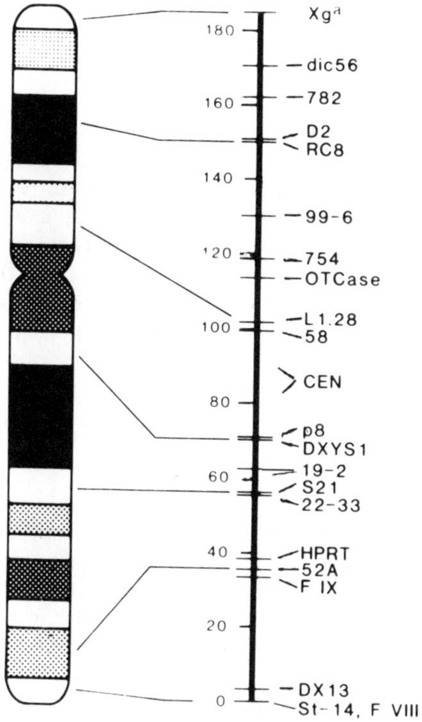

Figure 10 : Linkage map of the human X chromosome (Drayna and White, 1985).

Mapped genetic markers are shown on the right. Genetic distance is given in cM. Chromosome region/band locations of some markers are shown.

Murray and Buetow (in preparation) have constructed a map on the long arm of chromosome 4 with 10 markers, 8 of which are RFLPs. The map span is approximately 90 cM, extending from the centromere to band 31. The data for constructing the map were generated from large nuclear families, many with all four grandparents studied.

Leppert et al. (1985) have mapped the long arm of chromosome 13 with 7 RFLPs and one polymorphic enzyme marker. Large nuclear families, each with four grandparents, were the source for the mapping data. The map, extending from 13q12 to 13q33 spans 87 cM. A preliminary map of 6 markers has been constructed for the long arm of chromosome 22 (Julier et al., 1985); 5 of these markers are RFLPs. Other human linkage maps include the distal portion of the short arm of chromosome 11 (6 markers all assigned to band 15) and the short arm of chromosome 6 (8 markers) (White et al., 1985; Holm et al., 1985; Leach et al., 1986).

Diagnosis of genetic disorders by linkage

The idea of diagnosis of a genetic disorder by markers linked to its locus is attractive. In the ideal situation, it supposes one or more efficient genetic markers linked so closely to a locus of a deleterious (with respect to the disease) allele that the linked ensemble segregates as a unit with an acceptable probability. The marker(s) will faithfully trace the disease gene and so rarely be separated from it by recombination that it (they) will reliably identify individuals who will develop the disease. The at risk situations are well known, usually pertaining to prenatal diagnosis and, postnatally, to prediction of disease with delayed age of onset. The idea is not new, and prior to the availability of RFLPs, a few reports of prenatal diagnosis appeared (e.g., Insley et al., 1976).

The approach to diagnosis is similar but not identical to a linkage analysis of the family of the individual at risk, whose phenotype at the disease locus is unknown. At least one parent must be heterozygous for at least one marker and at the closely linked locus of the deleterious allele. Most patients with single locus determined genetic disorders have at least one parent heterozygous for the deleterious allele, and at risk sibling or offspring may be tested if the heterozygous parent is also heterozygous for the linked marker(s). This depends on the heterozygote frequency of the marker in the population. The diagnostic potential is favored if the linkage involves efficient markers. Thus, not all families of patients are eligible for diagnostic or predictive linkage studies. Eligibility will be highest for disease loci linked to markers with heterozygote frequencies approaching those of the HLA system and some exceptional RFLPs.

Despite parental double or multiple heterozygosity, some ambiguous results may be expected, especially with diallelic marker systems. In this context, an ambiguous result refers to poor discrimination by the linkage based test, i.e., an outcome indicating equal probabilities for being affected or unaffected. Phase information, about a doubly heterozygous parent or about the chromosome(s) carrying the deleterious allele(s), is important for the diagnostic test. The parents of the doubly heterozygous parent who carries an allele determining an autosomal dominant or X-linked disorder may be available to establish the phase of this individual. In the absence of the grandparents, parental phase may be inferred from previously affected offspring homozygous at the marker locus in the case of an autosomal dominant disorder. An unaffected parent homozygous at the marker locus also provides phase information. Previously affected offspring typed for the genetic marker will provide phase information about the chromosomes carrying the alleles for an autosomal recessive disorder.

A few examples illustrate the utility of phase information. In the case of an autosomal recessive disorder, diagnostic testing will be informative for only marker homozygous offspring when the mating is an intercross (both parents heterozygous) for the same two alleles at the marker locus and a previous affected offspring is also heterozygous. The probability that a marker homozygous offspring will be affected is low, roughly twice the recombination frequency for small values of θ . This is also true if one of the parents is homozygous for a marker allele; the risk to the marker homozygous offspring is close to θ . For an autosomal dominant disorder, a previously affected child, heterozygous for the marker, provides no phase information for diagnostic testing when the mating is a diallelic intercross. Unless phase of the affected parent is known, the diagnosis for any offspring in this family is ambiguous. If the unaffected parent is homozygous at the marker locus, phase information is available, and ambiguity is avoided. The probability of a marker heterozygous offspring being affected will be high, about $1-2\theta$, and of a homozygous offspring being affected will be low, roughly 2θ, for small values of θ . These examples also illustrate the advantages of using markers as closely linked as possible to the locus of the deleterious allele.

The additional information provided by segregation of three marker alleles in the family will prevent many but not all ambiguous outcomes, and with four marker alleles there is no ambiguity at all. Two or more markers closely linked to each other and to the locus of the deleterious allele improve the potential for more than two marker alleles (allelic haplotypes) to segregate in a family at risk. Ambiguous results should be encountered less frequently.

For close linkage between a genetic marker and the disease locus of an allele for an X-linked recessive disorder, ambiguity should not be encountered with linkage based diagnostic tests when phase information is available, e.g., from the marker genotype of the maternal grandfather or a previously affected male offspring.

Two or more closely linked marker loci provide the opportunity for markers to flank the disease locus. If the genotypes at the flanking marker loci are heterozygous and phase information is available, recombination occurring between one of the markers and the disease locus will be detected as a recombination between the flanking markers, which are typed for diagnostic testing. If the phase of the flanking markers of one of the haplotypes carried by the individual being tested is the same as that of the parental haplotype carrying the deleterious allele, the probability is minimized that recombination has separated this allele from the haplotype. For separation to occur, two crossover events flanking the disease locus would be required, the probability of which would be very low if flanking markers are closely linked. Markers flanking the disease locus can add to the accuracy of the diagnostic test. It is likely that the information provided by flanking markers will benefit diagnostic testing for autosomal dominant and X-linked disorders moreso than for autosomal recessive disorders, for which parental phase is more difficult to determine, especially with respect to the deleterious allele.

The use of efficient RFLPs as linkage markers for mapping and diagnostic testing enhance these procedures. The heterozygote frequencies for the RFLPs found to be linked to the loci of Huntington's disease (Gusella et al., 1984; Youngman et al., 1985), the fragile-X mental retardation syndrome (Oberle et al., 1986) and cystic fibrosis (White et al., 1985) range from 0.6 to 0.9. The locus for Huntington's disease is linked to a DNA segment containing several restriction site polymorphisms (D4S10) on the short arm of chromosome 4 (band 4p16). A recent report (Zabel et al., 1985) estimates the distance between marker and disease loci as about 5 cM (confidence limits not presented). The X-linked fragile site, FRAXQ27 or FRAXA, associated with a form of X-linked mental retardation, is flanked by two efficient RFLPs, DXS52, localized to band Xq28, and F9 (the gene for coagulation factor IX gene), localized to Xq27. The estimated recombination frequency between DXS52 and FRAXA is 0.10 (90% confidence limits: 0.04-0.18), between F9 and FRAXA is 0.12 (90% confidence limits: 0.04-0.22) and between DXS52 and F9 is 0.19 (90% confidence limits: 0.09-0.32) in families with affected individuals. The map distances between FRAXA and each of the single marker loci are too high for diagnostic testing. However, these markers flank FRAXA and can be used to detect crossing over between them. The probability of a double crossover event involving the intervals between FRAXA and F9 or DXS52 is of the order of 1-2 %, an error level which might be acceptable to some individuals. A single recombination event between the flanking markers is expected to occur in about 20% of meioses, and evidence of crossing over would indicate that the diagnosis is ambiguous. Thus the test could be useful for diagnosis of 80% of at risk males in informative families.

Very close linkage between the locus of the gene for 21 hydroxylase and flanking markers, HLA-A and B (distally) and HLA-DR (proximally), is the basis of a diagnostic test for congenital adrenal hyperplasia due to 21 hydroxylase deficiency (Mornet et al., 1986), an autosomal recessive disorder (Figure 3). The genetic distance between the HLA-DR and HLA-B loci is approximately 1 cM. This small distance indicates that a diagnostic error due to recombination between the 21 hydroxylase locus and either of the marker loci is likely to be very small indeed. The probability of a double crossing over event flanking this locus is even lower. Thus, this linkage group possesses characteristics favorable for diagnosis by linkage. The test is enhanced by the use of markers which are efficient. First trimester prenatal diagnosis was undertaken in seven pregnancies at risk for 21 hydroxylase deficiency. The fetal genotype at the 21 hydroxylase locus in each case was inferred from chorionic villi DNA probed for RFLPs associated with alleles at the marker loci. The prenatal diagnosis was confirmed by independent tests in 6 cases; the outcome of the seventh case is not yet known.

Recent data for the linkages between the cystic fibrosis locus and the RFLPs on the long arm of chromosome 7 (between bands 7q21-q31), at the met oncogene locus (White et al., 1985) and at the anonymous DNA segment pJ3.11 (Wainwright et al., 1985), have not been reported. However, the initial data suggest that very close linkage with each marker is possible. If these markers are indeed very closely linked and flank the cystic fibrosis locus, a useful diagnostic test could be available.

As basic information accumulates on a genetic disease, it sometimes becomes evident that the disorder represents a heterogeneity, i.e., a disease phenotype which is determined at one of several possible loci. Examples of such genetic heterogeneity are well known in medical genetics. It is reasonable to assume that the potential for genetic heterogeneity exists for most inherited disorders appearing to fit a single locus determination. The diagnosis or prediction of a genetic disease by linkage is limited in this respect, and it cannot be emphasized sufficiently that what is being tested is the genotype at a single disease locus (or, perhaps, at a group of closely linked loci). The test gives no diagnostic information whatsoever about a similar disease or a different form of the condition determined at an unlinked locus. Detection of close linkage between one or more genetic markers and a locus of a deleterious allele is encouraging for the development of a diagnostic test, but many families of patients, with different recognizable forms of the disease, must be studied to attempt to rule out heterogeneity in the recombination fraction between loci. In 1955, Morton, in an elegant demonstration of the power of linkage in studying disease, presented evidence for genetic heterogeneity in elliptocytosis, an autosomal dominant disorder of red blood cells, one form of which is determined at a locus which is linked to the complex Rh blood group locus on chromosome 1 (Morton, 1955). His analysis demonstrated that in some families of affected individuals there is no evidence of linkage with Rh, while in others the evidence is quite compelling. Thus, linkage analysis is a useful method for detecting genetic heterogeneity. One motivation for searching for linkage between RFLPs and a disease locus is the lack of basic information about the molecular pathogenesis. The concept of diagnosis by linked markers is appealing for such disorders. It is lack of basic knowledge about the disease which also could prevent geneticists and physicians from appreciating heterogeneity.

Experience is beginning to show that searching for linkage with a battery of genetic markers in a group of families in which a hereditary disorder is segregating is likely to demonstrate one or two markers linked to the locus of the deleterious allele. Further efforts at studying and refining this linkage will make use of the genetic map. The marker found to be linked to the locus of the deleterious allele will also be studied in the normal informative families of a reference panel for efficient and relatively rapid localization on the map. This approach is informative for the disease, because it will demonstrate other interests. The advantages of linkage with multiple markers has been discussed. In addition, some of these markers are likely to be more closely linked to the disease locus than the original marker. It is possible, indeed essential, to use the genetic map derived, in large part, from normal families to study the linkage relationships of a disease locus,

Multifactorial inheritance

Ordinarily, linkage between loci is not evident at the population level. Association of phenotypes at these loci is not usually noted in the population. Family studies are required to demonstrate co-segregation of the loci. The reason population association is not evident is that recombination tends to separate the various allelic combinations of the loci on the same chromosome; note that such allelic combinations are haplotypes. Over evolutionary time, one should find in a sufficiently large population all possible haplotypes representing all possible combinations of alleles from each locus. The frequency of each haplotype is expected to be the product of the frequencies of the component alleles in the population. This outcome of recombination between linked loci is known as linkage equilibrium.

Exceptions to linkage equilibrium are encountered, especially in the case of extremely close linkage, perhaps 1 cM and less. Separation by recombination of alleles at extremely close loci will occur relatively slowly over evolution giving rise, if enough time has not elapsed to permit sufficient exchange, to associations of alleles on haplotypes such that their frequencies will be higher than expected. Natural selection may contribute to the association of alleles by favoring the carriers of such haplotypes. These associations can be recognized at the population level. Linkage disequilibrium refers to associations of alleles from linked loci with frequencies which differ from the expected.

Linkage disequilibrium is probably the best explanation for population association of certain disorders and various HLA alleles (Svejgaard et al., 1983) (Table 1) . For instance, comparison of a group of patients with ankylosing spondylitis and a group of control individuals shows that the allele, HLA-B27, occurs in approximately 90% of the former and about 10% of the latter. The frequencies of the alleles, HLA-DR3 and DR4, are significantly increased, more than doubled, among patients with insulin dependent diabetes mellitus as compared to suitable control groups. The frequency of HLA-Cw6 is significantly higher in patients with psoriasis than the general population. The explanation usually given for these types of associations is that the locus of the HLA marker allele is close to that of a locus involved in determining the disease, and the resulting linkage disequilibrium is the basis for the population association. It is unlikely that the disease is directly determined by genotypes at the locus so detected, because these conditions do not show the formal genetic characteristics of single locus control, with the exception of 21 hydroxylate deficiency. Rather, they are thought to be determined by multifactorial inheritance, determined by genes at more than one locus in concert with environmental influences. The locus detected by an HLA association is considered to be one of the loci involved in determining the disorder. These associations are useful in defining at least one of the loci in the multifactorial determination of these diseases, and inferences about the nature of the pathogenesis may be made (cautiously), based on the location of the locus in a chromosomal region determining a particular function.

Table 1: Some significant HLA and disease associations

Disease	HLA	Patients	Controls	RR*
Ankylosing Spondylitis	B27	89%	9%	69.1
I.D.D.M.	DR3	46%	22%	3.3
	DR4	51%	25%	3.6
	DR3/DR4			14.3
Multiple Sclerosis	DR2	51%	27%	2.7
Myasthenia Gravis	B8	44%	19%	3.3
Psoriasis	CW6	56%	15%	7.5

*RR - Relative Risk

RFLPs, detected with probes from various HLA loci, are being used to refine the associations with disease (Cohen-Hagenauer et al., 1985; Marcadet et al., 1985). At the present state of knowledge, it is unlikely that most associations between HLA and disease provide the basis for widely used diagnostic tests.

Many other genetic disorders determined by multifactorial inheritance show no population associations with HLA or other genetic markers. Many congenital malformations, some forms of schizophrenia and common forms of arteriosclerotic heart disease are but a few examples of disorders falling in the multifactorial group of genetic diseases, which contribute significantly to morbidity and mortality in the population. At present, there is not enough information on the inheritance of these types of disorders; diagnosis by linkage is not a possibility. However, linkage analysis with batteries of efficient genetic markers of families with multiple affected individuals offers promise of localizing one or more genes involved. Evidence of coinheritance of the disease phenotype and a marker can be interpretated as localizing one of the genes in the multifactorial process as being linked to the marker locus. The more complete localization of such genes will involve use of the human genetic map, as discussed. Localization of a locus involved in multifactorial inheritance of a genetic disorder will be the first step in learning about its contribution to disease determination.

Perspective

Some limitations of diagnostic and predictive tests based on linkage have been presented. Ways to overcome some of the limitations, especially with efficient markers, are potentially available. Until these limitations are remedied, geneticists and physicians must be aware of them and consider them in presenting the pros and cons of the diagnostic test to the family at risk. Despite the limitations, such tests will provide diagnostic information to individuals at risk for the appropriate genetic disorder not available prior to the development of the test. Despite the exciting explosion of knowledge set off by the scientific revolution called molecular genetics, most inherited disease still have not been unravelled to the point where rational diagnostic and predictive tests can be designed. With map, linkage becomes a viable, realistic and practical basis for diagnosis and prediction. The direct detection of a specific disease gene by an oligonucleotide probe, available for some disorders, is predicated on much existing basic knowledge about the disorder, not available for most genetic diseases. The detection of linkage will not only lead to diagnostic tests, but also contribute to the molecular genetic analysis of many hereditary diseases.

References

Barker, D., Holm, T. and White, R.
A locus on chromosome 11p with multiple restriction site polymorphisms.
Am. J. Hum. Genet. 36, 1159-1171, 1984.

Bell, G.I., Karam, J.H. and Rutter, W.J.
Polymorphic DNA region adjecent to the 5' end of the human insulin gene.
Proc. Natl. Acad. Sci. USA 78, 5759-5763, 1981.

Botstein, D., White, R.L., Skolnick, M. and David, R.W.
Construction of a genetic linkage map in men using restriction fragment length polymorphisms.
Am. J. Hum. Genet. 32, 314-331, 1980.

Cohen-Haguenauer, O., Robbins, E., Massart, C., Busson, M., Deschamps, I., Hors, J., Lalouel, J.M., Dausset, J., Cohen, D.
A systematic study of HLA class II-ß DNA restriction fragments in insulin-dependent diabetes mellitus.
Proc. Natl. Acad. Sci. USA 82, 3335-3339, 1985.

Drayna, D. and White, R.
The genetic linkage map of the human X chromosome.
Science 230, 753-758, 1985.

Francke, U. and Pellegrino, M.A.
Assignment of the major histocompatibility complex to a region of the short arm of human chromosome 6.
Proc. Natl. Acad. Sci. USA 74, 1145-1151, 1977.

Gusella, J., Tanzi, R.E., Anderson, M.A., Hobbs, W., Gibbons, K., Raschtchion, R., Gilliam, T.G., Wallace, M.R., Wexler, N.S., Conneally, P.M.
DNA markers for nervous system diseases.
Science 225, 1320-1326, 1984.

Histocompatibility Testing 1984, Ed. Albert, E.D. et al., Springer-Verlag, Berlin, Heidelberg, 1984.

Holm, T., O'Connell, P., Leppert, M., Callahan, P., Lalouel, J.M. and White, R.
Parathyroid hormone and calcitonin are tightly linked and have been placed on the genetic map of chromosome 11p.
Human Gene Mapping 8 (1985).
Cytogenetics and Cell Genetics, Vol. 40, Nos. 1-4, p. 653, 1985.

Human Gene Mapping 8 (1985) : Eight International Workshop on Human

Gene Mapping.
Cytogenetics and Cell Genetics, Vol. 40, Nos. 1-4, 1985.

Insley, J., Bird, G.W.G., Harper, P.S. and Pearce, G.W.
Prenatal prediction of myotonic dystrophy.
Lancet i, 806, 1976.

Jeffreys, A.J., Wilson, V. and Thein, S.L.
Hypervariable minisatellite regions in human DNA.
Nature 314, 67-73, 1985.

Julier, C., Lathrop, M., Lalouel, J.M., Reghis, A., Szajnert, M.F. and Caplan, J.C.
New restriction fragment length polymorphisms on human chromosome 22 at loci SIS, MB and IGLV.
Human Gene Mapping 8 (1985).
Cytogenetics and Cell Genetics, Vol. 40, Nos. 1-4, p. 665, 1985.

Lathrop, G.M., Lalouel, J.M., Julier, C. and Ott, J.
Strategies for multilocus linkage analysis in humans.
Proc. Natl. Acad. Sci. USA 81, 3443-3446, 1984.

Lathrop, G.M., Lalouel, J.M., Julier, C. and Ott, J.
Multilocus linkage anlysis in humans : detection of linkage and estimation of recombination.
Am. J. Hum. Genet. 37, 482-498, 1985.

Leach, R., De Mars, R., Hasstedt, S. and White, R.
Construction of a map of the short arm of human chromosome 6.
Proc. Natl. Acad. Sci. USA, 83, 3909-3913, 1986.

Leppert, M., Callahan, P., Cavenee, W., Holm, T., O'Connell, P., Thompson, K., Lalouel, J.M. and White, R.
A genetic linkage map for human chromosome 13.
Human Gene Mapping 8 (1985).
Cytogenetics and Cell Genetics, Vol. 40, Nos. 1-4, p. 679, 1985.

Marcadet, A., Massart, C., Semana, C., Fauchet, R., Sabouraud, O., Marienne, M., Dausset, J. and Cohen, D.
Association of class II HLA-D Q ß-chain DNA restriction fragments with multiple sclerosis.
Immunogenetics 22, 93-96, 1985.

Mornet, E., Boué, J., Raux-Demay, M., Couillin, P., Oury, J.F., Dumez, Y., Dausset, J., Cohen, D. and Boué, A.
First trimester prenatal diagnosis of 21-hydroxylase deficiency by linkage

analysis to HLA-DNA probes and by 17-hydroxyprogesterone determination.
Hum. Genet. 73, 358-364, 1986.

Morton, N.E.
Sequential tests for the detection of linkage.
Am. J. Hum. Genet. 7, 277-318, 1955.

Morton, N.E.
Detection and estimation of linkage between genes for elliptocytosis and Rh blood type.
Am. J. Hum. Genet. 8, 80-96, 1956.

Morton, C.C., Kirsch, I.R., Nance, W.E., Evans, G.A., Korman, A.J.
Orientation of loci within the human major histocompatibility complex by chromosomal in situ hybridization.
Proc. Natl. Acad. Sci. USA 81, 2816-2820, 1984.

Muller, H.J.
The mechanism of crossing-over.
Am. Nat. 50, 193-434, 1916.

Oberlé, I., Heilig, R., Moisan, J.P., Kloepfer, C., Mattéi, M.G., Boué, J., Froster-Iskenius, U., Jacobs, P.A., Lathrop, G.M., Lalouel, J.M. and Mandel, J.L.
Genetic analysis of the fragile-X mental retardation syndrome with two flanking polymorphic DNA markers.
Proc. Natl. Acad. Sci. USA 83, 1016-1020, 1986.

Schumm, J., Knowlton, R., Braman, J., Barker, D., Vovis, G., Akots, G., Brown, V., Gravius, T., Helms, C., Hsiao, K., Rediker, K., Thurston, J., Botstein, D. and Donis-Keller, H.
Detection of more than 500 single-copy RFLPs by random screening.
Human Gene Mapping 8 (1985)
Cytogenetics and Cell Genetics, Vol. 40, Nos. 1-4, p. 739, 1985.

Svejgaard, A., Platz, P. and Ryder, L.P.
HLA and disease 1982. A survey.
Immunol. Rev. 70, 193-218, 1983.

Wainwright, B.J., Scambler, P.J., Schmidtke, J., Watson, E.A., Law, H.Y., Farrall, M., Cooke, H.J., Eiberg, H., Williamson, R.
Localization of cystic fibrosis locus to human chromosome 7cen-q22.
Nature 318, 384-385, 1985.

White, P., New, M. and Dupont, B.

HLA-linked congenital adrenal hyperplasia results from a defective gene encoding an cytochrome P-450 specific for steroid 21-hydroxylation.
Proc. Natl. Acad. Sci. USA 81, 7505-7509, 1984.

White, R., Leppert, M. Bishop, D.T., Barker, D., Berkowitz, J., Brown, C., Callahan, P., Holm, T. and Jeroninski, L.
Construction of linkage maps with DNA markers for human chromosomes.
Nature 313, 101-105, 1985.

White, R., Woodward, S., Leppert, M., O'Connell, P., Hoff, M., Herbst, J., Lalouel, J.M., Dean, M. and Van de Woude, G.
A closely linked genetic marker for cystic fibrosis.
Nature 318, 382-384, 1985.

Youngman, S., Harper, P., Sarfarazi, M., Quarrell, O. and Gusella, J.F.
Genetic linkage between the G8 locus (D4S10) and Huntington's Disease families in Britain.
Human Gene Mapping 8 (1985).
Cytogenetics and Cell Genetics, Vol. 40, Nos. 1-4, p. 786, 1985.

Zabel, B.U., Naylor, S.L., Sakaguchi, A.Y. and Gusella, J.F.
Regional localization of a DNA polymorphism (D4S10) linked to Huntington's Disease at 4p16-p15.
Human Gene Mapping 8 (1985).
Cytogenetics and Cell Genetics, Vol. 40, Nos. 1-4, p. 787, 1985.

IMPACT OF GENETIC COUNSELING AND PRENATAL DIAGNOSIS FOR DOWN SYNDROME AND NEURAL TUBE DEFECTS

Anne SWERTS

Center for Human Genetics, K.U.Leuven
Campus Gasthuisberg, Herestraat, B-3000, Leuven, Belgium

Abstract

In two parallel studies the impact of genetic counseling and prenatal diagnosis upon family planning decisions was evaluated for parents of a child with Down syndrome and for parents of a child with neural tube defect.

One hundred and nineteen parents of a child with standard trisomy 21 volunteered to participate in study I; 94 parents who had a neural tube defect child took part in study II. Each study included three groups of parents : one group received genetic counseling, another group had already an amniocentesis performed and a third group of parents had neither received genetic counseling nor had they an amniocentesis performed. Data collection took place by means of interviews by a social nurse at the parents' home. An exhaustive questionnaire was used to guide the interview and to assess the total impact of the birth of the affected child as completely as possible. Some years later additional follow-up information was gathered by sending a questionnaire to all families.

In both studies a significantly better recall of the relevant risk figures was found in the counseled group as compared with the group of parents who did not receive genetic counseling. The relationship between the recalled risk and its subjective interpretation was very complex. The information given during the counseling session(s) influenced more than half of the parents of a child with Down syndrome, to decide in favour of further pregnancies. In the group of parents having a child with neural tube defect the information received at the genetic counseling session(s) even had a more important effect : 80 percent decided to plan another pregnancy.

Birth Defects: Original Article Series, Volume 23, Number 2, pages 61–83

Results of both studies clearly indicate that for more than half of the families the availability of prenatal diagnosis was of crucial importance in the decision to plan future pregnancies.

Introduction

The remarkable evolution in the understanding of genetic mechanisms which took place during the last decades, has created the opportunity of offering genetic advice to a growing number of people. In 1975 the aims of genetic counseling were defined by the Committee on Genetic Counseling as follows :

"Genetic counseling is a communication process which deals with the human problems associated with the occurrence, or the risk of a genetic disorder in a family. This process involves an attempt by one or more appropriately trained persons to help the individual or family :

(1) comprehend the medical facts, including the diagnosis, the probable course of the disorder, and the available management;
(2) appreciate the way heredity contributes to this disorder, and the risk of recurrence in specified relatives;
(3) understand the options for dealing with the risk of recurrence;
(4) choose the course of action which seems appropriate to them in view of their risk and their family goals and act in accordance with that decision;
(5) make the best possible adjustment to the disorder in an affected family member and/or to the risk of recurrence of that disorder;"

From this definition it is obvious that genetic counseling sessions may result in informing the parents of a child with a genetic handicap about the disorder they are confronted with. Furthermore, discussing all options open to a couple, who is at risk for transmitting a genetic handicap, can be helpful when decisions about further pregnancy planning are to be reached.

The present investigation was set up to evaluate how genetic counseling offered in the Center for Human Genetics of Leuven is experienced by couples, who are at risk for a genetic handicap. It will also try to establish the influence of the counseling on their knowledge of the incidence and the recurrence risks and evaluate the impact of counseling on their decisions concerning further pregnancy planning.

A growing number of disorders can be detected prenatally through amniocentesis. This procedure already allows investigation of the condition of the unborn fetus early in the second trimester of the pregnancy. The examination of a sample of amniotic fluid, which contains both cells and biochemical components of fetal origin, can reveal the presence of a number of defects. Up to now this examination was mainly performed for the following reasons :

1. detection of chromosomal abnormalities (e.g., Down syndrome)
2. detection of multifactorially determined abnormalities (e.g., neural tube defects)
3. fetal sexing for X-linked disorders which cannot yet be detected in utero

More recently the use of recombinant DNA-techniques, which allow to study genes directly (e.g., hemophilia A) or indirectly by DNA-linkage (e.g., Duchenne muscular dystrophy), has widened the spectrum of defects detectable by either amniocentesis or chorionic villi sampling.

To make sure that an adequate volume of amniotic fluid is obtained, amniocentesis is usually delayed until the 16th to the 18th week of pregnancy. Performed by a skilled person and monitored under ultrasound visualization of the fetus, the risk for miscarriage caused by this procedure is estimated to be less than 1% (Turnbull, 1984). Much attention has been paid to the technical aspects of this method, the experience however of parents, who have used this possibility to obtain information about their unborn child, has not been evaluated thoroughly. Therefore, parents' attitudes towards amniocentesis and the impact of this technique on subsequent pregnancy planning were also evaluated.

A review of a number of follow-up studies investigating the impact of genetic counseling made it obvious that in order to make appropriate comparisons it is recommended to choose a population confronted with a single disease (Evers-Kiebooms and Van den Berghe, 1979). Down syndrome and neural tube defects are disorders for which at risk families often consult the Center for Human Genetics of Leuven. As both disorders constitute the most frequent indications for prenatal diagnosis, two parallel studies were set up with couples at risk for either one of these handicaps.

Down syndrome is the most common serious chromosome abnormality. The defect is caused in 95% of the cases by the presence of three chromosomes 21 (standard trisomy 21). The clinical characteristics of this disorder are moderate to severe mental retardation, typical mongoloid facial features and general growth retardation. Repeated lung infections and congenital heart diseases are also common in affected infants. The incidence of Down syndrome is about 1 per 1000 live births (Evers-Kiebooms et al., 1984b). After the birth of a child with standard trisomy 21, the empirical recurrence risk for parents with a normal karyotype is 1%. Analysis of chromosome preparations from cultured fetal cells obtained from the amniotic fluid already allows the detection of this disorder in an early stage of the pregnancy.

Neural tube defects appear to result from a defect in the closure of the neural groove. The most frequent types of neural tube defects (about 95% of all neural tube defects) are anencephaly and spina bifida, the closure defect being located respectively at the anterior or at the posterior portion of the neural groove. The occurrence of both defects is approximately equal. Anencephaly is a lethal disorder : all affected children are stillborn or die within hours after birth. The degree of the handicap of spina bifida children is very variable. A considerable number die soon after birth, while surviving children are often severely handicapped. Weakness or paralysis of the legs, urinary and faecal incontinence and hydrocephaly are the most typical features of this disorder. A number of children also become mentally retarded due to problems related to hydrocephaly.

While the cause of these defects is not yet known, the disorder is thought to be determined multifactorially. Environmental as well as hereditary factors are involved. The incidence of neural tube defects shows considerable geographical differences. In Great-Britain the incidence is 4 to 5 per 1000 births (U.K. Collaborative Study, 1977). In most other European countries a lower incidence is found. As no systematic registration of all children born with this defect is performed in Belgium, the incidence and recurrence rate in our population is not exactly known. Parents attending counseling sessions after the birth of one affected child are generally told that their recurrence risk is between 3% and 5%.

In 1972, Brock and Sutcliffe established the association between increased levels of alpha-fetoproteins in the amniotic fluid and the presence of open neural tube defects. Since, prenatal diagnosis of these defects by means of amniocentesis has become possible.

Sample composition

Families were selected that had been in contact with the Center for Human Genetics of Leuven since 1974. They consulted the Center after the birth of a child with standard trisomy 21 (parents of a child with Down syndrome with chromosomal mosaicism or translocation were not included in the study) or of a child with neural tube defect. To evaluate the impact of genetic counseling and of prenatal diagnosis on further family planning, parents were selected who were still expected to extend their family. Recent population surveys reveal that in Belgium about 95% of all children are born to mothers aged 35 years or less and that in most families only two or three children are born (Cliquet et al., 1983). Therefore only families meeting the following two criteria were included in the studies : first, maternal age at birth of the affected child had to be 35 years or less and secondly, the affected child had to be firstborn or secondborn.

One hundred and nineteen families with a child having Down syndrome and meeting these two criteria were willing to participate in study I. Ninety-four families having a child with neural tube defect took part in study II. Forty-four of them had an anencephalic child and to 50 a child with spina bifida had been born.

At the time the families were interviewed, 24 of the children with Down syndrome and 80 of the children with neural tube defect had died.

As a function of the research goals, the group of parents in both studies has been divided into three subgroups.

1. Families that had neither received genetic counseling nor had an amniocentesis performed.
2. Families that received genetic counseling at the Center for Human Genetics of Leuven. During these session(s) recurrence risks and the procedure for prenatal diagnosis were outlined in detail to the parents. None of the mothers in this group had an amniocentesis performed.
3. Families of which the mother had an amniocentesis performed for a pregnancy occurring after the birth of the index patient. Most families belonging to this group also attended one (or more) genetic counseling session(s) at the Center for Human Genetics. When analysing the impact of genetic counseling this group was divided into two subgroups in function of their attendance of the counseling session.

Initially we planned to include 40 families in each subgroup. This number, however, was not reached in families having a child with neural tube defect and no amniocentesis performed. As we wanted to ascertain the comparability of the moments at which the different subgroups handled the genetic problem, it was decided to pursue study II with reduced numbers in two of the subgroups. Table 1 gives an overview of the composition of the research sample.

Table 1 : Sample composition

	Down syndrome	**Neural tube defect**
GROUP 1 No genetic counseling, no amniocentesis	N = 40	N = 23
GROUP 2 Genetic counseling, no amniocentesis	N = 40	N = 29
GROUP 3 Amniocentesis performed, most families received genetic counseling	N = 39	N = 42
Total	N = 119	N = 94

In both studies the sociological characteristics of the group of families attending counseling sessions were essentially identical to these of the uncounseled group, except for the educational level of the parents. This level was substantially lower in the uncounseled group. Forty-seven percent of the mothers of a child with Down syndrome who attended genetic counseling had an educational level below high school, against 74% in the uncounseled group. The difference in paternal educational level was less important : 45% of the fathers in the counseled group had an educational level below high school against 63% in the uncounseled group (Table 2).

Table 2 : Educational level of Down syndrome parents

	Counseled group (N = 76)	**Uncounseled group** (N = 43)
MATERNAL educational level		
< High School	47 %	74 %
High School	39 %	16 %
> High School	13 %	9 %
PATERNAL educational level		
< High School	45 %	63 %
High School	26 %	26 %
> High School	29 %	12 %

Table 3 : Educational level of neural tube defect parents

	Counseled group (N = 63)	**Uncounseled group** (N = 31)
MATERNAL educational level		
< High School	46 %	55 %
High School	32 %	35 %
> High School	22 %	10 %
PATERNAL educational level		
< High School	38 %	48 %
High School	29 %	29 %
> High School	33 %	23 %

The same result was found in the group of parents having a child with neural tube defect although the differences were less extreme. Forty-six percent of the mothers, attending consultation, had an educational level below high school against 55% in the uncounseled group, while the educational level of 38% of the counseled fathers was below high school against 48% in the uncounseled group (Table 3).
This difference may be due to the tendency that families with a lower educational level attend existing medical services less frequently.

Methodology

In both studies parents were first contacted by letter and asked for their collaboration. Couples who agreed to participate were interviewed at home by a social nurse.
A very exhaustive questionnaire, identical in both studies, was used to guide the interview. It included questions with precoded answer categories as well as a number of open ended questions. The latter were used to allow the parents to express their personal opinions as accurately as possible.
Besides information about parents' attitudes toward genetic counseling and prenatal diagnosis and their knowledge about incidence and recurrence risks, the interview also covered a number of socio-economical characteristics of the parents, their reproductive history and their experiences with the index patient. In both studies the interview lasted on average about 2½ hours. Although attempts were made to have both parents present during the interview, this was only the case in 62% of the families in study I and in 33% of the families in study II. When only one of the parents was present the other partner was requested to fill out and return by mail that part of the questionnaire that related to his or her attitude towards the index patient.
Data collection took place during the years 1978-1981. To evaluate the long-term effects of counseling, follow-up data were collected more recently, namely in 1982 for the Down syndrome families and in 1984 for the neural tube defect families. To that end a questionnaire was sent to all families. Information was gathered about the parents' actual knowledge of recurrence risks, their reproductive plans, their intention to use prenatal diagnosis, their reproduction during the period following the interview, the use made of prenatal diagnosis in the same period and about some other issues. The response rate was high. Ninety-five out of the 119 families of study I returned the follow-up questionnaire. In the group of parents of a child with neural tube defect 86 out of the 94 families filled out the questionnaire.

RESULTS

An extensive report of the results of both studies will not be given. (The results of study I are outlined in detail in Evers-Kiebooms et al., 1984a). The emphasis will be placed on the findings of study II and for the most crucial results a comparison with the data of study I will be made.

1. Genetic counseling

a. Acquaintance with and attitudes towards genetic counseling

The existence of services for genetic counseling does not seem to be a matter of common knowledge. Only about one fourth of all families who had been confronted with the birth of a child with neural tube defect were to some extent informed about the existence of these services before being themselves referred to the Center for Human Genetics. Thirty-seven percent of the informed families obtained their information from the mass media (radio, television, newspapers), while family or friends were the second most important source of information (32%).

Thirty-seven of the counseled neural tube defect families came to the Center for Human Genetics only once. The remaining 26 families attended two or more counseling sessions.
All the counseled families had one (or more) specific expectation(s) when they first visited the Center for Human Genetics. Fifty-nine percent of these families expected to be informed about the nature of the disorder of their child. Advice about future pregnancies was requested by 56% of the counseled families. Thirty percent of them wanted to be informed about recurrence risks while explanation about the prenatal diagnosis of neural tube defects was expected by one fourth of them.
In both studies there seemed to be general satisfaction with the genetic counseling. For more than 90% of the counseled families the counseling was a positive experience. Eighty percent of the families reported that no questions remained unanswered. Up to 90% of the families found the information given during the counseling session(s) easy to understand and giving them more insight into the nature of the handicap and into risk figures.

b. Impact of genetic counseling on recall of risk figures

When the awareness of the recurrence risk is examined, the impact of attending genetic counseling becomes very obvious. Almost all neural tube defect families that received genetic counseling, knew they were still at risk to have another child with this anomaly. In the uncounseled group not less than 16% of the families were (almost) sure about the favorable outcome of a future pregnancy (Table 4).

Table 4 : Awareness of recurrence risk

	Counseled group (N = 63)	**Uncounseled group** (N = 31)
Still at risk	97 %	84 %
Probably no longer at risk	3 %	6 %
Definitely no longer at risk	-	10 %

When asked to give a numerical risk, about two thirds of the families that attended genetic counseling reported correctly that their recurrence risk was about 3% to 5%, against only 29% of the uncounseled families. (Two families, having two children with neural tube defect, thus in fact underestimated their recurrence risk). Despite this distinct better recall by the counseled families even in this group about one fourth of the parents could not give a numerical risk figure and 11% had an explicit misconception (Table 5).

Table 5 : Effect of genetic counseling on the recall of risk figures for neural tube defects

	Counseled group (N = 63)	**Uncounseled group** (N = 31)
No risk	0 %	10 %
<1%	3 %	6 %
1% - <3%	0 %	13 %
3% - 5%	65 %*	29 %*
>5% - 10%	3 %	0 %
>10% - 25%	3 %*	3 %
>25%	2 %	6 %**
No numerical risk figure	23 %	32 %

* To one of these parents twice a child with a neural tube defect had been born

** One mother with a closed spina bifida estimated her risk to be 100%

Comparison with the recall of risk figures in study I, makes it obvious that the knowledge of the recurrence rate of the handicap was in no way better in the Down syndrome families. Only about half of the counseled families and 21% of the uncounseled families knew their correct recurrence risk, while 21% of the parents who attended genetic counseling had an explicit misconception (Table 6).

Table 6 : Effect of genetic counseling on the recall of risk figures for Down syndrome

	Counseled group (N = 76)	**Uncounseled group** (N = 43)
Underestimation	14 %	21 %
Correct 1% risk	45 %	21 %
Overestimation	7 %	5 %
No numerical risk figure	34 %	54 %

Besides attendance to a genetic counseling session, the educational level of the parents was a second factor which clearly affected the knowledge of recurrence risks. In study II almost twice as many parents having an educational level above high school were aware of their correct numerical risk as compared with parents who did not have a high school degree (Table 7).
The same relationship was found in study I. Here only one fourth of the parents belonging to an educational level below high school were aware of their recurrence risk for Down syndrome against about half of the parents having more than a high school degree.

At the end of each interview the social nurse always mentioned the correct risk figure and if necessary, gave the parents additional genetic information to correct misconceptions. At the follow-up contact some years after the initial interview recall of the correct risk figures was nevertheless disappointing : only 30 out of the 76 families (39%) knew the correct recurrence risk of 3% to 5%. A substantially large amount of families had either a misconception or could not give a numerical risk figure (Table 8). Three families that had already been confronted twice with a pregnancy of a child with neural tube defect at the moment of the

Table 7 : Recall of risk figures and educational level of the parents

	Maternal educational level		
	< high school (N=46)	high school (N=31)	> high school (N=17)
< 3%	11%	16%	-
3% to 5%	37%*	61%*	82%
> 5%	11%	6%	6%
No numerical risk figure	41%	16%	12%

	Paternal educational level		
	< high school (N=39)	high school (N=27)	> high school (N=28)
< 3%	10%	19%	4%
3% to 5%	41%*	44%*	79%
> 5%	10%	7%	7%
No numerical risk figure	38%	30%	11%

* To one of these parents twice a child with a neural tube defect had been born

follow-up contact, knew correctly that their risk was higher than 5%, although two of them still overestimated their 10% recurrence risk. One mother had been pregnant three times with a child with neural tube defect at the time of the follow-up contact. This family estimated its recurrence risk at 50%. Reliable data, however, on recurrence risks for neural tube defects after three affected children were not found in the literature. (The four families with multiple neural tube defect pregnancies are not included in Table 8.)

Comparison between the risk figure recalled at the first interview and the one recalled at the follow-up some years later shows that fewer parents were aware of their 3% to 5% recurrence rate at the time of the follow-up. It is also clear that a number of shifts occurred from correct to incorrect answers and vice versa (Table 8).

The recall data were not any better in study I. Here, 34 of the 95 families (36%) that returned the follow-up list gave a correct answer. Although the overall knowledge was found to be very similar at the first interview and at the follow-up contact it must be emphasised that a relatively important number of shifts occurred from correct to poor knowledge and vice versa.

Table 8 : Comparison between the risk figures recalled at interview and at the follow-up contact

Risk recalled at interview	Risk recalled at follow-up contact				
	< 3%	3%-5%	> 5%	No numerical risk figure	Total (N=76)
< 3%	-	3%	1%	7%	11%
3% to 5%	1%	34%	12%	9%	56%
> 5%	1%	1%	3%	1%	6%
No numerical risk figure	4%	1%	4%	17%	26%
Total	6%	39%	20%	34%	100%

While the recalled recurrence risk figure will influence a couple's decision about pregnancy planning to a certain extent, the subjective evaluation of this recurrence risk may affect the decision process to a larger extent. Table 9 makes it clear that identical recurrence figures do not have the same meaning for the different families : e.g., a < 3% risk can be found to be a high or a low risk depending on the evaluating family. These differences in evaluation of identical recurrence numbers were also apparent during the follow-up contact. It is clear that a number of psychological mechanisms are playing a part in the interpretation of risk figures. A number of factors, such as the parents' anticipated idea about the recurrence rate, the manner in which the risk figure is presented to them, their subjective evaluation of the outcome and also a number of personality factors (Pearn, 1973) can affect the individual interpretation of a genetic risk.

It must be emphasised that during the interview, more than half of the neural tube defect families that knew their recurrence risk was between 3% and 5% found this a high or a very high risk. At the follow-up contact even as many as 66% of the families that thought their risk number was between 3% and 5% estimated this to be a high or very high recurrence rate.
In study I this complex relationship between the recalled numerical risk figure and the subjective evaluation of the risk was also present. More than half of the families that were aware of their correct 1% recurrence risk during the interview estimated this to be a high or very high risk.

Table 9 : Relationship between the subjective evaluation of the risk and the recalled numerical risk figure

	Recalled numerical risk figure			
Subjective evaluation	< 3% (N=7)	3% - 5% (N=48)	> 5% (N=8)	No risk figure (N=24)
High or very high risk	29%	56%	100%	37%
Medium risk	29%	19%	-	21%
Low or very low risk	43%	23%	-	25%
No subjective evaluation	-	2%	-	17%

When the importance of one's own recurrence risk is evaluated, information about the incidence of the handicap in the general population can also be an influencing factor. However, only 24% of the interviewed families knew the incidence of neural tube defects at birth in the general population (answers between > 0.01% and < 1%). Once again counseling clearly improved knowledge : almost half of the families in the counseled group knew the correct incidence rate against only 16% in the uncounseled group (Table 10).

Table 10 : Knowledge about the incidence of neural tube defects in the general population

	Counseled group (N = 63)	**Uncounseled group** (N = 31)
Underestimation	3 %	6 %
Correct	46 %	16 %
Overestimation	2 %	3 %
No numerical risk figure	49 %	74 %

When asked to compare the importance of their recurrence risk only with that of parents who did not give birth to a child with neural tube defect, 20% of the counseled families and as many as 62% of the uncounseled families seemed not to be aware of their increased risk (Table 11).

Table 11 : Awareness of increased risk for a child with neural tube defect compared to random families

	Counseled group (N = 61)	Uncounseled group (N = 26)
Own risk lower	-	8 %
Same risk	10 %	15 %
Own risk higher	80 %	38 %
No comparison	10 %	38 %

The previous data made it clear that the recall of the correct risk figures was substantially better in the counseled group than in the uncounseled group. A substantially large number of families, however, that attended consultation were found not to be aware of the correct recurrence and incidence figures. When the answers of the same parents on all knowledge-items were compared the degree of correct knowledge became even more disappointing. Only 17 out of the 63 neural tube defect families that attended consultation and one of the 31 families that did not receive genetic counseling answered all questions about risk figures correctly and thus reproduced the risk figures completely accurately. Even more striking was that a number of parents gave contradictory answers to the different questions such as being no longer at risk although knowing their correct 3% to 5% recurrence risk. Obviously a number of parents 'knew' risk figures but did not understand their meaning.

This poor knowledge of risk figures was also reported by other investigators (e.g., Veenema et al., 1981). Laurence and Morris (1981) who compared the recall of risk figures by parents interrogated before and after the introduction of amniocentesis, suggested that the poorer knowledge of risk figures after the introduction of amniocentesis was possibly related to the availability of this procedure. Knowledge of the exact risk figure becomes apparently less important when the defect can be detected prenatally.

c. Impact of genetic counseling on pregnancy planning

The influence of genetic counseling on family planning was established in all 51 families in which the mother was not pregnant at the time of the first counseling session. One mother decided not to have other children on the

basis of the information received during genetic counseling, although her husband seemed positive towards a future pregnancy. Not less than 80% of the parents reported that the information given during the counseling session(s) made them decide to have more children. Prior to counseling most parents hesitated to have other children. Based on the information received during the counselling session(s), a number even altered the decision to have no subsequent pregnancy (Table 12).
Fifty-five percent of the families having a child with Down syndrome reported that the information received during the counseling session(s) made them decide in favour of further pregnancies. The remainder of the families had already taken a decision about having other children before attending genetic counseling and they did not change their mind subsequently.

Table 12 : Impact of genetic counseling on family planning

	Percentage of families (N=51)
Undecided ---> decided to have no more children	2%
Undecided ---> decided to have more children	70%
Decided no more children ---> decided to have more children	10%
Still undecided	8%
No change of decision	10%

Table 13 clearly demonstrates that the influence of genetic counseling on the decision to have more children can be attributed mainly to the availability of prenatal diagnosis. Information concerning recurrence risks or the nature of the handicap influenced this decision to a lesser extent.
For Down syndrome families, information about the availability of prenatal diagnosis together with the knowledge of risk numbers were also important factors leading to a positive decision concerning future pregnancies.

Most neural tube defect families (86%) reported that they reached their decision concerning family planning almost immediately after the counseling session(s). Two thirds of the families that came to a decision about pregnancy planning after genetic counseling wanted to take this decision all by themselves. No family wanted the genetic counselor to decide for them.

Table 13 : Influence of different topics discussed during counseling on the decision to have more children

	Percentage of families (N=41)
Knowledge of risk (A)	2%
Prenatal diagnosis (B)	56%
Nature of handicap (C)	-
A + B	10%
A + B + C	32%

2. Prenatal diagnosis

a. Acquaintance with and attitudes towards prenatal diagnosis

The majority of neural tube defect families were informed about the availability of amniocentesis before the beginning of a pregnancy following the birth of the index patient. Only five out of the 94 families, all from the group which did not attend a genetic counseling session, were not informed about the possibility of prenatal detection of neural tube defects (Table 14).
Knowledge about the possibility of prenatal diagnosis by means of amniocentesis was also widespread in the Down syndrome families. Ninety-two percent of the families were aware of the availability of the procedure at the time they were interviewed, and 90% of the families even knew this before a pregnancy, subsequent to the birth of the index patient, occurred.

Almost half of the informed neural tube defect families that did not receive genetic counseling were told about the availability of this procedure by an obstetrician. It was also the obstetrician who mentioned the existence of this detection method to a great number of the parents in the counseled group. Once more, the mass media (radio, television, newspapers) seem to have played a substantial role in the spreading of information about this medical procedure (Table 15).

Table 14 : Source of information about the availability of prenatal diagnosis

	Counseled group (N=63)	**Uncounseled group** (N=26)	**Total** (N=89)
Geneticist	32%	-	22%
Obstetrician	27%	46%	33%
General practitioner	3%	4%	3%
Other (para)medical profession	6%	8%	7%
Communication media	22%	35%	26%
Study or work situation	5%	4%	4%
Relative, friend	5%	4%	4%

Table 15 : Time of information about the availability of prenatal diagnosis

	Percentage of families (N=94)
Informed before or during the pregnancy giving birth to the index patient	10%
Informed withing 6 months after the birth of the index patient	32%
Informed before the beginning of a pregnancy subsequent to the birth of the index patient	37%
Informed in the first trimester of the pregnancy subsequent to the birth of the index patient	5%
Informed after one or more pregnancies subsequent to the birth of the index patient	11%
Not informed	5%

Amniocentesis still carries some minor risks, especially the risk of miscarriage. Eighty-two percent of the neural tube defect parents, who were informed about the existence of this detection technique, knew that this method was not completely without risks. Twelve percent of these families still presumed that this method involved no risks at all, although in three cases the mother already had an amniocentesis performed. The remaining six percent had no idea about possible risks.

Most parents were aware of the fact that in their situation only neural tube defects and chromosomal abnormalities would be detected by this examination (in Leuven chromosome analysis is routinely performed on amniotic fluid even when the indication for the procedure is a neural tube defect). Most parents knew that a "good result" (a negative test result) did not guarantee the child to be without handicap (Table 16).

Table 16 : Meaning of a "good result" of the amniocentesis

	No neural tube defect (N=88)	**No chromosomal abnormality** (N=86)	**Completely without handicap** (N=84)
Yes	97%	78%	5%
No	2%	2%	83%
Do not know	1%	20%	12%

Most families (73%) reacted positively when they were informed about the availability of amniocentesis for the detection of neural tube defects. Fourteen percent of the families could not decide at once whether they wanted this examination during a subsequent pregnancy. Only nine percent of the families had a (rather) averse reaction to the first information about amniocentesis. The remaining families could not give a clear answer on this topic.
In study I an almost identical number of positive reactions was found : 72% of the Down syndrome families said that they had reacted positively when being informed about this diagnostic technique.

b. Impact of prenatal diagnosis on pregnancy planning

The possibility to detect neural tube defects prenatally seems to be an important element in the parents' decisions concerning further pregnancies. Almost one third of the families that knew it was possible to detect neural tube defects prenatally, and that knew this before starting a new pregnancy following the birth of the index patient, reported that this knowledge played a major favorable role in their decision about a future pregnancy. Another third of the families even said that it was an essential condition to start another pregnancy. Even in the group of families, that already had a pregnancy before being informed about this detection method, 20 % held the view that the possibility of having an amniocentesis was an essential condition to start a further pregnancy. The positive influence of the availability of prenatal diagnosis on the reproductive plans of a number of parents of a child with neural tube defect has also been

reported by other authors (e.g., Laurence, 1977; Hsia et al., 1979).
The importance of the availability of prenatal diagnosis on decisions about family planning is also obvious in the group of Down syndrome families. Half of the families that were informed about the availability of amniocentesis before the interview said that it was an important factor in their decision to have other children. For 16% it was even a conditio sine qua non for having other children.

At the time the interview data were collected, about two thirds of the neural tube defect families, that had not yet an amniocentesis performed, planned to have this examination should they become pregnant (Table 17). Twenty-seven percent of the families did not plan to make use of amniocentesis in case of a future pregnancy or had already rejected this possibility during a previous pregnancy. Only one out of the 42 families, that had an amniocentesis performed, had decided against this form of prenatal examination should a future pregnancy occur. However, this decision was probably due to the fact that the pregnancy for which an amniocentesis had been performed ended shortly afterwards in a miscarriage. Three families had not yet made up their mind whether they should have this examination performed or not.

Table 17 : Intention to use amniocentesis

Intentions at interview	**No amniocentesis performed** (N=52)	**Amniocentesis performed** (N=42)
Planned amniocentesis	69%	90%
Doubt	4%	8%
No amniocentesis	27%	2%

In the group of families having a child with Down syndrome and without a previous amniocentesis an almost identical percentage (62%), reported during the interview that they intended to make use of prenatal diagnosis. Thirty-four percent rejected prenatal diagnosis and four percent were still undecided.

The intention to use prenatal diagnosis was tested to the reality during the follow-up contact some years later. In 61 of the 80 neural tube defect families that returned the questionnaire at least one pregnancy had occurred after the interview. Forty-three mothers had an amniocentesis performed during this pregnancy while four mothers who intended to make use of it had an early miscarriage. During the interview 40 of these mothers (80%) had said they planned to have an amniocentesis and four of them had doubted whether to have this examination performed. Two mothers even expressed the intention not to use prenatal diagnosis while one mother previously had rejected amniocentesis because the obstetrician had advised her so. Only three of the mothers who planned an amniocentesis did not make use of it when pregnant. All three ultimately renounced to undergo prenatal diagnosis when pregnant because at that time their physician estimated it to be a superfluous examination.

In the 95 Down syndrome families that returned the follow-up list 35 mothers had at least one pregnancy after the interview. Thirty mothers had an amniocentesis performed during this pregnancy while another two who intended to use it had an early miscarriage. Twenty-seven of these 32 mothers (84%) had planned an amniocentesis at the time of the interview. The five remaining mothers had not indicated the intention to use prenatal diagnosis during the interview.

At the follow-up contact as much as 80% of the neural tube defect families and 81% of Down syndrome families reported that they planned an amniocentesis should a new pregnancy occur.

Moral and religious convictions and risks of the procedure, especially the risk for miscarriage and fear of harming the unborn child were the most frequent motives cited by the parents who rejected amniocentesis.

Conclusions

Notwithstanding the fact that most parents evaluated the genetic counseling as a positive experience, their awareness of recurrence figures was rather disappointing. Only about half of the neural tube defect families knew the 3% to 5% recurrence rate, while in study I even as few as one third of the families were aware of their 1% recurrence rate.

Attending a genetic counseling session clearly improved the knowledge. Two thirds of the neural tube defect families that received genetic counseling knew the correct recurrence rate against only about one third of the uncounseled families. In the group of Down syndrome families correct knowledge of recurrence risks was found in about half of the uncounseled families only as compared with the counseled ones.

In both studies there was an obvious positive correlation between the educational level of the parents and their knowledge of recurrence figures. Nearly twice as many parents with a higher education knew the correct recurrence rate as compared with parents who did not have a high school degree.

The relationship between the recalled risk figure and the parents' subjective evaluation of the risk level seems to be very complex. Nevertheless more than half of the families knowing their correct recurrence risk (between 3% and 5% for neural tube defects and 1% for Down syndrome) found this to be a high or very high risk. While it is obvious that a number of psychological factors are influencing the transfer of information and the evaluation of genetic risks, further research is needed to unravel the determining psychological mechanisms.

Genetic counseling and the possibility to detect these defects prenatally play an important part when deciding on further pregnancies. Half of the counseled Down syndrome families and up to 80% of the families with a child with neural tube defect that attended consultation reported that they were positively influenced in their decision to have more children by the information received during the counseling session(s). Especially the possibility of detecting the disorder prenatally was of crucial importance for pregnancy planning. More than half of the Down syndrome families and as much as about two thirds of the neural tube defect families reported that the availability of prenatal diagnosis played a major role in their decision in favour of a future pregnancy.
Most families reacted positively the first time they were informed about the availability of prenatal diagnosis. In both studies about two thirds of the families that had not yet an amniocentesis performed at the time of the interview, planned to have it done should a pregnancy occur. At the follow-up contact even as many as 80% of all families returning the questionnaire said that they would ask for this examination should they become pregnant. Parents who rejected amniocentesis most often cited moral convictions or fear for the risks of the procedure as reasons for not using this detection technique.
When the intentions to use amniocentesis were tested with reality during the follow-up contact it was clear that most families that planned this examination also made use of it when a pregnancy occurred.

References

Brock, D.J.H. and Sutcliffe, R.G.
Alpha-fetoprotein in antenatal diagnosis of anencephaly and spina bifida.
Lancet ii, 197-199, 1972.

Cliquet, R.L., Debusschere, R., Deven, F., Delmotte, G., Van Maele, C. and Wyewickrema, S.
Gezinsvorming in Vlaanderen. Resultaten van de nationale enquête gezinsontwikkeling 1975-1976 (Nego III).
(Family building in Flanders. Data from the 3rd survey on family development.)
C.B.G.S. report 58, Population and Family Study Center, Brussels, 1983.

Committee on Genetic Counseling

Genetic Counseling.
Am. J. Hum. Genet. 27, 240-242, 1975.

Evers-Kiebooms, G. and Van den Berghe, H.
The impact of genetic counseling : a review of published follow-up studies.
Clin. Genet. 15, 465-474, 1979.

Evers-Kiebooms, G., Vlietinck,R., Fryns, J.P. and Van den Berghe, H.
Impact on family planning of the birth of a child with 21 trisomy.
In : Perspectives and Progress in Mental Retardation (ed. Berg, M.J.) vol II, 323-333, University Park Press, Baltimore, 1984a.

Evers-Kiebooms, G., Vlietinck, R. and Van den Berghe, H.
The impact of the present change of childbearing age on the incidence of trisomy 21 : a review of the literature and an empiric investigation in Belgium, 1960-1978.
C.B.G.S. Document nr. 6, Population and Family Study Center, Brussels, 1984b.

Hsia, Y., Leung, F. and Carter, L.
Attitudes toward amniocentesis : Surveys of families with spina bifida children.
In : Service and education in medical genetics (Porter,J. and Hook,E., eds). Academic Press, New York and London, 1979.

Laurence, K.M.
The impact of antenatal diagnosis for central nervous system malformation in high-risk pregnancies and pregnancy screening in a high-risk community.
Zeitschrift für Kinderchirurgie und Grenzgebiete 22, 383-395, 1977.

Laurence, K.M. and Morris, J.
The effect of the introduction of prenatal diagnosis on the reproductive history of women at increased risk for neural tube defects.
Prenatal Diagnosis 1, 51-60, 1981.

Pearn, J.H.
Patients' subjective interpretation of risks offered in genetic counseling.
J. Med. Genet. 10, 123-134, 1973.

Turnbull, A.C.
Amniocentesis.
In : Antenatal and neonatal screening (ed. Wald. N.Y.) Oxford University Press, 1984.

U.K. Collaborative study on alpha-fetoprotein in relation to neural tube defects.
Maternal serum alpha-fetoprotein measurement in antenatal screening for anencephaly and spina bifida in early pregnancy.
Lancet i, 1323-1332, 1977.

Veenema, H., Ouboter-Kooij, E.C. de B. and van Holthe tot Echten, J.E.
Genetisch advies bij defecten van de neurale buis; een vervolgonderzoek.
(Genetic counseling in neural tube defects; a follow-up study).
Nederlands Tijdschrift voor Geneeskunde 125, 1492-1496, 1981.

GENETIC COUNSELING IN HUNTINGTON'S CHOREA

Audrey TYLER

Department of Medical Genetics, University of Wales College of Medicine
Heath Park, Cardiff, CF4 4XN, United Kingdom

Disease characteristics

Huntington's chorea (HC) is an autosomal dominant hereditary disorder, which means that men and women are equally affected and that the disease is carried on a single gene. All the children of an affected parent have a 50% chance of inheriting the gene, and, since it has complete penetrance, of developing the disease themselves. The new mutation rate is not precisely known but is extremely low.

The characteristic symptoms are neurological degeneration which usually results in involuntary movements (chorea) and intellectual impairment, commonly called dementia. The clinical manifestations vary widely but are often severe and accompanied by mental features such as irritability and lability of mood and more florid psychiatric manifestations, often of a schizophreniform nature.

The disease runs a prolonged course, often over 15-20 years or longer, and is slowly and relentlessly progressive. Onset can be at any age from early childhood to over 70 years but is commonly in middle life, between the ages of 35-55 years. There is no treatment which can influence the underlying course of the condition and the effect of drugs to relieve symptoms is often uncertain.

Developments in prediction

Until recently, there was no way of predicting gene-carriers until symptoms appeared. Now the position has changed because a marker for the HC gene has been identified.

Birth Defects: Original Article Series, Volume 23, Number 2, pages 85–95

Genes are the basic units of inheritance and are made up of deoxyribonucleic acid (DNA). Each cell in the body contains an identical set of genes, which are arranged in a specific order on structures known as chromosomes. There are 46 chromosomes arranged in 23 pairs and one of each person's pair is contributed by the mother and the other by the father. A genetic linkage study, using a DNA probe called G8, recently localized the HC gene to the short arm of chromosome 4 (Gusella et al., 1983). It must be stressed that the HC gene itself has not yet been found but, since the G8 locus is close to the HC gene and appears to be transmitted with it over 90% of the time, it can be used to infer its presence in family studies. This is possible because G8, on laboratory analysis, shows variations (called polymorphisms) which can be classified as haplotypes A, B, C and D. These can be used to distinguish the chromosome 4 which comes from the affected side of the family from the chromosome 4 which comes from the unaffected side of the family. Thus, one of the clinical applications of the probe is in genetic prediction for families where HC is known to be present (Harper, 1983). The conditions under which this is possible are as follows :

1. Family studies can be performed : usually three generations of a family, in the direct line of descent, need to be available from which blood samples for DNA extraction and analysis can be obtained.

2. The distribution of genotypes (gene characteristics) is favourable. It is mandatory that the relevant parent of the proband (the person seeking prediction) is heterozygous for the marker and has a different genotype from their spouse and grandparent(s).

Three examples are presented :

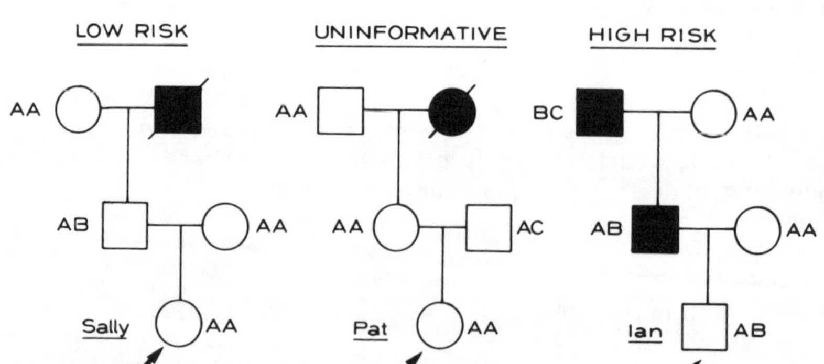

Since it is clear that Sally received the A from her father which could only have come from the unaffected grandmother she can be deemed to be at very low risk. Pat is uninformative since there is no way of knowing which haplotype was contributed by her father and which by her mother. Ian has received the B haplotype, shared by two affected family members, and thus is at very high risk.

The limitations and problems of the marker test

1. The diagnosis of HC must be accurate and, wherever possible, validated by a post mortem. Since G8 is present in everyone it is only of predictive use in families where the disease is already known to be present.

2. There is an error rate of approximately 5% in the test, which allows for the possibility of the separation of the marker from the gene and of recombination taking place. This means that a few people predicted to carry the gene will never show symptoms and vice versa. Thus, until the HC gene itself is found, it is not possible to predict gene-carriers with certainty : it is only possible to raise the risks for an individual to a maximum of 95%.

3. Without the right family structure and genotype distribution no form of prediction is possible, as already indicated. If DNA is not available from key family members the genotype which denotes high risk cannot be identified. However, in some families, usually containing several affected members, it may be possible to make a prediction even if grandparents are not available.

4. Genetic heterogeneity is theoretically possible. The HC gene may have mutated at more than one locus and, in fact, also be present on another chromosome. To date, no evidence for this has been found, though a considerable number of large families, in different parts of the world, have now been studied.

Types of prediction possible

The finding of a marker close to the gene for HC has profound implications for genetic counselling. The first question to be asked is : do families want to make use of genetic prediction before effective treatment is available? Several surveys have been carried out to test family attitudes, notably in the USA (Stern & Eldridge, 1975), Australia (Teltscher & Polgar, 1981), UK (Tyler & Harper, 1983) and Belgium (Evers-Kiebooms et al., 1985).

The results have been variable, but consistently appear to show that a significant proportion of those questioned would wish to take a test. However, a survey carried out in South Wales in 1985 showed that "the overall pedigree structure of affected families imposed limitations on prediction using any linked DNA marker, quite apart from the limitations imposed by the marker itself" (Harper & Safarazi, 1985). This survey was carried out in an area where complete ascertainment of the disease has been attempted and families followed up for over eleven years. Under 20% of subjects at high risk had at least one grandparent living to allow prediction for themselves and the number with affected siblings was also small, 10,5%. Admittedly this position will change for the next generation as DNA banking from affected and unaffected relatives is now being undertaken. Also, the HC gene itself may well be discovered in the foreseeable future. But, for the present, it appears that individual prediction will be available only for a few.

Examples of pregnancy exclusion testing are as follows :

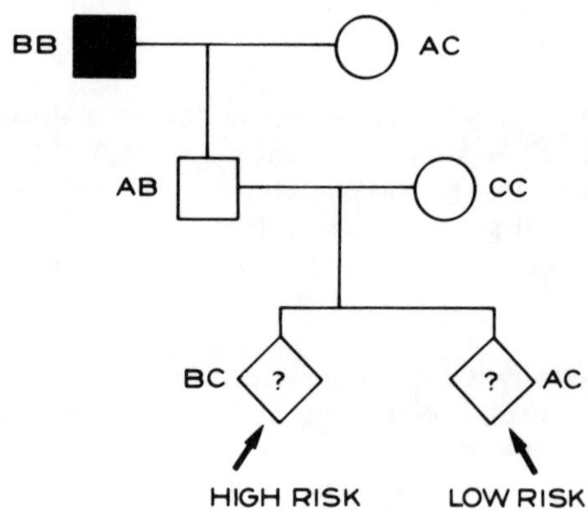

By contrast G8 can be used to allow an individual at 50% risk to have children who, themselves, will be virtually free from risk. This is called exclusion testing in pregnancy as the disorder can be excluded but not predicted in the fetus and the risk to the parent does not change. Again, three generations are required but, as the fetus is the third generation, it is much more likely that the criterion will be met. The only constraint of this form of testing is distribution of genotypes : however it is estimated that over 2/3 of couples will be informative at present, and, as more polymorphisms (or markers) at the G8 locus are identified this proportion will rise.

It is very important to realize that, in these cases, the disorder can either be excluded from the fetus (in the absence of recombination) or its risk raised to the level of the parent i.e., from 25% to 50%.

In this situation it is known that it is the B haplotype which has been received by the at-risk father from the affected grandfather but what is not known is whether the HC gene has been transmitted with it (it could equally well have been transmitted with the other B haplotype). Therefore, if the fetus receives the B haplotype it will be known to be at the same risk as the father. If the fetus receives the A haplotype, which is known to come from the unaffected grandmother, then HC can be excluded.

Safeguards

Clearly these new developments extend the choices open to at-risk individuals but their application needs careful planning and scrutiny. Considerable discussion has already taken place in many countries concerning the conditions under which the test should be administered and the safeguards necessary. Some of the main recommendations which have been made are :

1. Some degree of "quality control" over the test results should be exercised : one possibility is that every test should be run in two different laboratories which could check each others results. Present thinking is that testing should only be entrusted to certain "approved" centres which have developed not only the necessary technical expertise but which also can offer skilled counselling to applicants.

2. No one should be compelled to take a test : it should always be the free choice of the individuals concerned.

3. Applicants should always be allowed adequate time for consideration of all the issues involved before the testing is undertaken.

4. Skilled counselling should be available both pre and post test and adequate provision should be made for follow-up counselling.

5. The confidentiality of the results should be guaranteed.

6. Only applicants over the age of 18 years should be tested, except in very exceptional circumstances. Parents should not be given information about their minor children. Only persons capable of giving informed consent should be tested except, again, in very exceptional circumstances.

Predictive test counselling and protocols

The test has not yet been brought into clinical use and families are, at present, being studied for research purposes only. One of the centres which has been selected for these studies is in South Wales where we are in an advantageous position because we have had considerable experience in counselling HC families and have known many of them for at least eight years. Therefore the diagnosis has already been confirmed and the pedigrees documented for most of our HC population. Also genetic counselling has been offered to all persons at high risk and reinforced on follow-up, so that the great majority are conversant with the mode of inheritance and the genetic implications. In addition, as the National Health Service in the UK is free, no charge is made for counselling, for the taking of blood samples, or for the storage and testing of the DNA.

It is clearly essential that families are studied intensively during the research stage and that demographic information is collected, on all applicants, to include such areas as employment, education and past medical history. A psychological evaluation will also be carried out in some centres. The purpose is to try to ascertain which factors may predict a good outcome to testing and the optimum conditions under which testing should take place.

Counselling will obviously be of the utmost importance. The purpose of counselling will be to enable the individual (or couple) to reach the decision which is the right one for them. In order to be able to do this they must thoroughly understand the nature of the test and its limitations and written material should be made available to them. Also, the motivation of all applicants and the impact which the disease has had on them needs to be thoroughly explored, so that they can understand the consequences to them of being tested, whatever the result may be. Apart from these general areas there are aspects of counselling specific to the exclusion test in pregnancy and specific to presymptomatic testing.

Counselling for the pregnancy exclusion test

We advise couples to think about a pre-natal test as an option well before a pregnancy is planned. Undoubtedly this will be a difficult and painful area for some and they will need time to consider what is the right decision for them without any feeling of pressure. The test procedure will not be initiated when a pregnancy is already under way.

Couples need to understand that termination is strongly recommended if the result of the test on the fetus shows it to be at high risk. Otherwise, if the parent develops symptoms the child will be predicted also to be a gene-carrier and this is considered unacceptable. The preferred method of sampling the fetal cells will be by chorion villus biopsy. The advantage of this procedure is that it can be performed at eight weeks of pregnancy and thus termination can be carried out within the first trimester. This allows the couple to keep the pregnancy private, if they wish, and to defer bonding to the embryo. The disadvantage of chorion biopsy is that it carries with it a 5% risk of miscarriage.

The couple also need to explore, with the counsellor, their attitude towards childbearing and the history of the marriage so that areas of conflict (if any) can be identified and the impact of the test can be anticipated.

If a suitable couple choose a pre-natal test, obviously there may be a considerable time lag before pregnancy is actually achieved. Follow up in this period is considered essential because new factors can emerge, attitudes can change, and information about the test may need to be reiterated. It is also possible that the at-risk partner will develop signs of HC which would influence counselling.

When a pregnancy occurs it will be essential to enquire again into their attitude towards testing. However, thoroughly they have been prepared it is recognized that a pregnancy could alter their previous decision.

Where a miscarriage occurs or the fetus is shown to be at high risk and a termination is undertaken bereavement counselling must be offered. There is already evidence available that women undergoing termination for genetic reasons or spontaneous abortions can suffer considerable grief afterwards which, if unresolved, can affect their health and attitudes towards any further children (Donnai et al., 1981; Morgan, 1986).

Counselling in pre-symptomatic testing

Undoubtedly pre-symptomatic testing will cause the greatest anxiety, both for the testing team and for those to be tested. We have not yet finalized our protocol but it is clear that applicants for prediction for themselves should be led through all the possible ramifications of the test results, including effect on employment prospects, insurance matters, and related social and legal concerns. The stratagems already developed to deal with the anxiety engendered by the knowledge of being at risk for HC need to be known and the formal and informal support systems available to them.

The timing of the test also will need to be carefully thought out. The period between the taking of blood samples and the giving of results will be a time of great anxiety and probably should not coincide with other periods of stress such as starting a new job. It is also recommended that applicants bring a companion on some clinic visits as travelling could be hazardous in certain circumstances.

In the research stage post-test counselling for all applicants will be mandatory, whatever the result, and will cover such areas as :

1. Their understanding and interpretation of the test results.

2. Their attitude towards the test now and how it compares with that previously expressed.

3. How have their attitudes towards further childbearing been affected? (Where applicable).

4. The impact of the loss of pregnancy. (Where applicable).

5. Any evidence of positive effects on their lives?

6. Any evidence of adverse effects on their lives?

7. Have they and/or did they have any needs related to the test procedure which were not and/or are not being met?

It is thought that all applicants will go through a period of stress after hearing the results, even those who are deemed to be at very low risk, and that much support and counselling will be needed in this period of adjustment. Who is to provide this support when the test is released for clinical use is a matter for much debate : also it is not known how much follow-up families will need and tolerate.

Areas of potential controversy

Undoubtedly any procedure which alters the risk for the individual in a lethal disease such as HC will arouse much controversy. From discussion with family members it is already apparent that there are areas of potential disagreement between applicants and the testing centres, surrounding the conditions under which the test will be administered. One of these has already been touched on, e.g., in discussion of the age constraints on who should be tested.

Others relate to the responsibility of the testing centre to try to ensure that test results will be used constructively versus the right of the individual to decide for himself if and when he is tested. Undoubtedly some degree of what may be considered paternalism will be inevitable in the research stage : for example, individuals who are considered clinically depressed or severely unstable mentally may well be advised to seek treatment before being tested.

There is also the question of to whom do the test results belong? Many families feel that they belong to the individual alone and are not necessarily, to be shared with a partner. This is entirely understandable, particularly if marital problems already exist. However, in practice, this attitude could lead to great difficulties particularly if the partner disagreed and testing could well be postponed until the disagreement is resolved.

Preliminary data

Some preliminary data on approximately 50 Welsh couples and individuals with whom the predictive test has been discussed is presented. Roughly, half were not interested in an exclusion test in pregnancy because they were opposed either to termination per se or to termination where the fetus had a fifty-fifty chance of being healthy. One or two women refused on the grounds of their age : had they been younger they could have afforded the loss of a pregnancy but, at over 30 years, they felt they could not. One or two husbands felt they could not subject their wives to the procedure of chorion biopsy. Approximately 20 have continued to express interest in being tested and say they will discuss the situation further when they are planning a pregnancy, though a few have wondered whether they will be able to go through with testing when the pregnancy actually occurs. Several couples were extremely ambivalent and needed considerable time and discussion before they could make up their minds about what was the right decision for them. The persons who most welcome the exclusion test appear to be those who want children but have had considerable doubts about starting a family in view of the risks involved.

Prediction for the individual was discussed with all of them. The majority were positive that they did not want it as either they could not imagine how they could cope with an adverse result or the error rate in the test was unacceptable. A few felt that they <u>would</u> wish to know : if the results were favourable they would be freed from an immense burden of anxiety and could make plans with confidence. If unfavourable, they could use their remaining years of health to fulfil cherished ambitions and/or to make provision for the future. Others simply felt that any result which altered their risk would be preferable to their current state of uncertainty and one man, who was certain that he carried the gene, wanted the status of a sick person. The remainder were uncertain, feeling that the question was an impossible one to answer and even among those who gave a positive answer ambivalence was often apparent on discussion and attitudes could and did easily change. The results seem to suggest that an exclusion test in pregnancy will be more popular than a presymptomatic test for the individual.

In conclusion, predictive testing will pose many problems. Its effects are unknown at present, particularly for those whose risk is raised, as the age of onset cannot be estimated for the individual and the effects of early dementia are uncertain and unpredictable. In addition, there are significant social and legal implications to be clarified : for example the position of employment agencies who may currently be within their rights to demand proof that applicants are at low risk before accepting them as employees, and insurance companies who may base their premiums on the applicant's degree of risk.

However, the new genetic developments also bring with them a message of hope, not just for individuals who will be predicted to be at low risk or who can go forward with a pregnancy with little fear of passing on a destructive gene. The main purpose of the research is to identify the HC gene and then to try to understand the nature of the biochemical defect, so that an effective treatment can be developed for this devastating disease.

Acknowledgements

The author thanks Professor P.S. Harper and Dr. Oliver Quarrell for helpful comments.

References

Donnai, D., Charles, N. and Harris, R.
Attitudes of patients after "genetic" termination of pregnancy.
Brit. Med. J. 282, 621-622, 1981.

Evers-Kiebooms, G., Cassiman, J.J. and Van den Berghe, H.
Attitudes towards predictive testing in Huntington's disease : a recent survey in Belgium
J. Med. Genet. (in press), 1985.

Gusella, J.F., Wexler, N.S., Conneally, P.M., Naylor, S.L., Anderson, M.A., Tanzi, R.E., Watkins, P.C., Ottina, K., Wallace, M.R., Sakaguchi, A.Y., Young, A.B., Shoulson, I., Bonilla, E. and Martin, J.B.
A polymorphic DNA marker genetically linked to Huntington's disease.
Nature 306, 234-238, 1983.

Harper, P.S.

A genetic marker for Huntington's chorea.
Brit. Med. J. 287, 1567-1568, 1983.

Harper, P.S. and Safarazi, M.
Genetic prediction and family structure in Huntington's chorea.
Brit. Med. J. 290, 1929-1931, 1985.

Morgan, C.
Bereavement counselling for genetic terminations of pregnancy.
Unpublished paper presented to the 1986 meeting of The Genetic Nurses and Social Workers Association. University Hospital of Wales, Cardiff.

Stern, R. and Eldridge, R.
Attitudes of patients and their relatives to Huntington's disease.
J. Med. Genet. 12, 217-223, 1975.

Teltscher, B. and Polgar, S.
Objective knowledge about Huntington's disease and attitudes towards predictive tests of persons at risk.
J. Med. Genet. 18, 31-39, 1981.

Tyler, A. and Harper, P.S.
Attitudes of subjects at risk and their relatives towards genetic counselling in Huntington's chorea.
J. Med. Genet. 20, 179-188, 1983.

DNA DIAGNOSIS OF AUTOSOMAL DOMINANT AND RECESSIVE DISEASES

Jean-Jacques CASSIMAN

Center for Human Genetics, K.U. Leuven
Campus Gasthuisberg, Herestraat, B-3000 Leuven, Belgium

Recombinant DNA technology has revolutionized the analysis and diagnosis of inheritable disorders. Using fairly simple techniques, a growing number of genetic defects can be detected directly at the DNA level.

The basic principles of this technology will be briefly reviewed first. The application of this technology to two hitherto undetectable disease states, the dominantly inherited Huntington's chorea and Cystic Fibrosis, a recessive trait, will be illustrated on the basis of studies performed at our Center in Leuven.

1. DNA STRUCTURE AND ITS ANALYSIS BY RECOMBINANT DNA TECHNIQUES

1.1. DNA

The structure of DNA is essentially the same throughout the world of living organisms. Four building blocks, the nucleotides adenosine-tri-phosphate (ATP), thymidine-tri-phosphate (TTP), cytosine-tri-phosphate (CTP) and guanosine-tri-phosphate (GTP), are linked by phosphodiester bonds to form long chains of polynucleotides containing sequences of these building blocks, unique for each organism.

The typical conformation and structure of these nucleotides, allows them to form pairs, held together by hydrogen bonds, either between the bases adenine and thymine or between cytosine and guanine. The DNA double helix therefore is composed of two antiparallel nucleotide strands twisted around each other at about 11 nucleotides per turn. The nucleotides of each strand are perfectly complementary to each other.

Birth Defects: Original Article Series, Volume 23, Number 2, pages 97–114

This property, the complementarity of the two strands, provides the key to the understanding of DNA replication at the time of cell division and of RNA transcription for protein synthesis.

Indeed, each single strand of the DNA double helix can serve as a template for the synthesis of a complementary strand; the net result being the semi-conservative replication of the whole DNA molecule, essentially without loss or gain of nucleotides and of their sequence. At the time of RNA synthesis, stretches of a single DNA strand can be copied based on the same principle of complementarity. The thus formed single stranded RNA can then leave the nucleus carrying nucleotides which perfectly match the original DNA strand. Its sequence will determine, in blocks of three (codons), the nature and order of the aminoacids in the proteins which will be synthesized in the cytoplasm or on the endoplasmic reticullum.

1.2. Human DNA and chromosomes

Sperm and egg contribute the same amount of genetic information (DNA) to the fertilized egg. Each gamete contains 23 DNA molecules with a total of 3 x 10^9 base pairs (bp) each. The total length of this gamete-DNA is 120 cm. Semiconservative DNA synthesis will maintain the DNA content of each daughter cell of the fertilized egg to 6 x 10^9 bp, with an identical sequence of nucleotides throughout life. Analysis of the DNA of an individual should therefore yield identical results whatever its age or the nature of the tissue studied.

The number of genes (DNA stretches coding for a particular polypeptide) in the human genome is estimated at 10-50,000 with a length varying from 100 to 100,000 bp. This represents at best 10% of the DNA. The remainder contains repetitive sequences, sequences controlling DNA and RNA synthesis; sequences with an unknown function. A particular cell will express at best only 10% of all its genes (1% of the DNA) at any time of its life cycle. Differential activation of genes appears therefore to contribute the basis for cell differentiation and tissue specificity. In a few instances, such as the development of B and T cells from the immune system, rearrangement within the DNA leads to the construction of unique sequences which characterize the differentiation of a particular cell type.

After DNA replication, the total genetic information must be passed-on to two daughter cells. Each of these should contain genetic information, which is identical to its sister and to the parental cell. The entangled DNA molecules, 480 cm or 2 x 6 x 10^9 bp long after duplication, are maximally condensed into proteinaceous structures known as chromosomes. Each of these 46 bi-armed structures contains 2 identical DNA molecules, one in each sister chromatid, which upon dissolution of the centromere are transmitted to the appropriate daughter cell where they loose their extremely contracted state.

1.3. Recombinant DNA and DNA probes

Stretches of DNA isolated from any living organism or synthesized in vitro (between 100 and 10,000 bp) can be inserted enzymaticelly in different types of vectors. Bacteriophages, such as the lambda phage, thus manipulated will infect host bacteria and replicate their own and the inserted DNA to form multiple copies of the foreign DNA. Plasmids, circular DNA molecules which replicate as independent DNA molecules in bacteria, can be readily isolated, manipulated and reinserted in the host bacteria. Cosmids, constructs of phages and plasmids, will take large foreign DNA inserts and replicate them in the bacteria. The net result in each instance is the production of a large number of copies of the DNA insert. Through density centrifugation or HPLC the vector or its insert can be purified and labeled with radioactive or biotinylated nucleotides so as to be identifiable by autoradiography or avidin-labeled probes. Alternatively the DNA insert can be modified chemically and visualized by antibodies directed against the modified nucleotides. In each instance the cloned DNA can be selectively detected in a mixture of unlabeled DNA fragments.

1.4. Restriction enzymes

A few hundred enzymes which can cleave or hydrolyse a single or double DNA strand have been isolated from bacteria. Each of these enzymes recognizes a specific nucleotide sequence of 4 to 6 bases and is capable of nicking the DNA in this nucleotide stretch. The total DNA of a human cell contains 6×10^9 bp; composed of only four different bases. The nucleotide sequence recognized by a particular enzyme will therefore reoccur many times in the DNA, which will be cleaved in as many fragments. Moreover, a single base substitution in a cleavage point will result in differential fragmentation of this DNA stretch compared to DNA derived from an homologous chromosome or from cells from another individual without the substitution. The fragments can be separated by size in an electric field, e.g., by electrophoresis in agarose or polyacrylamide gels.

1.5. Southern Blotting and hybridization

Electrophoretically separated fragments are depurinated and treated with high salt in the gels to obtain single stranded fragments, which are then blotted onto a nitrocellulose or nylon membrane by capillarity. The blot is incubated with a labeled single stranded probe under circumstances (temperature, salt concentration) which will allow the association of DNA strands with a high proportion of sequence homology only. Usually, only

a few of the immobilized DNA strand show sufficient homology with the probe under stringent conditions to form hydrogen bonds, which will resist removal by stringent washes.
Autoradiographic or enzymatic visualization of the bound probe will visualize the homologous fragments clearly.

Heritable variation in the size of particular fragments, restriction fragment length polymorphism, or RFLP, allows one to study heritable or mutational change in a particular DNA stretch (gene or random fragment) and by doing so identify heterozygotes or homozygotes for a particular disease by studying the gene directly or by analyzing closely linked DNA fragments (see H. Cann, this symposium).

An essentially similar procedure can be used to visualize RNA sequences homologous to a DNA probe or vice versa. Also, unfragmented DNA spotted onto a membrane can be hybridized under similar circumstance to DNA probes containing unique sequences; the presence or absence of this sequence in the DNA e.g., Y-chromosome specific sequences, can then be established in a rather simple fashion.

2. STUDY OF HUNTINGTON DISEASE FAMILIES USING RFLP

First recognized by G. Huntington in 1872 as a distinct entity, Huntingon's chorea is a severe dominant condition which manifests only during or after the age of reproduction. It is characterized by unvoluntary choreic movements and mental deterioration. The prevalence is estimated at 1 in 25,000 birth. The age of onset varies between 6 and 70 years with a mean around 42 years. While the fundamental gene defect remains unknown, selective degeneration of the nerve cells in the basal ganglia has been established for long as being the first pathological change in the brain. In Belgium about 200 families which carry the trait have been identified.

Analysis of a large Venezuelan kindred with random DNA probes (Gusella et al 1983), provided the first breaktrough in the study of this disease. Using the random DNA probe G-8, a polymorphism detectable after digestion of the DNA with the restriction enzymes Eco RI or Hind III could be shown to be within an estimated 10 centimorgan ($10x10^6$ bp) of the gene. Using a set of human x mouse cell lines and subsequently <u>in situ</u> hibridisation, the G-8 fragment and therefore the HD gene could be mapped to the short arm of chromosome 4 at 4p16→pter (Wang et al., 1985).

In an effort to confirm and verify the nature of the linkage between the G-8 fragment and the gene, as well as to rule out heterogeneity in the genotype and the existence of other HD genes, a large number of families with verified Huntington's chorea were examined throughout the world.

Our own experience with this polymorphism on Belgian families will be summarized briefly.

2.1. Set-up of the study

The information available from the study by Gusella et al (1983) and from similar studies on European families was thoroughly discussed with representatives of the Belgian Huntington League at their request.
The following decisions were taken at this meeting : (1) limited numbers of families would be contacted by the league for DNA analysis. Representatives of these families would be fully informed about the nature of the study, and the identity of the family members participating in the study would be kept from the investigators. For this purpose the samples would be taken by nurses from the league and coded appropriately before reaching the laboratory. (2) The results of the investigations would be presented to the family representatives and the decision to apply the test and make the results known to the individual members of a family, who would wish so, would be discussed at that time, taking into account the results of similar studies and discussions occurring in other countries. (3) The members of a family submitting to the DNA test would be asked to fill out a questionnaire concerning their understanding of the DNA typing and its possible repercussions on their perception of the at risk-status. (G. Evers-Kiebooms, this symposium)

2.2. Methodology

Peripheral blood samples, 10 to 40 ml, were collected on EDTA from 146 individuals derived from 8 families (Table 1).
DNA was prepared by standard methods (Kunkel et al., 1977). Five to 8 micrograms of DNA was digested to completion with the restriction enzymes Eco RI, Hind III or Bgl II; the resulting fragments were separated by electrophoresis on a 1.2 % agarose gel and transferred to a nylon membrane (Zetaprobe-Biorad) by southern blotting (Southern, 1975).
The southern blot was hybridized overnight at 42°C, as described by the manufacturer, with 2 nanograms/ml of radiolabeled probe. The probes G-8 and λ G-8 were made available by P. Pearson (Leiden) and R7 by J. Gusella (Massachussets). The plasmids or λ phages containing the inserts were labeled by random oligonucleotide primed synthesis (Feinberg et al., 1984) with ^{32}P-dCTP (800 Ci/mMol) and ^{32}P-dTTP (800 Ci/mMol) both from NEN (Dupont) to a specific activity of 5-12x10^8 dpm/µg.

After hybridization, the membranes were washed at 60°C to a final salt concentration of 0.15M NaCl in 0.1 % sodiumdodecylsulphate.

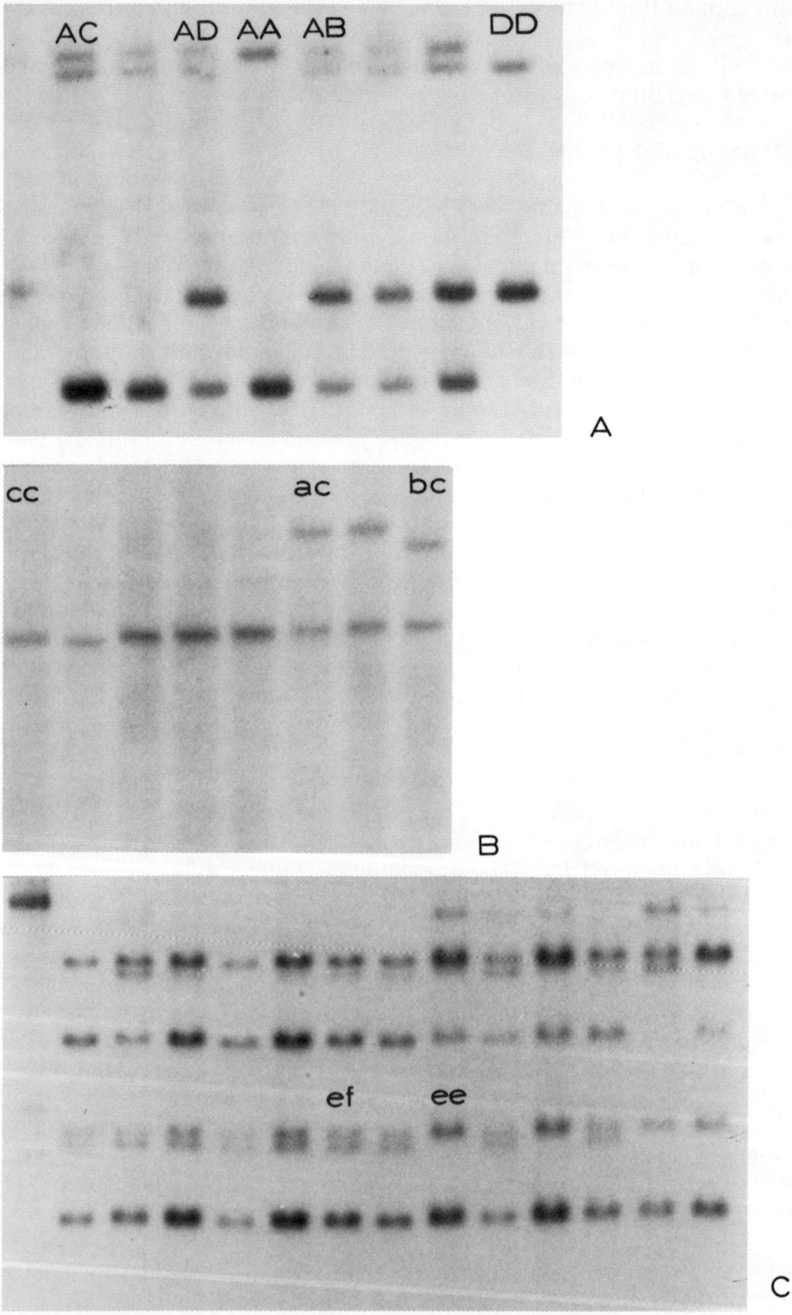
AC AD AA AB DD
A
cc ac bc
B
ef ee
C

Autoradiography with dual intensifying screens (Dupont) was performed on Kodak X-omat AR film at -70°C for 48 or 72 hours.

The G-8 probe detects a Hind III polymorphic locus with 17.5-3.7 kilobase (kb); 17.5-4.9 kb; 15-3.7 kb and 15-4.9 kb alleles designated A,B,C,D respectively. The λG8 probe detects an Eco RI polymorphic locus with 3 alleles designated a,b,c. The R7 probe detects a Bgl II polymorphic locus with 2.0 and 1.7 kb alleles designated e,f (Fig.1).

2.3. Results

In the present limited study, the alleles A and e were present in about 60 % of the individuals; while b and c distributed almost equally around 50 % (Table 2). The most frequent haplotype being Ace. The HD gene segregated in 3 families with A and b, in 2 families with A and c, in one family with D,c in another with D,b and one with C,b. The two largest families, which were studied for the R7 polymorphism showed segregation of the gene with the haplotype D,c,f in the first and A,b,e in the other (Table 1, Fig. 2).

Lod scores calculated for the combined G8 results by M. Conneally (Indianapolis) are given in Table 3. The maximal lod score for the 8 families was 3.39 at a recombination fraction of 0.00. For comparison, the total lod scores calculated for 49 families by Conneally et al. (1986) are given in Table 3. The maximum lod is 71.69 with a recombination fraction of 4 cM in males and 5 cM in females. The 95% confidence intervals are estimated from these data at 2.5 and 6.7 cM while no evidence for locus heterogeneity could be found (Tanzi et al., 1986). Interpretation of the data presented here assuming tight linkage between the probes and the HD gene would allow us to predict carrier status in 17 of the 77 at risk individuals tested, and non-carrier status in 46 of the 77. For 14 individuals or 18% of the at risk individuals, the haplotypes tested were not informative (Table 1). For family G in particular, lack of informative polymorphism would make it impossible to give a precise risk figure to any of the 4 at risk individuals.

Figure 1 : Representative Southern blots obtained in Huntingtons' Disease families. (p. 102)

a. Hind III digestion followed by hybridization with G8 detects the four haplotypes A, B, C and D as indicated.

b. Eco RI digestion followed by hybridization with λG8 detects the haplotypes a, b, c as indicated.

c. Bgl I digestion followed by hybridization with R7, detects the haplotypes e and f as indicated.

Table 1 : RFLP in Belgian Huntington families

Family	Persons (HD)	at risk	Segregation of G8 Hind III	Eco RI	R7 Bgl I	Informative carr.	norm.	Non-inform.
A	8(1)	4	C	b	-	2	2	0
B	28(5)	16	D	c	f	2	10	4
C	21(3)	12	A	c	-	2	9	1
D	24(2)	14	D	c	-	5	9	0
E	12(2)	7	A	b	-	3	2	2
F	37(6)	18	A	b	e	3	12	3
G	11(4)	4	A	b	-	0	0	4
H	5(2)	2	A	c	-	0	2	0
Total	146(25)	77				17	46	14(18%)

Table 2 : Haplotype frequencies of the restriction fragments in Huntington Disease Families

	Haplotype frequencies	Heterozygote frequency	
Hind III G8	A 0.60	AB 0.096	BC 0.04
(n=138)	B 0.08	AC 0.312	BD 0.006
	C 0.26	AD 0.048	CD 0.02
	D 0.04		
Eco RI G8	a 0.024	ab 0.022	
(n=144)	b 0.479	ac 0.023	
	c 0.496	bc 0.475	
Bgl I R7	e 0.59	ef 0.48	
(n=58)	f 0.41		

Table 3 : Lod scores for HD versus G8

	θ	0.00	.01	.02	.03	.04	.05	.06	.07	.10
Belgian families	Lod	3.39	3.32	3.24	3.17	3.10	3.02	2.95	2.87	2.64
International total for 49 families			66.85	70.09	71.33	71.67	71.55	71.23	70.38	67.37

Data analysed and computed by M. Conneally and presented at the Hereditary disease foundation workshop, Stanford, april 19-20, 1986.

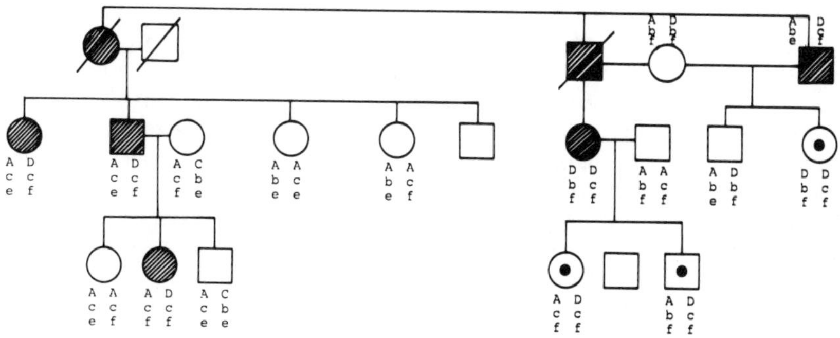

Figure 2 : Representative part of a pedigree of an HD family.
Segregation of the HD gene occurs apparently with the Dcf haplotype. Hatched symbols represents a known affected individual. A slash indicates that the individual is decreased. The central dot indicates the likely carrier status of the individual.

2.4. Discussion and conclusion

The results presented here illustrate how linkage analysis using RFLP might be used in the future for the identification of carriers of the Huntington's disease gene. Carrier detection, once established as a reliable technique, should be possible at any stage of the life of an individual after conception. Prenatal detection would thus become available for pregnancies in at risk families, as well as for premarital counseling of at risk individuals. As a consequence, the relatively abstract risk of 50% for a descendant of an Huntington parent, providing an accurate diagnosis of this parent, will increase to 99 or 100% or decrease to 1 % or less for his or her being carrier of the gene and thus presenting the first signs of the disease presumably around the age of 40. The consequences of such a test for at risk individuals identified as carriers of the gene both prenatally and postnatally are dramatic. Their impact will be discussed more extensively in other presentations at this symposium (G. Evers-Kiebooms, and A. Tyler). It should also be stressed that linkage analysis at the DNA level must be carefully examined before close linkage can be accepted (H. Cann, this symosium). The present study, while illustrating the possible use of this approach for carrier detection, is indeed too limited to allow one to decide that linkage is established or to calculate appropriate confidence intervals. Pooling of the data collected in different laboratories using the same probes is the only reasonable way to obtain sufficient information on the quality of the probes, pitfalls in the technique and meaningful results about linkage and locus heterogeneity (Tanzi et al., 1986).

At the present time, the pooled results suggest an error rate of about 5%, due to crossing-over, for individuals informative with restriction fragment length study, while about 20% individuals remain non-informative. Further efforts to develop probes which detect additional polymorphisms more closely linked to the gene or situated at the other side of the gene are necessary. Until such probes become available we feel, in communion with the members of the families, which collaborated in this study, that application of the available probes to the detection of carriers should be postponed. In the mean time, DNA from patients with Huntington's disease and their spouses is systematically collected in Belgium as to preserve it for the possible benefit of their descendants in the future.

3. CYSTIC FIBROSIS

Cystic fibrosis (CF) is the most common of the genetic diseases with a chronic debilitating course known in North European populations. The incidence at birth varies, but is estimated at 1 :3600 for Belgium with a carrier frequency of 1 :30. The fundamental defect and the pathogenesis remain unknown. Anion transport across membranes is clearly abnormal (Quinton et al., 1983); a possible explanation for the significantly elevated sweat chloride levels, which provide the only reliable diagnostic test.

The untreated disease is characterized by repeated bronchial and pulmonary infections and poor degradation of the food in the alimentary tract. Untreated CF will rapidly lead to bronchial obstruction and wasting resulting in heart failure and death. During the last ten to 15 years agressive medical and physical therapy treatment has progressively shifted the mean age of survival to 20 years and older. The general condition of the adults is good to fair but biliary atresia and hepatic cirrhosis as well as diabetes are major complications of the disease.

Carrier detection for CF is inexistant, (Qureshi and Punnett, 1985) while prenatal diagnosis, based on decreased digestive enzyme levels, carries a false negative rate of 5 or more. Screening for genetic linkage with random DNA probes provided the first indication for the localization of a CF gene on chromosome 7. Subsequently five DNA probes derived from chromosome 7, which recognize restriction fragment length polymorphism (RFLP's) were reported (Wainwright et al., 1985; Scambler et al., 1985; White et al., 1985; Tsui et al., 1985; Knowlton et al., 1985). Three of these probes pJ3.11 (Wainwright et al., 1985), pMet H and pMet D (White et al., 1985) appeared tightly linked to CF and mapped the gene to chromosome 7q2.1-2.2. In an effort to confirm and extend the linkage results with these probes, a study of Belgian families with one or more CF children was undertaken in collaboration with the Belgian CF foundation.

3.1. Materials and methods

Families

Table 4 : RFLP in CF families

Family	Individuals	CF	Sibs	Informative sibs	crossing-over
B	5	2	1	1	-
D	4	1	1	0	pMet H
E	5	2	1	1	-
G	7	3	2	0	CF all probes
L	9	2	3	2	-
LO	6	2	2	0	2x pMet H
LW	4	2	-	-	-
N	28	2	16	13	pJ x pMet H
VD	7	2	3	3	-
VL	5	2	1	1	pJ x pMet H
81	5	2	1	1	
88	6	2	2	2	
82	5	2	1	1	
83	4	2	-	-	
Total	100	28	34	25 (73%)	6 (9%) uncorrected for paternity

14 families, or a total of 100 individuals including 28 CF children and 34 sibs graciously provided their collaboration to the study (Table 4). One family (G) had 3 CF children and 2 normal sibs. In 2 families the CF children were first cousins. One of these families (N) was extensively analysed over three generations, the CF cousins belonged to the third generation. All individuals studied were amply informed about the preliminary nature of these investigations and about the uncertainty of being able to use the results for their own offspring.

DNA hybrisidation analysis

DNA was prepared from venous blood as described higher and digested with mspl or Taql to completion. Southern blotting, hybridisation and autoradiography were as described in the HD study except that 0.8% agarose gels were used for the separation of the fragments.
The probe pJ3.11 was obtained from J. Schmidtke (Gottingen), the Met H and Met D probes from G. Vande Woude (Frederic Cancer Institute). The plasmids were labelled by random oligonucleotide primed synthesis with ^{32}PdCTP (800Ci/mMol) and ^{32}PdCTTP (800Ci/mMol) to a specific activity of 5-12 x10^{8} dpm/µg
Representative autoradiographs for each of the probes are given in Figure 3.

3.2 Results

The combination of 3 probes and two restriction enzymes detected 4 pairs of polymorphic alleles (Table 5). Except for the pMet D probe, the allele frequencies of the other polymorphic sites were around 0.5 (Table 5), giving values of around 0.5 for the heterozygote frequencies.

Of the 35 normal sibs of CF patients examined, 25 (73 %) could be classified either as heterozygotes or as homozygote normal. The remainder 8 sibs were non-informative either due to the homozygote status of one of the carrier parents or due to an anomaly in the segregation of one or more of the alleles (Table 4, Fig. 4). In one CF patient clear crossing-over between the CF gene and all probes occurred. In 2 families abnormal segregation of pJ 3.11 and pMet H - pMet D occurred. Finally, in three cases recombination between the polymorphic pMet H - Msp I sites and the pMet H - Taq I sites seemed to have occurred. Whether the CF gene was involved in the recombination events could not be determined.

The presumed crossing-over cases will have to be reexamined and confirmed on fresh samples, while non-paternity will have to be ruled out using other polymorphic probes. If confirmed however, they would provide extremely valuable material to walk towards the CF gene, particularly if it would appear that the CF gene is flanked on either side by the J3.II and Met fragments. The unusually high number of crossing-overs in the Met H fragment are intriguing and will have to be confirmed, particularly since similar findings do not appear in other surveys (Wainwright, personal communication).

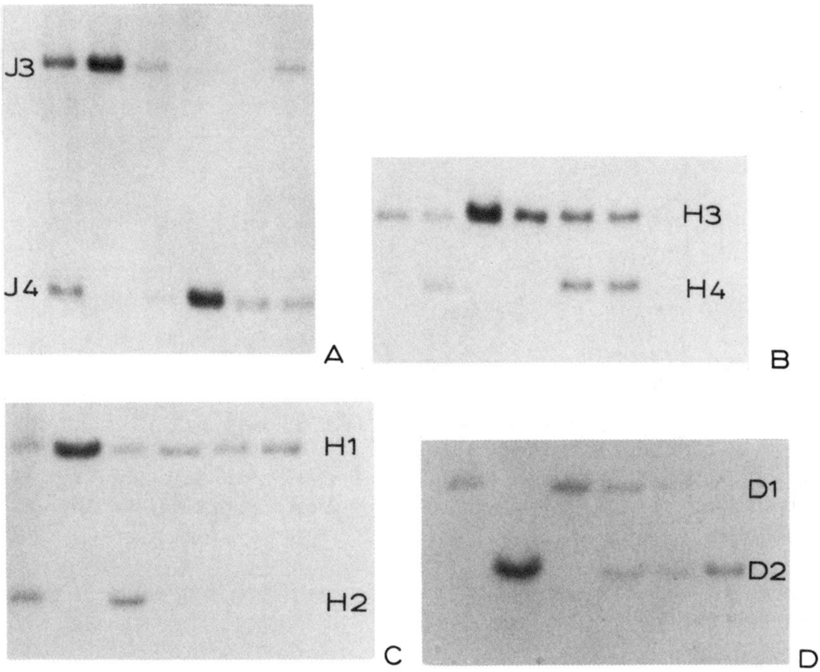

Figure 3 : Representative restriction pattern in Cystic Fibrosis families.

a. Msp I digestion followed by hybridization with PJ 3.11 detects the haplotypes J3 and 4 as indicated.

b. Msp I digestion followed by hybridization with pMet H detects the haplotypes H 3 and 4.

c. Taq I digestion followed by hybridization with pMet H detects the haplotypes H 1 and 2.

d. Taq I digestion followed by hybridization with pMet D detects the haplotypes D 1 and 2.

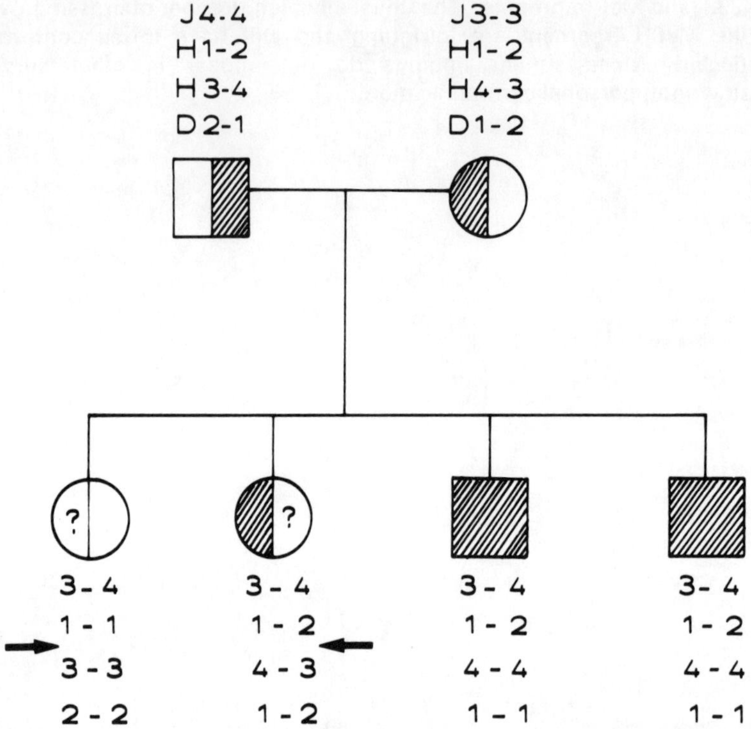

Figure 4: Representative pedigree of a CF family illustrating two presumed cross-over events (indicated by arrows) in the Met H fragment.

Table 5 : Haplotype frequencies of the restriction fragments in Cystic Fibrosis families

	Size kb	haplotype frequency		heterozygote frequency
msp I pJ 3.11	4.2	J3	0.495	0.499
(n=100)	1.8	J4	0.505	
msp I pMet H	2.3	H3	0.551	0.494
(n=98)	1.7	H4	0.449	
Taq I pMet H	7.0	H1	0.591	0.482
(n=98)	4.2	H2	0.408	
Taq I pMet D	5.0	D1	0.831	0.279
(n=98)	4.0	D2	0.168	

3.3. Conclusion

Presumed close linkage between the CF gene and two sets of DNA fragments has been described (Wainwright personal communication). The global results from all the surveys, which have since taken place, must be awaited before the quality of this diagnostic system can be convincingly evaluated. Only then will it be possible to provide sibs and parents of CF children with precise error rates of the procedure.

Moreover, since this particular test system can only be used in families with a living CF child, additional efforts will have to be made to get to the gene before screening of the population at large will become a reality.

While prevention of CF, mainly through prenatal diagnosis, will undoubtedly become feasible in the near future, and provide the opportunity for many CF families for low-risk parenthood, it should be kept in mind that the first concern in these families remains the cure or improved treatment of their affected child. For them, the search for the CF gene will only be succesful when it will have provided both diagnostic and curative possibilities.

GENERAL CONCLUSION

The technology for DNA diagnosis has progressively found entrance in many genetic centres around the world. Almost weekly, new DNA probes are found to be linked to a particular gene. In only a few instances however, direct analysis of the gene itself is possible (such as hemoglobunopathies or hemophilia) and the error rate of the whole procedure limited to laboratory errors. Without any doubt more genes will be cloned in the coming years, providing the genetic centres with more work than they might bargain for.

In addition, DNA diagnosis is also reaching into the field of somatic disease and will become an important diagnostic tool in the establishment of predispositions for cardiovascular and malignant diseas and for the precise identification of the nature of a particular tumor.

The impact of this diagnostic technology on genetic counseling will not only be qualitative but also quantitative. Many genes which cannot be traced prenatally at the present time will be detectable by DNA analysis long before the gene product will be known. If this service is to be provided to the community, one will have to solve the problem of the enormous costs of these procedures either by automating or simplifying them or by finding the necessary funds. In Belgium, for example, all genetic services, including DNA analysis, are reimbursed by the social security as long as they are performed in one of the eight academic centers.

But even more considerable will be the repercussion on society. Being labeled as a carrier of a recessive trait, even though asymptomatic, might be stressful for some; to have the certainty of developing a neurodegenerative disease later in life might be unbearable.

Information of the families concerned, of society and its political leaders, of the full significance of this technological revolution will become a major task for the genetic centers. Evaluation of the impact of genetic counseling, of the perception of risk and of the ways used to make decisions will provide invaluable information on how to inform and counsel individuals and families.

REFERENCES

Conneally, M.
Hereditary disease foundation workshop, Stanford, April 19-20, 1986.

Feinberg, A.P., Vogelstein, B.
A technique for radiolabelling DNA fragments to high specific activity.
Anal. Biochem. (addendum) 137, 266-267, 1984.

Gusella, J.F., Wexler, N.S., Conneally, P.M., Naylor, S.L., Anderson, M.A., Tanzi, R.E., Watkins, P.C., Ottina, K., Wallace, M.R., Sakaguchi, A.Y., Young, A.B. Shoulson, I., Bonnilla, E., Martin, J.B.
A polymorphic DNA marker genetically linked to Huntington's disease.
Nature 306, 234-238, 1983.

Knowlton, R.G., Cohen-Haguenauer, O., Van Cong, N., Frezal, J., Brown, V.A., Barker, D., Braman, J.C., Schumm, J.W., Tsui, L.-C., Buchwald, M., and Donis-Kelle, H.
A polymorphic DNA marker linked to cystic fibrosis is located on chromosome 7.
Nature 318, 380-382, 1985.

Kunkel, L.M., Smith, K.D., Boyer, S.H., Borgoankar, S.D., Wachtel, S.S., Miller, O.J., Breg, W.R., Jones, H.W., and Rary, J.M.
Analysis of human Y-chromosome specific reiterated DNA in chromosome varients.
Proc. Natl. Acad. Sci. USA 74, 1245-1249, 1977.

Quinton, P.M., Bijman, J.
Higher bioelectric potentials due to decreased chloride absorption in the

sweat glands of patients with cystic fibrosis.
New. Engl. J. Med. 308, 1185-1189, 1983.

Qureshi, A.R., Punnett, H.H.
Carrier detection in Cystic Fibrosis.
J. Pediatr. 106, 913-917, 1985.

Scambler, P.J., Wainwright, B.J., Farrall, M., Bell, J., Stanier, P., Lench, N.J., Bell, G., Kruyer, H., Ramirez, F. and Williamson, R.
Linkage of COL1A2 collagen gene to cystic fibrosis, and its clinical implications.
Lancet ii 1241-1242, 1985.

Southern, E.
Detection of specific sequences among DNA fragments separated by gel electrophoresis.
J. Mol. Biol. 98, 503-514, 1975.

Tanzi, R., Haines, J., Wexler, N., Harper, P., Folstein, S., Cassiman, J.J., Myers, R., Young, A., Hayden, M., Falek, A., Tulosa, E., Crespi, S., Campanella, G., Holmgren, G., Anvret, M., Kanazawa, I., Gusella, J., Conneally, M.
Linkage of G8 (D4S10) to Huntington's disease (HD); no evidence for locus heterogeneity.
Abstract submitted for the 7th International Congress of Human Genetics, Berlin, 1986.

Tsui, L.-C., Buchwald, M., Barker, D., Braman, J.C., Knowlton, R., Schumm, J.W., Eiberg, H., Mohr, J., Kennedy, D., Plasvic, N., Zsiga, M., Markiewicz, D., Akots, G., Brown, V., Helms, C., Gravius, T., Parker, C., Rediker, K., and Donis-Keller, H.
Cystic Fibrosis locus defined by a genetically linked polymorphic DNA marker.
Science 230, 1054-1057, 1985.

Wang, H.S., Greenberg, C.R., Hayden, M.
Subregional assignment of a DNA marker (G8) linked to Huntington disease by in situ hybridization.
Am. J. Hum. Genet. 37, A121, 1985.

Wainwright, B.J., Scambler, P.J., Schmidtke, J., Watson, E.A., Law, H.-Y., Farrall, M., Cooke, H.J., Eiberg, H. and Williamson, R.
Localization of cystic fibrosis locus to human chromosome 7cen-q22.
Nature 318, 384-385, 1985.

White, R., Woodward, S., Leppert, M., O'Connell, P., Hoff, M., Herbst, J.,

Lalouel, J.-M., Dean, M., and Vande Woude, G.F.
A closely linked genetic marker for cystic fibrosis.
Nature 318, 382-384, 1985.

DECISION MAKING IN HUNTINGTON'S DISEASE AND CYSTIC FIBROSIS

Gerry EVERS-KIEBOOMS

Center for Human Genetics, K.U. Leuven
Campus Gasthuisberg, Herestraat, B-3000 Leuven, Belgium

Abstract

Developments in genetic technology create increasing possibilities to alleviate human suffering through the prevention of the birth of handicapped children. The application of recombinant DNA research also entails new possibilities for heterozygote carrier detection (e.g. cystic fibrosis) and presymptomatic diagnosis (e.g., Huntington's disease). With these promising new developments comes also the burden of very complex and often painful decisions. This is illustrated by the results of interviews with cystic fibrosis families and also by a survey about the predictive test for Huntington disease.

Interviews with parents of an affected cystic fibrosis child revealed that the birth of a CF-child has a very considerable effect upon further family planning decisions. Specific attention is hereby paid to the role of the parental awareness of the 25% risk (which was satisfying in our group of respondents) and of the (future) availability of prenatal diagnosis. Since the recessive hereditary transmission was only superficially understood it was difficult for many parents to have a concrete idea of the risk that other family members could have the mutant gene. The knowledge of the risk to have another affected child is reported to have a very important effect upon family planning decisions.
The attitudes towards heterozygote carrier detection for cystic fibrosis for specific groups of persons are also investigated The relation between these attitudes and the knowledge of the increased risk for specific persons to be a carrier is also studied, as well as the association with some socio-demographic factors.

The decision to take a test for presymptomatic diagnosis of Huntington's disease is a difficult decision with far-reaching consequences. We

Birth Defects: Original Article Series, Volume 23, Number 2, pages 115–149

observed that the percentage of at-risk individuals who plan the test is smaller than in many other studies published previously. The main difference between at-risk individuals and their partners was that the partners were more in favour of taking the test as soon as it would be available. There was no association between the intention to take the test and some socio-demographic variables. The pattern of correlations with a number of other variables (e.g., presence or absence of children) was different for the at-risk persons and the partners. Since the difference in intention between an at-risk individual and his or her partner will be a source of additional stress in the decision making process to take the test we also investigated the agreement within a number of married couples.

Introduction

The new genetic technology which has emerged with tremendous speed is thrusting people into the position of having more control in matters that had previously been considered outside of their control. An increasing number of autosomal recessive diseases, of X-linked recessive diseases and of autosomal dominant diseases are detectable by DNA-diagnosis. In some cases the gene sequence itself has been cloned, in other cases carrier identification is possible by means of DNA-linkage. So prenatal diagnosis can be offered for a steadily increasing number of disorders.
All these developments are very important. They do not only increase the responsibility of individuals and families, but they also entail the burden of difficult and/or painful decisions. This is true for decisions concerning further pregnancies when there is an increased risk to have a child with a hereditary disease. This is also the case for couples who are deciding whether they want to make use of prenatal diagnosis, (either by amniocentesis or by chorion villi sampling) or not. It is even more true after the discovery of a fetal defect, when the very painful decision to abort or not is required. At that time the wish to avoid the anticipated burden of bearing a defective child is usually stronger than the desire for a child and may lead a couple to interrupt pregnancy even in the face of preexistent moral or religious objections to abortion. Depression may be the price of this internal psychic transaction (Blumberg, 1984).

The discovery of a fetal defect leads to an inescapable awareness that a similar outcome is possible in any subsequent pregnancy. The recognition that their own undesirable attributes (carrier status) have been responsible for the fetal abnormalities may lead to a sense of guilt. In autosomal recessive conditions the parents of an affected child may share a sense of genetic responsibility. If they are well informed, their feelings of guilt will be less pronounced because they realize that in their situation the birth of an affected child is the result of the combination of genes. Therefore the carrier status for autosomal recessive diseases as such is less stigmatizing. Guilt feelings may be particularly damaging in the case of X-linked disorders. In this situation the mother may be blamed or blame herself for the anomaly in her sons. For a discussion of the decision to make use of prenatal diagnosis and to abort when an X-linked fetal defect is detected in the fetus we refer to Beeson and Golbus (1985). The most difficult situation in prenatal diagnosis seems to occur when one parent suffers from an autosomal dominant disease, which leads to the decision to interrupt a pregnancy. Here the feelings of self-worth in the affected parent are strongly affected, this in addition to the guilt feelings associated with the transmission of a genetic disease. The availability of DNA-tests which lead to the diagnosis, in asymptomatic at-risk individuals, of late-onset serious disorders, for which there is no real treatment, also creates a difficult situation which is so far unique in medical history. It is obvious that the decision to make use of such a test is a very difficult decision with far-reaching consequences. The psychological implications and ethical aspects of presymptomatic diagnosis for autosomal dominant disorders for which there is no real treatment have already been discussed long before DNA-diagnosis by means of linkage was possible. (Stevens, 1971; Rothstein, 1972; Hayden, 1980; Thomas, 1982; Wexler, 1984)

The first part of our paper is a brief report of the results of a recent survey in Belgium on the attitudes towards predictive testing for Huntington's disease (HD) in asymptomatic at-risk persons. This study started some months after the occurrence of new perspectives for predictive testing.
In the second part of our paper we will present the results of a study on the impact of the birth of a child with cystic fibrosis (CF) on further pregnancy planning. Specific attention is hereby paid to the impact upon pregnancy planning of the risk to have another affected child and to the expectations towards prenatal diagnosis. Prenatal diagnosis of cystic fibrosis was not yet available in 1984, when most families were interviewed.

1. The decision to make use of predictive testing for Huntington's disease

Huntington's disease is a serious, lethal neurological disorder with autosomal dominant transmission. No real treatment exists for this disease. If one of the parents is affected, every child has a 50% risk to become affected. Although there is much variability in the age at onset, the first symptoms usually appear between 30 and 40 years of age. As a consequence, most at-risk individuals do not know whether they have inherited the disease or not at the time they have to make very important decisions about studies, career, marriage and children. Therefore the need for a reliable predictive test has often been expressed since many years.

In 1983 Gusella et al. published evidence for the existence of a DNA polymorphism closely linked to the gene for Huntington's disease. Although additional research is needed before this marker or any other can be put into clinical use, it is clear that in the near future predictive testing for Huntington's disease will be technically possible (Wexler et al., 1985; Merz, 1986). The prospect that asymptomatic persons can be tested for the presence of this disorder with onset in middle age, and for which there is no real treatment, creates a very difficult situation. After the communication of the results of predictive testing, the "risk status" of half of the persons at-risk is suddenly replaced by a "carrier status". Being told of the carrier status includes the knowledge of being in the presymptomatic phase of Huntington's disease, although there is no way to predict when the first symptoms will appear. There is no escape after predictive testing. Once a person receives the information, there is no way of obliterating the knowledge. Therefore, a careful analysis of all the implications of predictive testing is necessary on the individual level as well as on the population level. It also requires new evaluation of attitudes towards predictive testing, which will become a realistic possibility in the near future. The attitudes towards predictive testing were studied in a recent survey in Belgium in a group of people that are at-risk for Huntington's disease and in a smaller group of their partners.

1.1. Sample composition and methodology

In March 1984 the Center for Human Genetics of the University of Leuven organized an information meeting in collaboration with the Belgian Huntington Association for a limited number of persons. The purposes of this meeting were : (1) to explain the recent findings on the linkage of a DNA polymorphism with Huntington's disease and its implications for possible predictive testing, and (2) to ask for the cooperation of persons at-risk and their partners in a research project. The primary aim of this project was the investigation of the prevalence of DNA polymorphism in Belgian Huntington's disease families in order to explore the possible use of this polymorphism in a predictive test. From all cooperating individuals - those present at the meeting as well as other individuals in these families - a blood sample was taken for DNA-analysis and a questionnaire* was given to the at-risk persons and to the partners of affected individuals and at-risk individuals. We refer to the presentation of J.J.Cassiman for a discussion of the results concerning DNA-diagnosis.

* A copy of the questionnaire (in Dutch) is available upon request from the author.

1.2. Results

For a detailed discussion of all results we refer to Evers-Kiebooms et al. (1986). In this paper only the results concerning the intentions towards the use of a predictive test for the 41 individuals who are at 50% risk and 19 of their partners are discussed briefly. The results in table 1 reveal that almost the same percentage of at-risk persons and partners are in favour of using the predictive test. The main difference is that relatively more partners are in favour of testing immediately when available, instead of postponing the test.

Table 1 : Attitudes towards the use of a predictive test for Huntington's disease

	Individuals at 50% risk (N=41)		**Their partners** (N=19)	
Take the test immediately when available	17 (42%)	59%	11 (58%)	58%
Take the test undecided when	1 (2%)		0	
Take the test but not immediately	6 (15%)		0	
Undecided about the test	8 (20%)		5 (26%)	
Not take the test	9 (22%)		3 (16%)	

The percentage of at-risk individuals, who plan to take the test is smaller than in some of the studies published previously (Barette and Marsden, 1979; Schoenfeld et al., 1984; Stern and Eldridge, 1975; Teltscher and Polgar, 1981; Tyler and Harper, 1983). To get more insight into the motivation for wanting a predictive test, we asked the at-risk individuals and their partners to give us the reasons why they wanted a predictive test or not. It is necessary to keep in mind that this was formulated as an open-ended question, to have a spontaneous answer and to exclude any suggestions. The main reasons to want a test are : to have "certainty" instead of uncertainty and anxiety and secondly to make decisions concerning further children. The latter seems to be less important for the at-risk individuals than for the partners. The need for "certainty" as main reason for predictive testing was also reported by Mastromauro et al. (1986). These authors also discuss data suggesting that "many of those individuals who previously expressed a desire to learn whether or not they are likely to develop HD may indeed come forward to be tested, and that many will want to be tested shortly after gene linkage testing becomes available".

We also investigated if there is any association between the intention to take the predictive test and some social and demographic variables. To this means we calculated rank correlations (Kendall tau). For the group of at-risk individuals there seems to be no association with sex, age, educational level, and with the presence or absence of children. The lack of association with socio-demographic variables was also demonstrated by Schoenfeld et al. (1984). There is an association between the plans to take the test and the presence or absence at the information meeting (tau = .52, p <.001). The fact that the individuals present at the meeting are active members of the Huntington Association is probably one of the factors that is responsible for this association. There is also a negative correlation with the age at onset of HD in the affected parent (tau = -.35, p = 0.02) : the younger the father or mother of an at-risk individual has become affected the stronger seems the intention to take the test. Of course we are aware that a younger age at onset may imply a much stronger influence on the life of the children, so that it may not be the age as such but other associated factors that are responsible for this difference.

The pattern of correlations is different for the partners. Here we find a significant negative correlation with educational level (tau = -.44, p=0.03) and a positive correlation with the presence of children (tau = .43, p = 0.06). Partners with a lower educational level are more in favour of a predictive test for their at-risk husband or wife. The presence or absence of children also plays an important part in the attitude of the partners towards predictive testing . If they have children they are more in favour of a predictive test immediately when available. In contrast to the results for the at-risk individuals themselves we do not find an association with the presence or absence at the information meeting.

Additional research on a large sample of at-risk individuals and their partners to get more insight into the intentions and motivation to want a predictive test and also to assess the attitudes towards prenatal diagnosis is still going on. In this new survey, the role of their personal experiences with the affected parent will also be assessed. In this study we also explore the very intruiging finding that more than half of the respondents do not agree that the decision to take the test should be taken after consultation with experts. Even completely respecting the freedom of decision, we feel that the implications of taking a predictive test are so important that the development of an appropriate support program is indispensable to help the at-risk individuals and their partners to make the appropriate decision.

2. Decisions about subsequent pregnancies after the birth of a child with cystic fibrosis

Cystic fibrosis is the most frequent autosomal recessive disorder in white (Caucasian) children, for which about one person in 30 is a heterozygous carrier. It is a serious chronic disorder in which there are abnormalities of several exocrine secretions, including pancreatic and duodenal enzymes, sweat chlorides and bronchial secretions. The thick viscid mucus produced by the bronchi is particularly serious, since it makes the affected children highly susceptible to pneumonia. Physiotherapy plays an important part in the daily life of the CF patient. Even in face of medical treatment, regular physiotherapy and an appropriate diet the life expectancy of CF patients is limited and the implications for the family are very considerable. For a detailed discussion of the psychosocial impact of cystic fibrosis we refer to Falkman (1977), De Wet and Cywes (1984) and Denayer et al. (in preparation).

In 1984 the Genetics Centre of the University of Leuven has set up a research project in collaboration with the Belgian Cystic Fibrosis Association with the aim of collecting detailed information about CF by means of the following questions :

1. To what extent are parents conscious of the hereditary aspects of CF ?
2. What is the impact of the diagnosis of CF in their child and of the learning of the risk of recurrence in subsequent offspring upon the future reproductive plans ? pregnancies ?
3. Will the availability of prenatal diagnosis be an important element in the planning and to what extent will it be used ?
   It should be noted that at the time of the study prenatal diagnosis was not yet available; the first reports of the discovery of genetic markers for the cystic fibrosis gene were published in October 1985 in JAMA Medical News and were confirmed afterwards (Pembrey and Malcolm, 1986; Super, 1986; Brock and Van Heyningen, 1986).
4. What is the opinion of parents of a CF-child about carrier identification ?
   (it should be noted that at the time of the study heterozygous carrier detection was not available at all).

2.1. Sample composition and methodology

From the total population of parents who are members of the Belgian CF Association, we randomly selected families that met two additional criteria :

1. the affected child must be born in 1976 or later and must be alive at the time of interview
2. parental age at the birth of the child must not exceed 30 years

As a first step parents were contacted by phone asking for their collaboration. Only a few families were not ready to participate in the study. A group of 105 families was interviewed at home by a social worker of the Belgian CF Association using a standardized questionnaire to guide the interview. The questionnaire consisted of 5 parts : socio-demographic data, detailed description of the pregnancies, awareness of the hereditary aspects of CF, effect upon the planning of further pregnancies, expectations and attitudes towards prenatal diagnosis and carrier detection*.

The majority of the 105 families were interviewed in the second semester of 1984. All provinces were represented so that 61 Dutch-speaking and 44 French-speaking families participated in the study. The mother was interviewed without the father in 45 cases, the father without the mother in 2 cases and both parents in 58 cases (the father was only present during a part of the interview in 7 of these cases). So the answers of 103 mothers and 53 fathers were available for data analysis. The average duration of the interviews was 91 minutes.

We will now give a brief socio-demographic description of the children and the parents. At the time of the interview an average period of 4.9 years had elapsed since the families' first confrontation with the birth of a CF-child. This CF-child was firstborn in 66% of the families. The birth rank was two in 30% of the cases and it was the third child in 5% of the families. At the birth of this child the mean maternal age was 23.9 years (minimum 17, maximum 29 years) and the mean paternal age was 25.7 years (minimum 19, maximum 30 years). In 98 families one affected child was born, in 6 families 2 affected children were born and in one family 3 affected children were born. At the birth of the first affected child an average time of 3 years elapsed since marriage.
At the time of their marriage most parents had a concrete or a vague idea of the number of children they would like to have. In our study group about 20% of the mothers reported that initially they had no concrete number of children in mind. At first, more than half of the families planned to have 2 or 3 children (Table 2). These figures roughly correspond to the data for a ramdom sample from the population of the mothers of the same age-groups (Cliquet and Debusschere, 1984).
At the time of the interview an average period of 7.9 years elapsed since marriage. Four of the 105 couples were divorced or lived separated at the time of the interview.

All socio-economic classes are represented in the sample; this is obvious

---

* Copies of the questionnaire (in Dutch and in French) are available upon request from the author.

from the distribution of the final educational level that was reached (Table 3).

Table 2 : Initially planned number of children at the time of marriage

	Mothers (N=103)	Fathers (N=50)
No concrete idea	20%	26%
No children	1%	0%
One child	5%	4%
Two children	38%	42%
Three children	27%	20%
Four or more children	8%	4%

Table 3 : Parental educational level (N=105)

	Mothers	Fathers
Primary School	18.1%	8.6%
< High School	28.6%	35.3%
High School	27.6%	29.5%
> High School	18.1%	15.2%
University degree	6.7%	9.5%
(No information)	(0.9%)	(1.9%)

The distribution of the socio-economic classes in our sample corresponds roughly to the data for the total population in the same age-groups.

Of course a correct diagnosis must be established before information on the hereditary aspects of CF may be given. Therefore it is worth noting that the average age of the children at the moment of diagnosis was approximately 3 months. About one fourth of the children was only diagnosed when the child was one year or older. As a consequence the first information concerning the implications for future pregnancies could only be given very late (even too late) to a considerable number of families. For more details about the age at the moment of diagnosis we refer to table 4. In two families the diagnosis was only established after the birth of a second affected child. These two families are not represented in table 4.

Table 4 : Age at diagnosis (N=103)

	Frequencies	Cumulative %
two days or less	8	7.8%
3 - 7 days	6	13.6%
8 days - 1 month	18	31.0%
2nd - 3rd month	25	55.3%
4th - 6th month	11	66.0%
7th - 12th month	11	76.7%
between 1 - 2 years	11	87.4%
between 2 - 3 years	5	92.2%
between 3 - 4 years	4	96.2%
between 4 - 5 years	1	97.1%
between 5 - 6 years	2	99.0%
8 years	1	100.0%

2.2. Results*

2.2.1. Knowledge about the hereditary aspect of Cystic Fibrosis

It was rather exceptional that parents knew about the existence of CF before the diagnosis was established in their child : less than 20 % knew anything at all about this disease. The first information - however vague - about the consequences for further pregnancies was given together with the diagnosis in 85% of the families, usually by the paediatrician. The way the attitude towards future pregnancies of the person who gave the first information was perceived, varied from one person to another. Sixty-one percent of the mothers and 56% of the fathers had the impression that this person dissuaded them from having subsequent pregnancies.

A detailed series of 13 questions was formulated to measure the understanding of the autosomal recessive transmission mode and the awareness of the incidence of the disease in newborns and the frequency of heterozygous carriers. Of course it is of utmost importance that the parents of an affected child know their risk of having another CF-child in subsequent pregnancies. The parental awareness of the 25% risk is rather satisfying : about 3 out of 4 parents knew the correct risk figure (Table 5).

* For all the analyses the SAS-system was used (see references).

Table 5 : Parental awareness of the 25% risk in future pregnancies

	Mothers (N=103)	**Fathers** (N=53)
Overestimation of the risk	16%	13%
Correct 25% risk	76%	74%
Underestimation of the risk	4%	2%
No numerical answer	5%	11%

This knowledge, however, seems to be rather superficial. A correct explanation of the meaning of this risk could only be given by 2 out of 3 parents who knew the numerical 25% figure. The increased risk that specific family members are heterozygous carriers of the CF gene is less well reproduced by most parents. Only one out of 103 mothers and 4 out of 53 fathers knew that "normal" sibs of the CF-child have 2 chances out of 3 to be carrier of the mutant gene. Notwithstanding the mothers' and fathers' poor knowledge of the 50% risk that their own brothers and sisters are carriers, 59% of the mothers and 70% of the fathers were aware of the fact that the risk to have a CF-child is smaller for their brothers and sisters than for themselves (half of them were not able to give an explanation why). The approximate incidence of CF in newborn children is known by 63% of the mothers and 57% of the fathers. The approximate risk that any individual in the population is a heterozygous carrier is given by 35% of the mothers and 34% of the fathers. Only 16% of the mothers and 21% of the fathers are familiar with the terminology "recessive disease". An overview of the percentage of correct answers to the 13 items measuring the knowledge about the hereditary aspect of CF is given in table 6.

For seven of the knowledge-items we asked the parents to indicate on a four-point scale how certain they felt that the answer they had given was correct. For five items there was a significant rank correlation between the correctness of the answer and the degree to which they felt sure about their answer and this as well for the mothers as for the fathers. For the two items concerning the risk for specific family members to be a carrier this association did not exist.

Since the "knowledge-items" are intercorrelated, a maximum likelihood factor analysis was performed to detect the basic dimensions of the parental knowledge on the hereditary aspect of CF. This analysis was limited to 11 of the 13 knowledge-items. The answers were used in a dichotomous form (correct or not). Item 4 of table 6 was not used because the answers were identical to the answers of item 3; item 8 was omitted because there was almost no variability in the answers. The resulting 3-factor solution after oblique rotation by the Harris-Kaiser method is given in table 7 for the mothers and in table 8 for the fathers.

Table 6: An overview of the knowledge about the genetics of cystic fibrosis. Percentage of correct answers.

	Mothers (N=103)	**Fathers** (N=53)
1. 25% risk for parents of a CF-child	76%	74%
2. explanation of this 25% risk	50%	55%
3. risk after 1 CF-child followed by 2 normal children	61%	62%
4. risk after 2 normal children followed by 1 CF-child	61%	62%
5. risk to be a heterozygous carrier for brothers and sisters of the parents	18%	24%
6. relative risk to have a CF-child compared with brothers and sisters of the parents	59%	70%
7. explanation of this relative risk	27%	32%
8. risk to be a heterozygous carrier for "normal" sibs of the CF-child	1%	8%
9. incidence of CF in newborn children	63%	57%
10. risk to be a heterozygous carrier for any individual in the population	35%	34%
11. terminology "recessive"	16%	21%
	Mothers and/or Fathers (N=105)	
12. risk of a mating carrier - non carrier	26%	
13. risk of a mating carrier - carrier	55 %	

Table 7 : Factorloadings of the 11 knowledge-items (N=103 mothers)

	UNDERSTANDING the autosomal recessive transmission	**MEMORY** for numbers	Use of the **PROBABILITY CONCEPT**
1. 25% risk for parents of a CF-child	0.73	0.27	0.26
2. explanation of this 25% risk	0.58	-0.03	0.16
3. risk after 1 CF-child followed by 2 normal children	0.87	0.19	0.11
5. risk to be a heterozygous carrier for brothers and sisters of the parents	0.40	0.00	0.02
6. relative risk to have a CF-child compared with brothers and sisters of the parents	0.10	0.08	0.98
7. explanation of this relative risk	0.22	0.22	0.47
9. incidence of CF in newborn children	0.19	0.89	0.05
10. risk to be a heterozygous carrier for any individual in the population	0.43	0.36	-0.00
11. terminology "recessive"	0.37	0.16	-0.00
12. risk of a mating carrier - non carrier	0.40	-0.20	-0.20
13. risk of a mating carrier - carrier	0.75	0.15	0.20

The factors could respectively be interpreted as "understanding of the autosomal recessive character", "memory for numbers" and "use of the probability concept". The factorscores for the mothers and the fathers were used for further analysis (instead of the total series of knowledge-items).

As could be expected, giving a correct answer is related to the parental educational level for some of the knowledge-items. When a significant rank correlation - at least at the 5% level - was found, either for the fathers or for the mothers, the result is shown in table 9. For the mothers we found a significant rank correlation with the factors "understanding of the autosomal recessive transmission" and "memory for numbers"; the relationship with the third factor "use of the probability concept" was not significant.

Table 8 : Factorloadings of the 11 knowledge-items (N=53 fathers)

	UNDERSTANDING the autosomal recessive transmission	**MEMORY** for numbers	**Use of the PROBABILITY CONCEPT**
1. 25% risk for parents of a CF-child	0.79	0.12	0.27
2. explanation of this 25% risk	0.66	0.08	0.25
3. risk after 1 CF-child followed by 2 normal children	0.90	0.05	0.14
5. risk to be a heterozygous carrier for brothers and sisters of the parents	0.22	0.22	0.23
6. relative risk to have a CF-child compared with brothers and sisters of the parents	0.20	-0.02	0.98
7. explanation of this relative risk	0.30	0.17	0.39
9. incidence of CF in newborn children	0.03	0.99	- 0.01
10. risk to be a heterozygous carrier for any individual in the population	0.25	0.37	0.07
11. terminology "recessive"	0.25	0.15	0.18
12. risk of a mating carrier - non carrier	0.42	-0.10	0.02
13. risk of a mating carrier - carrier	0.56	-0.13	0.25

A multivariate analysis of variance was also performed to test the hypothesis that respectively maternal and paternal educational level had an effect on the three factorscores. The overall effect was highly significant for the mothers ($F=3.04$, $p<0.001$) but not significant for the fathers ($F=1.26$, $p=0.25$). The result for the mothers could be attributed to the highly significant effect of educational level on the factor "understanding of the autosomal recessive transmission" (see table 10 for the results of the univariate analysis of variance). The effect of the educational level on the other two factors "memory for numbers" and "use of the probability concept" was not significant.

Table 9 : The knowledge about the genetics of CF in relationship with the educational level (Kendall tau rank correlations)

	Mothers (N=103)	Fathers (N=53)
1. 25% risk for parents of a CF-child	.26 (p=0.003)	.21 n .s.
2. explanation of this 25% risk	.28 (p=0.001)	.19 n .s.
3. risk after 1 CF-child followed by 2 normal children	.40 (p<0.001)	.35 (p=0 .004)
4. risk after 2 normal children followed by 1 CF-child	.40 (p<0.001)	.35 (p=0 .004)
8. risk to be a heterozygous carrier for "normal" sibs of the CF-child	-.05 n.s.	.40 (p=0 .001)
9. incidence of CF in newborn children	.08 n.s.	.20 (p=0 .02)
10. risk to be a heterozygous carrier for any individual in the population	.24 (p=0.006)	.12 n.s.
11. terminology "recessive"	.42 (p<0.001)	.30 (p<0.001)
13. risk of a mating carrier - carrier	.38 (p<0.001)	.28 (p=0.001)
Factor "understanding of autosomal recessive transmission"	.34 (p<0.001)	.17 n.s.
Factor "memory for numbers"	.15 (p=0.04)	-.03 n.s.

The parents also indicated all sources of information contributing to their actual knowledge on the hereditary aspect of CF. In 51% of the cases a medical specialist, usually a paediatrician, was reported to be the main source of information. The Cystic Fibrosis Association also played a very important part, so that it was considered to be the main source of information for 29% of the families (the journal of the association for 16%, the visits of the social worker for 9% and the meetings for 4%). The other parents reported that they obtained most of the information by self-study (12%) or else they could not give a main source of information (8%).

Table 10 : The effect of maternal educational level on the factorscores for "understanding of the autosomal recessive transmission"

Source of variance	df	SS	F	p
Educational level	4	21.57	7.58	0.0001
Error	97	69.03		

Mean factorscore per educational level :

Primary school	(N=18)	-0.73
< High school	(N=30)	-0.25
High school	(N=29)	0.35
> High school	(N=18)	0.27
University degree	(N=7)	0.86

In our study the awareness of the 25% risk to have another affected child was rather satisfying. This may be due to the fact that our data were collected from members of the Cystic Fibrosis Association, who get regular information about the genetics of the disease. Their knowledge however was rather superficial. This finding is compatible with the results of a number of published follow-up studies concerning the understanding of the genetics of CF (McCrae et al., 1973; De Wet and Cywes, 1984 and Passarge et al., 1984). The data of Passarge et al. (1984) also indicate that genetic counseling in cystic fibrosis is not given or is ineffective in a high proportion of families. In the study of Kaback et al., (1984) the knowledge of risk percentages was better than in our study. We guess that parents had the opportunity to consult some information sources, since in this study mailed questionnaires were used (while we used the interview method).

2.2.2. Pregnancy planning after the birth of the CF-child

2.2.2.1. The 'global' effect of the birth of the CF-child on planning another pregnancy

The effect of the birth of the CF-child on further pregnancy planning and further reproduction was assessed in 103 of the 105 interviewed families. In the two remaining families the situation was very specific, because in the former the diagnosis CF was only established after the birth of two affected children and in the latter it was even worse ... the diagnosis was only established after the birth of three affected children (the first and the third child in this family were healthy, the second and the fourth child were affected and died in the neonatal period).
The large majority of mothers and fathers stress the influence of the birth of the CF-child on further pregnancy planning. The degree of influence is variable : undecision about further pregnancies, decreasing the number of children or postponing pregnancies and for the most important group not planning any subsequent pregnancy (Table 11).

Table 11 : The global effect of the birth of the CF-child upon further reproductive plans

	Mothers (N=103)	**Fathers** (N=53)
No influence upon subsequent planning	15 (14.6%)	4 (7.5%)
Influence upon subsequent planning		
- undecided about further pregnancies	19 (18.4%)	7 (13.2)
- same number planned but postponed	10 (9.7%)	4 (7.5%)
- number has decreased	3 (2.9%)	3 (5.7%)
- no subsequent pregnancies wanted	54 (52.4%)	32 (60.4%)
No answer	2 (1.9%)	3 (5.7)

For 48 couples the answers of both partners with regard to the global effect of the birth of their CF-child on further pregnancy planning were available. Forty-three of them agreed completely on the effect of the CF-child on their plans; in the other 5 couples only one of the partners decided to stop further reproduction because of the birth of the CF-child, while the other partner was still undecided or still wanted a subsequent pregnancy. The interpretation of the answers with regard to the "global" effect upon pregnancy planning in the total group is complicated for two reasons : the initially planned number of children may already be reached at the time of the birth of the CF-child and secondly the mother may become pregnant again before the diagnosis of CF is established (in both instances this may lead to the answer "no influence"). Therefore we analysed the global effect on the subgroup of families in which the initially planned number of children was not yet reached and in which no subsequent pregnancy was started before the establishment of the diagnosis of CF in their affected child. The results concern 72 mothers and 37 fathers and are shown in table 12. They are rather similar to the results for the total group.

Table 12 : The global effect of the birth of the CF-child upon further reproductive plans in a well-defined subgroup*

	Mothers (N=72)	**Fathers** (N=37)
No influence upon subsequent planning	6 (8.3%)	2 (5.4)
Influence upon subsequent planning		
- undecided about further pregnancies	17 (23.6%)	7 (18.9%)
- postponed or decreased	11 (15.3%)	7 (18.9%)
- no subsequent pregnancies wanted	38 (52.8%)	21 (56.8%)

* in which the initially planned number of children was not yet reached and in which the CF-diagnosis was established before the start of a subsequent pregnancy

For this subgroup we also investigated if the global effect of the birth of the CF-child was correlated with the following variables : parental age at birth, the first reactions (negation, shock and guilt), the birth rank of the CF-child and the age of the child when the diagnosis was established. Neither for the 72 mothers nor for the 37 fathers a significant rank correlation on the 5% level was found. In both groups however a borderline significant correlation with birth rank was found (tau=0.20, p=0.07 for the mothers and tau=0.29, p=0.06 for the fathers) : the higher the birth rank of the CF-child, the more pronounced is the effect of this child on the planning of further pregnancies.

2.2.2.2. The role of the risk to have another affected child on pregnancy planning

In this study we have paid special attention to the influence of the information about the 25% risk to have another affected child upon further pregnancy planning. To this means we first describe the parents' subjective interpretation of the level of their risk in future pregnancies. It is clear from table 13 that 75% of the mothers and 65% of the fathers felt their risk was high or even very high. The educational level does not influence the subjective interpretation of the risk level (the rank correlation is +0.008 for the mothers and -0.14 for the fathers and is not statistically significant).

Table 13 : Subjective interpretation of the risk level in future pregnancies

	Mothers (N=103)	**Fathers** (N=53)
Very high	51.5%	43.4%
High	23.3%	22.6%
Medium	12.6%	15.1%
Low	3.9%	5.7%
Very low	1.0%	1.9%
(No clear answer)	7.8%	11.3%

We also asked explicitely to what extent the "risk in future pregnancies" had played a part in the planning of a future pregnancy. For 64% of the mothers and for 60% of the fathers the risk-factor has played a very important part in further pregnancy planning (Table 14).

Table 14 : The influence of the risk to have another affected child upon the planning of further pregnancies

	Mothers (N=103)	**Fathers** (N=53)
Very important role	66 (64.1%)	32 (60.4 %)
Rather important role	9 (8.7%)	7 (13.2%)
Rather unimportant role	8 (7.8%)	6 (11.3%)
No role	10 (9.7%)	2 (3.8%)
(No answer)	10 (9.7%)	6 (11.3%)

In 38 out of the 44 cases in which the answers of both partners were available, both agreed on the importance of the risk as a factor influencing pregnancy planning. In five of the six remaining couples the risk played a more important part for the father than for the mother.
As could be expected there is a significant rank correlation between the subjective evaluation of the risk level and the influence of the risk as a factor upon planning, as well for the mothers (tau=0.25; p=0.01) as for the fathers (tau=0.29; p=0.03). This means that the higher the risk level is evaluated subjectively, the more important is its effect upon pregnancy planning.

2.2.3. Reproduction after the birth of a CF-child

In paragraph 2.2.2. we discussed "reproductive decision making", reproductive plans after the birth of the CF-child. Now we present results about "reproduction", the occurrence of pregnancies after the birth of the affected child. Although it should be used with much care, we first give an overview of all pregnancies after the birth of the CF-child. Twenty-five of the 103 families had one subsequent pregnancy after the birth of the CF-child, five families had two subsequent pregnancies and only one family had three subsequent pregnancies. We also calculated the interval between the birth of the CF-child and the immediately following pregnancy for this subgroup of 31 families (Table 15).

Table 15 : Interval between CF and the beginning of the subsequent pregnancy

	f (%)
< 1 year	10 (9.7%)
> 1 year - < 2 years	7 (6.8%)
> 2 years - < 3 years	6 (5.8%)
> 3 years - < 4 years	4 (3.9%)
> 4 years - < 5 years	2 (1.9%)
> 5 years	2 (1.9%)
(no subsequent pregnancy before the time of interview)	(72) (69.9%)
	103 (100%)

The interval between the birth of the CF-child and the follow-up interview was different from one family to another (average interval = 4.9 years, SD=2.6 years). Therefore, it was impossible to assess in a simple way the impact of the birth of the CF-child on the occurrence of a subsequent pregnancy for the total group. For that reason we analysed our data by successively considering overlapping subgroups with an increasing follow-up interval (respectively one year or more, two years or more ..... five years or more). As a consequence these subgroups become smaller in size.

For all families in which the follow-up interval was at least one year, we examined if the beginning of a subsequent pregnancy was situated within a year of the birth of the CF-child. For the smaller subgroup with a follow-up interval of at least two years, we examined if the beginning of a subsequent pregnancy was situated within two years of the birth of the CF-child. We used the same methodology for the smaller subgroups that could be followed respectively three years, four years and five years (Table 16).

Table 16 : Occurrence of a subsequent pregnancy as a function of the time elapsed since the birth of the CF-child

	Time between the birth of the CF-child and the interview				
Subsequent pregnancy started	At least 1 year (N=97)	At least 2 years (N=87)	At least 3 years (N=75)	At least 4 years (N=61)	At least 5 years (N=53)
within 1 year	10 (10.3%) 4/10 a.d.				
within 2 years		16 (18.4%) 5/16 a.d.			
within 3 years			19 (25.3%) 7/19 a.d.		
within 4 years				20 (32.8%) 9/20 a.d.	
within 5 years					18 (34.0%) 9/18 a.d.

a.d. = after the diagnosis was established in the CF-child.

For 53 couples 5 years or more elapsed since the birth of their child with CF. During this period 34% of them started a subsequent pregnancy. For nine of these 18 families the diagnosis of CF was not yet established in the affected child before the start of this pregnancy. For an additional number of families the interval between the birth of the CF-child and the interview was shorter. In 33 % of the 61 families that were interviewed at least four years after the birth of the CF-child a pregnancy started within 4 years. Of the families interviewed at least 3 years after the CF-birth, 25% started a new pregnancy within 3 years. Of the 87 families that were interviewed at least 2 years after the CF-birth, 18% started another pregnancy within 2 years. Only 10% of the group of 97 families that were contacted at least 1 year after the birth of the CF-child started a new pregnancy within one year. It is worth noting that in only 4 of these 10 families the diagnosis of CF was already established at that time. Moreover, one of these 4 families seemed to have wanted an abortion because of the risk involved. It should be noted that in table 16 we only discussed the immediately subsequent pregnancies. We did not consider the second pregnancy after the CF-child in the five families that had two subsequent pregnancies, nor the second and third pregnancy after the CF-child in the only family that had three subsequent pregnancies. In table 17 we present the number of subsequent pregnancies as a function of the birth rank.

Table 17 : Number of subsequent pregnancies as a function of the birth rank of the CF-child

	Firstborn	**Secondborn**	**Thirdborn**	**Total group**
No subsequent pregnancy	43 (63.2%)	24 (80.0%)	5 (100%)	72
One subsequent pregnancy	20 (29.4%)	5 (16.7%) **11 a.d.**	0 **4 a.d.**	25
Two subsequent pregnancies	4 (5.9%)	1 (3.3%) **1 a.d.**	0 **0 a.d.**	5
Three subsequent pregnancies	1 (1.5%)	0 **1 a.d.**	0	1
	68 (100%)	30 (100%)	5 (100%)	103

a.d. = after the diagnosis was established in the CF-child.

When the affected child was firstborn, no subsequent pregnancy occurred in 63.2% of the families. The remaining families had one or more subsequent pregnancies.

When the affected child was secondborn, only 20% had a subsequent pregnancy. None of the 5 families in which the CF-child was thirdborn attempted a subsequent pregnancy. It is very striking that twelve of the 25 families that attempted a subsequent pregnancy after a firstborn CF-child did so before the diagnosis was established in their CF-child. Of the 6 families that attempted another pregnancy after a secondborn CF-child two did so before the establishment of the diagnosis in their affected child. So the family size-reducing effect of the birth of a CF-child is even much more important than the data reveal at first sight. It is also worth noting that of the 17 pregnancies started after the diagnosis of CF was established, three were due to failure of contraception and two of them probably resulted in abortion because of the risk involved. Of the 14 mothers that started a subsequent pregnancy before the diagnosis was established, two still had a second subsequent pregnancy after the establishment of the diagnosis.
We also explored to what extent the start of a new subsequent pregnancy within a fixed interval - successively from one year to five years - was related to the parental age, the parental educational level, the birth rank of the CF-child, the awareness of the risk (in three levels : "underestimated", "correct 25% risk", "overestimated") and the subjective interpretation of the risk level. We also studied the relationship of the start of a pregnancy within a fixed interval with the experienced effect of the risk as a factor influencing pregnancy planning, the experienced effect of the past problems with the CF-child as a factor for pregnancy planning and the fear for future problems with the CF-child as a factor for planning. As could be expected, there is a significant negative rank correlation between the birth rank of the CF-child and the occurrence of a new pregnancy within a fixed interval (Table 18) : the higher the birth rank the less probable a new pregnancy is started.

Table 18 : Rank correlations between the birth rank of the CF-child and the beginning of a subsequent pregnancy within a given interval

	Rank correlation tau	
Pregnant or not within 1 year (N=97)	-0.24	(p=0.02)
Pregnant or not within 2 years (N=87)	-0.24	(p=0.02)
Pregnant or not within 3 years (N=75)	-0.36	(p=0.02)
Pregnant or not within 4 years (N=61)	-0.28	(p=0.03)
Pregnant or not within 5 years (N=53)	-0.26	(p=0.05)

No association was found (= no significant rank correlation at the 5% level) with parental age, parental educational level and awareness of the risk, neither for the mothers nor for the fathers. Some significant correlations were found with the other variables. They are shown in table 19 for the mothers and in table 20 for the fathers.
The higher the mothers' subjective interpretation of the risk level, the less probable was the start of a new pregnancy within 4 or 5 years. In the same line is the negative correlation between the fathers' reported importance of the risk as a factor influencing pregnancy planning and the start of a new pregnancy within 2, 4 or 5 years. The reported importance of past problems with the CF-child as a factor influencing planning also correlates negatively with the start of a new pregnancy, as well for the mothers as for the fathers. The more important the past problems were experienced, the less probable was the start of a new pregnancy. A similar relationship, however less pronounced, existed with the reported influence of the fear for future problems.

All these findings suggest that most couples stop having children after an offspring is identified with CF and they are made aware of the risk of recurrence. Of course this is a description of the situation before the availability of prenatal diagnosis.

Table 19 : The start of a new pregnancy in relationship with a number of variables (tau rank correlations for the mothers)

	Pregnant within 2 years	**Pregnant within 3 years**	**Pregnant within 4 years**	**Pregnant within 5 years**
Reported importance of the risk level for pregnancy planning	-	-	-0.26 (p=0.04) N=57	-0.33 (p=0.02) N=50
Reported influence of past problems with CF-child upon planning	-0.30 (p=0.004) N=77	-0.35 (p=0.002) N=67	-0.33 (p=0.008) N=55	-0.31 (p=0.02) N=48
Reported influence of fear for future problems upon planning	-	-0.35 (p=0.002) N=67	-0.31 (p=0.01) N=55	-

Table 20 : The start of a new pregnancy in relationship with a number of variables (tau rank correlations for the fathers)

	Pregnant within 2 years	**Pregnant within 3 years**	**Pregnant within 4 years**	**Pregnant within 5 years**
Subjective interpretation of the risk level upon planning	-0.31 (p=0.05) N=39	-	-0.39 (p=0.04) N=27	-0.49 (p=0.02) N=26
Reported influence of past problems with CF-child upon planning	-0.31 (p=0.04) N=39	-0.41 (p=0.002) N=33	-	-
Reported influence of fear for future problems upon planning	-	-0.33 (p=0.04) N=34	-	-

2.2.4. Attitudes towards prenatal diagnosis

Although prenatal diagnosis for cystic fibrosis was not yet available at the time the families were interviewed, the majority of the issues which were discussed during the interviews do not become less important; even the opposite is true. The opinions of the parents about the necessity of prenatal diagnosis for CF were very clear. Ninety-four percent of them held the opinion that the efforts to offer prenatal diagnosis should be continued.
Since the attitude towards prenatal diagnosis may be related to the parental attitude towards abortion, we first describe the attitude of the parents towards abortion in general. Eighteen percent of the mothers felt that abortion in general was completely acceptable, 24% rather acceptable, 22% rather unacceptable and 36% completely unacceptable. In the group of fathers the percentages were similar : 20% completely acceptable, 22% rather acceptable, 28% rather unacceptable and 30% completely unacceptable. The attitude towards abortion in general was negatively correlated to religiousness, as measured by the regularity of practicing of the mothers (tau=-0.18, p=0.02) as well as of the fathers (tau=-0.32, p=0.007). The higher the educational level of the fathers, the more positive is the attitude towards abortion in general (tau=+0.25 p=0.04). This association did not exist for the mothers.

Retrospectively, we asked the parents of CF-children if they would have used prenatal diagnosis and if it would have influenced their reproductive plans, had it been available. It is clear from table 21 that 77% of the mothers and 72% of the fathers reported that they obviously would have used it, had a pregnancy occurred. Twenty-six percent of the mothers and 19% of the fathers even told us that they would have a subsequent pregnancy (a pregnancy which they did not want without prenatal diagnosis), as can be seen in table 22. For many others it would have made the decision to have another child much easier.

Table 21 : Suppose prenatal diagnosis had already been available after the birth of your affected child, would you have used it ?

	Mothers (N=102)	Fathers (N=47)
Yes, obviously used	77%	72%
Probably used	9%	13%
Doubts, don't know	6%	6%
Probably not used	2%	2%
Certainly not used	6%	6%

Table 22 : Had prenatal diagnosis been available after the birth of your CF- child, would it have influenced your pregnancy planning ?

	Mothers (N=101)	Fathers (N=47)
No influence	41%	38%
Decision to have another pregnancy would be easier	33%	43%
Would have decided to have another pregnancy (and otherwise not)	26%	19%

We investigated the relationship between the opinion about the use of prenatal diagnosis - supposed that it had been available in the period after the birth of the CF-child - and educational level, religious convictions (regularity of practicing) and the first reactions (negation, shock and guilt) after the birth of the CF-child. We found no correlation at all with educational level nor with religious convictions. For the mothers we found a positive rank correlation between the retrospectively expressed intention to make use of prenatal diagnosis for CF and the intensity of the feelings of negation after the birth of the CF-child (tau=+0.17, p=0.03). In the group of fathers a highly significant correlation with the intensity of the feelings of guilt was found (tau=+0.35, p=0.004). We also calculated the same series of rank correlations with the retrospectively expressed influence of prenatal diagnosis for CF (had it been possible) on pregnancy planning. No significant correlation was found for the fathers. For the mothers the only significant correlation concerned educational level (tau=0.21, p=0.02). The higher the educational level the more important was the influence of the availability of prenatal diagnosis on pregnancy planning.

In addition to the retrospective data concerning the use of prenatal diagnosis - had it been available - we also measured the intentions towards the future use of prenatal diagnosis, should it become available (and now it already is). We only describe these results for the subgroup of couples who can still have further pregnancies (no sterilization performed, neither in the mother nor in the father). The results are very clear : 81% of the mothers and 88% of the fathers will obviously use it, if a pregnancy occurs (Table 23).

Table 23 : Suppose prenatal diagnosis becomes available in the near future, will you use it should you become pregnant ? *

	Mothers (N=78)	**Fathers** (N=41)
Yes, obviously use it	81%	88%
Probably use it	9%	10%
Doubts, don't know	5%	2%
Probably not use it	3%	0%
Certainly not use it	3%	0%

* this analysis is limited to the subgroup of couples in which no sterilization has been performed, neither in the mother nor in the father.

The effect of the availability of prenatal diagnosis on future pregnancy planning is also striking. Twenty-six percent of the mothers and 18% of the fathers would plan another pregnancy should prenatal diagnosis become available, and otherwise not. For 31% of the mothers and 27% of the fathers the decision to plan a subsequent pregnancy would be facilitated by the availability of prenatal diagnosis. For the others there would be no influence upon planning. The relationship between the intended use of prenatal diagnosis in the future - should it become available - and the variables religious practicing, educational level, first reactions ("negation" feelings, "shock" feelings and "guilt" feelings) after the birth of the CF-child was also studied in this subgroup. The intended use of prenatal diagnosis was positively correlated with these first reactions in the mothers. Although no correlation existed with the estimation of the risk percentage, a positive correlation was found with the subjective interpretation of the risk level (Table 24). For the fathers we did not find any significant correlation with the above variables. The intended use of prenatal diagnosis is clearly not related to religiousness, neither in the mothers nor in the fathers.

Table 24 : Intended use of prenatal diagnosis in relationship with the maternal first reactions and subjective risk evaluation

		Rank correlation	**(Kendall tau)**
Feelings of negation	(N=76)	+ .20	(p=0.02)
Feelings of shock	(N=76)	+ .24	(p=0.009)
Feelings of guilt	(N=76)	+ .20	(p=0.02)
Subjective interpretation of the risk level	(N=73)	+ .21	(p=0.05)

We did not find any correlation between the same series of variables and the effect of prenatal diagnosis on the future planning of a subsequent pregnancy, neither for the mothers nor for the fathers.

All parents were asked if they would choose to interrupt the pregnancy should prenatal diagnosis reveal a fetus affected with CF. It is clear that 57% of the mothers and 73% of the fathers would choose to interrupt when CF is detected (Table 25).

These figures reveal that the attitude towards abortion in general is quite different from the attitude towards abortion because of a genetic indication. The latter seems to be more accepted as well by parents of affected children as by the population in general (Evers-Kiebooms and Delmotte, 1984). The intention to have an interruption of the pregnancy when prenatal diagnosis reveals that the fetus has CF, is positively correlated with the maternal educational level and with the intensity of feelings of shock and guilt in the mothers (Table 26).

Table 25 : Would you choose to interrupt the pregnancy when prenatal diagnosis reveals that the fetus is affected with CF ?

	Mothers (N=102)	**Fathers** (N=44)
Pregnancy interruption when CF	47%	48%
Probably interruption	10%	25%
Don't know	18%	14%
Probably no interruption	6%	2%
No pregnancy interruption	20%	11%

Table 26 : The mothers' intention towards therapeutic abortion in relationship with some variables

		Rank correlation	**(Kendall tau)**
Educational level	(N=102)	+0.22	(p=0.009)
Feelings of shock	(N=98)	+0.16	(p=0.04)
Feelings of guilt	(N=98)	+0.16	(p=0.04)

No correlation was found in the group of fathers. It is worth noting that, as opposed to the attitude towards abortion in general, the intention to interrupt a pregnancy because of the detection of a fetal defect is not correlated with religiousness as measured by the regularity of practicing.

2.2.5. Attitudes towards carrier detection

At the time of the interview 94% of the mothers and 96% of the fathers held the opinion that an effort should be made to ensure that carrier detection becomes available. A content analysis of all answers to the open-ended question "Why is future carrier detection important ?" reveals that one or more of the following elements were present in at least 10% of the answers :

- to know the risk, to inform people correctly about the risk (so that they can take into account this information for decisions about marriage and children) was mentioned by 30.7% of the mothers and 32% of the fathers
- to prevent problems : no marriage between carriers and/or no children when both parents are carriers was mentioned by 12% of the mothers

and 18% of the fathers
to avoid the birth of CF-children was mentioned by 15% of the mothers and 14% of the fathers.

It is clear from table 27 that almost all parents stress the necessity of carrier detection in brothers and sisters of the CF-child and also, to a slightly lesser extent, in other relatives. Carrier detection in any individual in the population seems indicated for about 3/4 of the parents (Table 27).

Table 27 : Percentage of parents who find that carrier detection is indicated for specific groups

	Mothers	Fathers
Brothers and sisters of the CF-child	97%	98%
Brothers and sisters of the parents of the CF-child	91%	96%
Children of brothers and sisters of the parents of the CF-child	87%	92%
Any individual in the population	79%	70%

We studied the relationship between the opinion about the need for carrier identification in specified relatives and the knowledge about the hereditary aspect of the disease. For the fathers we did not find a significant rank correlation with the factor "understanding of the recessive transmission mode" nor with the factor "memory for risks", nor with the factor "understanding of the concept probability". For the mothers we found a slightly positive correlation between their degree of "understanding of the recessive transmission mode" and the fact that they feel carrier detection is indicated or not in the children of their brothers and sisters (tau=+0.17, p=0.04).
We also analysed the correlation between the opinion about the need for carrier detection in an arbitrary individual and the knowledge about the hereditary aspect of CF (3 dimensions), the educational level, the knowledge of the exact risk to be a carrier for an arbitrary person in the population and the consequences of a marriage between a carrier and a non-carrier. There was no correlation at all, neither for the mothers, nor for the fathers. It is clear that the attitude towards carrier identification is

determined by factors that were not measured in our survey. There is a need for further exploration of this topic.

2.3. Conclusions

The parental awareness of the 25% risk was rather satisfying in the group of interviewed parents : 3 out of 4 parents reproduced the correct risk figure. It should be noted, however, that the knowledge of the autosomal recessive transmission seemed to be rather superficial. This finding is compatible with the results of most studies published previously. Some aspects of the knowledge of the genetics of cystic fibrosis are related to the parental educational level.

The birth of a child with cystic fibrosis has a major impact on the further reproductive plans. More than half of the families did not want any subsequent pregnancy. This finding is compatible with the results of Kaback et al. (1984), Passarge et al. (1984), De Wet and Cywes (1984) and McCrae (1973). We paid specific attention to the factors influencing the decision making concerning further pregnancies. The risk level, which was evaluated as high or even very high by the majority of the families, is a very important factor influencing the planning of a subsequent pregnancy. The decision making process about further pregnancies is very complex and research is going on with the ultimate purpose of helping parents in their decision making.

Although many couples decided to stop reproduction after the diagnosis of CF in their affected child, a considerable number of unplanned pregnancies occurred due to failure of contraception. Nevertheless the birth of a CF-child has an important family size reducing effect : we found that only 34% of the families that could be followed at least five years had a subsequent pregnancy. Moreover it is important to stress that for half of them the diagnosis of CF was not yet established at the time of the start of this pregnancy. The start of a new pregnancy within a given interval is related to the subjective evaluation of the risk level and also to the reported influence of problems with the CF-child in the past and to the reported influence of the fear for future problems with their affected child.

Almost all parents of children with cystic fibrosis interviewed in our study felt that prenatal diagnosis for CF should be made available. It is very clear from our results that the availability of prenatal diagnosis will have a major effect upon family planning : for about 60% of the interviewed families the decision to have a subsequent pregnancy would be facilitated (even stronger : when prenatal diagnosis is available a pregnancy will be planned and otherwise not). Our data do not only confirm the results of Kaback et al. (1984), but the attitude towards prenatal diagnosis is even more positive. We also investigated the intended use of prenatal diagnosis in all parents who didn't have a sterilization performed : 85% of the parents have the intention to make use of prenatal diagnosis should a pregnancy occur. The intended use of prenatal diagnosis is clearly not related to religiousness, but seems to be related to the subjective interpretation of the risk level and to the first reactions after the birth of the child.

Almost all interviewed parents held the opinion that an effort should be made to ensure that carrier detection becomes available and found that carrier detection is indicated for specific groups of relatives. Three out of four parents also found that it is indicated for every individual in the population. The attitude towards carrier detection did not seem to be related to the knowledge of the genetics of cystic fibrosis nor to the parental educational level.

2.4. References

Barette, J. and Marsden, C.D.
Attitudes of families to some aspects of Huntington's chorea.
Psychol. Med. 9, 327-336, 1979.

Beeson, D. and Golbus, S.
Decision making : Whether or not to have prenatal diagnosis and abortion for X-linked conditions.
Am. J. Med. Genet. 20, 107-114, 1985.

Blumberg, B.
The Emotional Implications of Prenatal Diagnosis.
in : Emery A.E.H. & Y. Pullen (Eds) Psychological Aspects of Genetic Counselling, Academic Press, London 201-217, 1984.

Brock, D.J. and Van Heyningen, V.
The facts on cystic fibrosis testing (letter).
Nature 319, 184, 1986.

Cliquet, R.L. and Debusschere, R. (Eds)
Relationeel en reproductief gedrag in Vlaanderen. (Partner relations and family building in Flanders. Results of the 1982-1983 survey) with English summary.
C.B.G.S. Monografie, No 1. Population and Family Study Center, Brussels, 1984.

Denayer, L., Evers-Kiebooms, G., Cassiman, J.J. and Van den Berghe, H.
De geboorte van een kind met mucoviscidose : de gevolgen voor latere

zwangerschappen. (The birth of a child with cystic fibrosis : consequences for subsequent pregnancies) (in preparation), 1986.

De Wet, B. and Cywes, S.
The psychosocial impact of cystic fibrosis. A review of research literature.
S. Afr. Med. J. 65, 526-530, 1984.

Evers-Kiebooms, G. and Delmotte, G.
Preventieve instelling ten aanzien van zwangerschappen. (Preventive attitude concerning pregnancies).
C.B.G.S. Monografie No 1, 63-80. Population and Family Study Center, Brussels, 1984..

Evers-Kiebooms, G., Cassiman, J.J. and Van den Berghe, H.
Attitudes towards predictive testing in Huntington's disease : a recent survey in Belgium.
J. Med. Genet. (in press), 1986.

Falkman, C.
Cystic fibrosis. A psychological study of 52 children and their families.
Acta Paediat. Scand., Supplement 269, 1977.

Freund, R.J. and Littell, R.C.
SAS for linear models. A guide to ANOVA and GLM procedures.
Cary, North Carolina, SAS Institute Inc., 231 pp, 1981.

Gusella, J.F., Wexler, N.S., Conneally, P.M., Naylor, S.L., Anderson, M.A., Tanzi, R.E., Watkins, P.C., Ottina, K., Wallace, M.R., Sakaguchi, A.Y., Young, A.B., Shoulson, I., Bonilla, E., Martin, J.B.
A polymorphic DNA marker genetically linked to Huntington's disease.
Nature 306, 234-238, 1983.

Hayden, M.R.
Social perspectives in Huntington's Chorea.
S.A. Med. J. 58, 201-203, 1980.

Kaback, M., Zippin, D., Boyd, P., Cantor, R., Lewiston, N, Davi, S.B., Dooley, R., Giammona, S., Harwood, I., Kagan, B., Kurland, G., Osher, A., Rucker, R., Stiehm, R., Wang, C.
Attitudes toward prenatal diagnosis of cystic fibrosis among parents of affected children.
In : Lawson d (ed), cystic fybrosis : horizons. John Willey and Sons, NY, 1984.

Mastromauro, C., Myers, R.H. and Berkman, B.
Letter to the Editor : Change in Attitudes toward Presymptomatic Testing

in Huntington Disease.
Am. J. Med. Genet. 24, 369-371, 1986.

McCrae, W.M., Cull, A.M., Burton, L. and Dodge, J.
Cystic fibrosis : parents' response to the genetic basis of the disease.
Lancet ii, 141-143, 1973.

Merz, B.
Screening for Cystic Fibrosis & Huntington's disease begins (news)
JAMA 255, 1826-1827, 1986.

Passarge, E., Eckerland, B. and Stephan, U.
Genetic counseling in cystic fibrosis. Results of a survey of 572 families.
Eur. J. Pediatr. 143, 54-57, 1984.

Pembrey, M.E. and Malcolm, S.
Genetic prediction of cystic fibrosis (letter).
Nature 320, 114, 1986.

Rothstein, E.
Huntington's Chorea : optimistic View (Letter to the Editor).
New Engl. J. Med. 285, 13, 751, 1972.

SAS Institute Inc. SAS User's Guide : Basics
Cary, North Carolina, SAS Institute Inc., 923 pp, 1982.

SAS Institute Inc. SAS User's Guide : Statistics
Cary, North Carolina, SAS Institute Inc., 584 pp, 1982.

Schoenfeld, M., Myers, R.H., Berkman, B. and Clark, E.
Potential Impact of a Predictive test on the Gene Frequency of Huntington's Disease.
Am. J. Med. Genet. 18, 423-429, 1984.

Stern, R. and Eldridge, R.
Attitude of patients and their relatives to Huntington's disease.
J. Med. Genet. 12, 217-223, 1975.

Stevens, D.L.
Test for Huntington's Chorea (Letter to the Editor)
New Engl. J. Med. 285, 7, 413-414, 1971.

Super, M.
Prenatal diagnosis of cystic fibrosis (letter).
Lancet i, 510, 1986.

Teltscher, B. and Polgar, S.
Objective knowledge about Huntington's Disease and attitude towards predictive tests of persons at-risk.
J. Med. Genet. 18, 31-39, 1981.

Thomas, S.
Ethics of a predictive test for Huntington's Chorea.
Brit. Med. J. 284, 1383-1385, 1982.

Tyler, A. and Harper, P.S.
Attitudes of subjects at-risk and their relatives towards genetic counseling in Huntington's Chorea.
J. Med. Genet. 20, 179-188, 1983.

Wexler, N.S.
Huntington's Disease and Other Late Onset Genetic Disorders.
in : Emery A.E.H. & I. Pullen (Eds) Psychological Aspects of Genetic Counselling, Academic Press, London 125-146, 1984.

Wexler, N.S., Connealy, P.M., Housman, D. and Gusella, J.F. (Editorial)
A DNA-Polymorphism for Huntington's disease marks the future.
Arch. Neurol. 42, 20-24, 1985.

THE AMNIOCENTESIS DECISION : TEN YEARS OF DECISION ANALYTIC EXPERIENCE

Susan P. PAUKER and Stephen G. PAUKER

Harvard Community Health Plan, Massachusetts General Hospital, Harvard Medical School
New England Medical Center, Tufts University School of Medicine, Boston, Massachusetts, USA

SUMMARY

Over the past decade we have used a decision analytic model to counsel 849 patients (468 women, 381 men, 432 couples) about amniocentesis for prenatal diagnosis. The model explicitly considers the possibilities of miscarriage (both after amniocentesis and spontaneously), an affected child (as a function of maternal age), and various diagnostic errors. Prospective parents are shown the model after routine counseling is used to explain the options and potential outcomes. Using the lottery technique (in which they are asked to choose between therapeutic abortion and carrying a pregnancy to term without the benefit of amniocentesis, where the likelihood of an affected child is varied in a structured sequence), prospective parents expressed their attitudes on a utility scale, where zero corresponds to an unaffected child and where 100 corresponds to an affected child. On that scale, the mean assessed disutility of therapeutic abortion was 33.7±32.6 (35.8±32.1 among women, 30.9±32.9 among men).

The decision model encourages couples to confront their attitudes toward specific reproductive outcomes, to clarify their values and to incorporate them, along with their current risks, into a logical decision about prenatal diagnosis.

INTRODUCTION

Prior to the 1970's, most patients expected their physicians to make therapeutic or diagnostic decisions for them. In a session with a genetic clinician, patients expected to receive relevant information. When these patients asked how best to proceed with further evaluation, they were

Birth Defects: Original Article Series, Volume 23, Number 2, pages 151–169

generally counseled in a non-directive fashion (Beeson & Golbus, 1979; Evers-Kiebooms et al., 1980; Grobstein, 1979; Murphy & Chase, 1975; Pauker, 1982; Pearn, 1977). Perhaps because many genetic diagnostic decisions involve abortion-related issues, or perhaps to avoid the possibility of passing moral judgment, the genetic philosophy led to a preference for leaving the decision process to the patient. This left the patient with the dilemma of trying to resolve difficult, emotionally-charged choices without adequate guidance from genetic professionals and under the unfamiliar conditions of uncertainty.

Increasingly, patients expect to be active participants in the decision making aspects of their genetic counseling sessions (Pauker et al., 1982; Pauker et al., 1981). They no longer anticipate that their geneticist or obstetrician will provide them with the "right" answer to a pre-natal diagnostic decision. They expect their own values to be the basis upon which they will act. Consider the following cases :

> It took Attorney C.A. (Case #689755) 7 years to conceive her current pregnancy at the age of 34 years. This was clearly a precious pregnancy. Although she and her husband, a 40 year old attorney, did not wish to pose any risk to their fetus by performing an amniocentesis, they were anxious to avoid a Down syndrome baby, which would be inconsistent with their chosen lifestyles. They had delayed their amniocentesis decision as long as they could and requested genetic counseling to go beyond the usual non-directive information from their obstetrician.
>
> Mrs. S.T. (Case #927534) had lost her last pregnancy following an amniocentesis through an anterior placenta. At age 37 years, she had waited nine years to have a second child and now faced a 1/200 risk of having a Down's baby. For her, this was an unacceptably high risk, given her exposure to her Down syndrome cousin. At 11 weeks gestation, she requested help resolving her conflicting attitudes in time to schedule a possible amniocentesis.

In response to cases such as these, we developed a decision analytic model in 1975 (Pauker & Pauker, 1977; Pauker & Pauker, this symposium) and began to help patients consider their personal attitudes about the relative burden to themselves and to their prospective families of such pregnancy outcomes as elective abortion, spontaneous abortion, and an affected newborn (Pauker & Pauker, 1979).

Decision analysis is a formal technique which allows the genetic clinician to incorporate patient values with individualized risks in a logical framework to derive the best possible choice under conditions of uncertainty. Patients are usually eager to have their own values be the basis for a decision process which is tailored to their own current circumstances. Without promising a perfect answer or revealing the clinician's own values to the patient, formal decision analysis can provide the patient with a clearer path through the apparent maze.

Of the 849 genetics patients we have counseled using decision analysis since 1975, 468 females, 381 males (including 432 couples) have presented with the question of whether or not to utilize amniocentesis for the prenatal diagnosis of advancing maternal age-related chromosomal abnormalities of the fetus, particularly Down syndrome. In addition, 26 patients presented for prenatal diagnosis counseling for other birth defects such as meningomyelocele, hemophilia, or Duchenne muscular dystrophy. This counseling was also augmented by the use of formal decision analysis.

As new prenatal diagnosis techniques become more widely available and affordable, patients are becoming more anxious about the options they face. They hear about chorionic villous sampling, DNA testing, alpha-fetoprotein screening, and fetal umbilical venous sampling. They are confused about how much risk is too much, how accurate the tests are, and how to balance the risk of testing the fetus against the potential burden of having an affected child. These difficult and complex choices lend themselves quite nicely to our present model and similar approaches to decision support.

The purpose of this paper is to demonstrate that it is possible to help patients assess their values or utilities about specific outcomes of their current or planned pregnancies in a quantitative way and to use those utilities in a formal decision analytic model to derive the most logical choice under the circumstances. The final choice about prenatal testing rests where it can only be - in the hands of the potential parents, whose own values have driven the decision.

METHODS

The first step in the design of our decision analytic model was the construction and pruning of the decision tree reproduced in Figure 1. On the far left, the square node represents the key choice the prospective parent or couple faces. If they choose not to have an amniocentesis, they expose themselves to a chance event over which they have no control, i.e., the possibility of the pregnancy's continuing to term versus the possibility of having a spontaneous abortion. This and other chance events are depicted as open circles.
If the pregnancy continues, it can result in a child affected or unaffected by a particular problem, such as Down syndrome or meningomyelocele.

If patients choose amniocentesis for the prenatal diagnosis (lower branch of decision node), they face the chance that the pregnancy will spontaneously abort following the procedure or that it will continue toward term. The next node on the lowest branch of the tree represents the chances that the fetus will appear on amniocentesis to be unaffected or affected by the problem under discussion. If the amniocentesis is positive, that result may be a true positive or a false positive; similarly, if the amniocentesis is negative, it can be a true or a false negative result.

The likelihood of any of the eight possible outcomes of the decision is equal to the product of the probabilities along the path leading to that outcome. The resolution of the decision tree is totally dependent on the potential parents' assessed attitudes toward these various outcomes of the pregnancy.

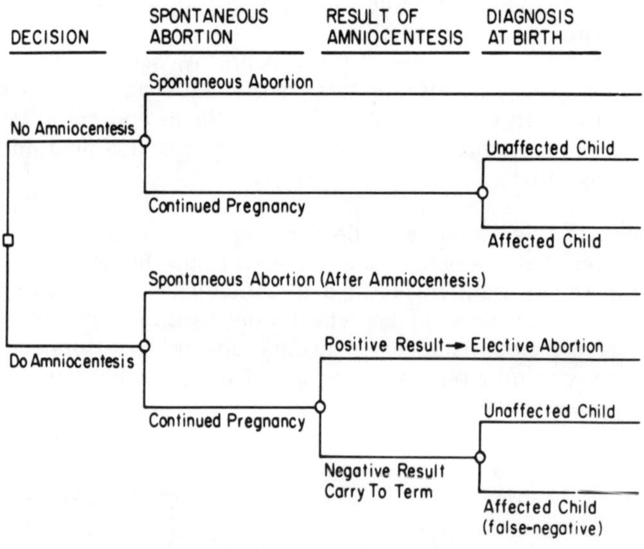

Figure 1 : A Decision Tree of the Amniocentesis Decision. Reprinted from Pauker and Pauker (1979).

To assess their attitudes or utilities toward these outcomes, the prospective parents must assign a relative value, representing the relative desirability or burden of each alternative. These utilities are expressed on a single consistent scale : in this model, ranging from zero to one-hundred, where zero represents the best possible outcome and one-hundred the worst. Most parents would choose giving birth to an unaffected fetus as the best possible outcome. The birth of an affected fetus would usually be the worst. The values of spontaneous abortion and elective abortion of affected and unaffected fetuses are of intermediate utility, between zero and one-hundred.

In a routine genetic counseling session for prenatal diagnosis of birth defects and hereditary illnesses, patients were asked about family history of hereditary disorders, complete pregnancy history including the nature of previous pregnancy losses, and the relative "preciousness" of the pregnancy based on whether the pregnancy was desired and how long it took the couple to conceive.

The risk to the patients of having an affected or an unaffected child was presented in terms of odds, framing the risk in both positive and negative terms (McNeil et al., 1982). For all women 35 years and older, the risks of Down syndrome and other maternal age-related chromosomal anomalies were discussed. The baseline probability of 3-4 % of having a child with some birth defect was always given.

The risks and benefits of amniocentesis were discussed, including the possible complications of fluid leakage, cramping, spotting, infection, and a 0.3 % or less chance of abortion following the procedure. The decision tree was often shown to patients to augment their understanding of the amniocentesis choice.

The use and value of diagnostic ultrasound and the possibility of dealing with a twin gestation were discussed. Patients were informed of the possibility of false positive and false negative test reports and of the possibility of unanticipated cytogenetic results such as 47,XYY. Techniques for mid-trimester abortion were presented along with the option of placing affected newborns for adoption. The long- and short-range significance of having a Down syndrome newborn was discussed at some length with advanced maternal age parents.

Amniocentesis was presented as a technique which could provide reassurance for parents and not necessarily lead to abortion.

After routine counseling, some potential parents were certain of their choice about whether or not to avail themselves of amniocentesis for prenatal diagnosis; decision analysis was not offered to these patients. For patients having trouble deciding about amniocentesis under the presented conditions of uncertainty, decision analysis was offered as one way to help them appreciate their own values and make a rational choice.

Utility assessment

In order to ascertain where on the arbitrary scale (ranging from zero to 100) any given patient's values regarding the possible outcomes of pregnancy belong, patients were asked to imagine that they faced a 50 % risk for having an affected baby and that prenatal diagnosis were not available. In the case of Down syndrome risk, patients were asked,

> "If your risk for Down syndrome were 50-50 in this pregnancy, would you carry the pregnancy to term, or do you think you would elect to abort the pregnancy?"

If patients had difficulty with odds assessment, other terms were used, such as "one out of two risk," "50 % risk", or "a room with two children, one of them has Down syndrome." If patients easily answered this question and said that they would carry the pregnancy to term, the next question was :

> "If there were a 90 % chance of Down syndrome, that is 10 % chance that this would not happen, would you still be willing to carry to term?"

If "yes", the risk was changed to 99 %, and then 100 %. If "no", the risk was changed to 75 % to search for the "point of indifference" where the patient could not decide between abortion and carrying on the pregnancy.

If the answer to the first question was that the patient would readily abort at a 50 % risk, the next question posed a 10 % risk then a 25 % risk, depending on the answers until the "point of indifference" was ascertained.

Patients who could not choose between abortion and continued pregnancy at the 50 % risk (first question), were asked if they would abort if they knew they were carrying a Down's baby (i.e., a 100 % risk) to determine if 50 % were truly their "point of indifference" or simply represented an anchoring effect.

This process of utility assessment is called the lottery technique and has been described elsewhere in this volume and in the literature. In effect, the patient is being asked to compare a certain hypothetical outcome (e.g., therapeutic abortion) to a gamble between two outcomes, one better and one worse. The probability of a good outcome of that gamble (e.g., carrying the pregnancy to term) is then varied in a systematic fashion until the patient is indifferent between the two choices, i.e., until both are equally burdensome. In that case, the utility of the intermediate outcome just balances the utility of the gamble (see Figure 2). At that point, the expected utility of the gamble can be calculated as the weighted average of the utilities of having an affected child and having an unaffected child.

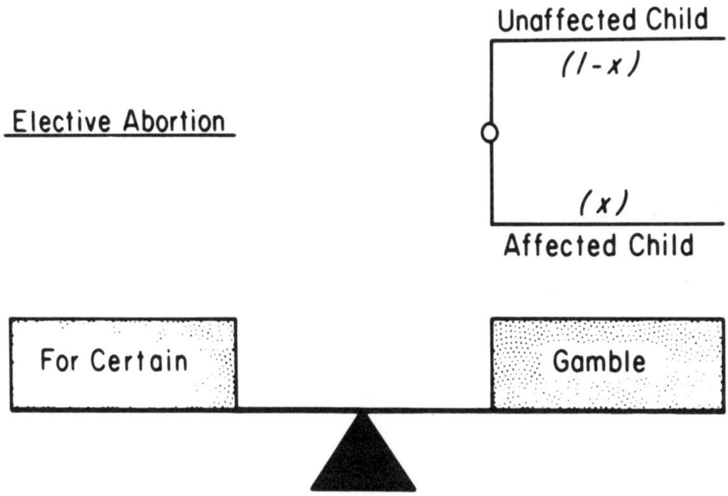

Figure 2: The balance representation of the lottery for therapeutic abortion. Reprinted from Pauker and Pauker (1979).

Providing advice

Initially we used a hand-held programmable computer to calculate the decision threshold for each patient or couple. Later, we developed a decision diagram (see Figure 3) which summarized the effect of maternal age on the risk of Down syndrome and the risk and potential errors associated with amniocentesis. Each patient could be placed on that diagram. If the point corresponding to maternal age and attitudes toward abortion fell above the sigmoid curve, then the analysis would demonstrate that amniocentesis would not be optimal. If the point fell below the curve, then amniocentesis would be recommended. If the age-utility pair fell within the grey zone, then the couples were advised that their attitudes did not support a clear cut choice.

The decision diagram and the plotted age-value pair was shared with the patient with an interpretation as to whether the values fell into the range of advising or not advising an amniocentesis. The phraseology for sharing the analysis with the patient was usually :

> "Using this decision analytic model, your own values, given your current risk, would indicate that an amniocentesis might

not be (might be) a wise choice for you at this time. The final choice is yours alone, although we will support you however you decide".

In the case of couples, utilities were derived individually and privately, if desired. If their values resulted in different recommendations, we suggested that they reconsider the risks and their values while they schedule an amniocentesis to reserve the option.

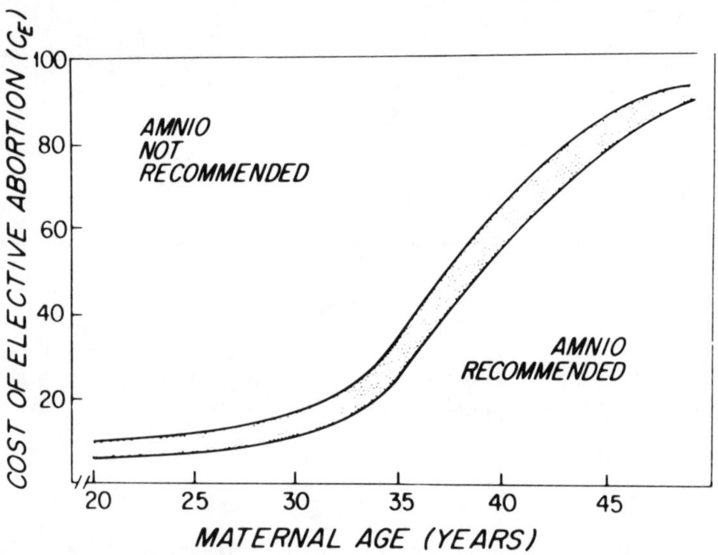

Figure 3: Decision diagram of the amniocentesis decision for Down Syndrome. Reprinted from Pauker and Pauker (1979).

When the result of the analysis was different from what the patients may have anticipated prior to the counseling, extra attention was given to repeating the information to be sure that comprehension was good.

Decision analysis usually added 10 minutes to the average 50 or 60 minutes counseling session. Occasionally, an additional counseling session was helpful to allow patients time to consider and reconsider their values.

RESULTS

Most of the patients who presented for genetic counseling were members of the Harvard Community Health Plan, the oldest and largest health maintenance organization in New England, which served a population of from 50,000 to 218,000 members during the time of the study. Patients tended to live in Eastern Massachusetts and most joined through their employers. Other patients were seen at the Genetics Clinic at Massachusetts General Hospital on referral from the New England States.

Many patients had already decided to have or not to have prenatal testing prior to the counseling session and decision analysis was not offered. Some patients wanted to discuss amniocentesis but absolutely could not consider abortion for any indication, due often to religious beliefs (usually Catholic and rarely Orthodox Jewish). Others were adamant that they would abort for almost any abnormality in a fetus and demanded amniocentesis regardless of indication.

Patients often said that the outcome of a pregnancy was "God's will", or "Nature's way" and were opposed to intervention, including testing.

Of the 849 patients for whom decision analysis was indicated, most were debating the use of amniocentesis for the mid-trimester diagnosis of chromosome abnormalities in advancing maternal age. Most presented as couples and were referred in the first trimester because the woman was age 35 years or over. Others were referred in the pregnancy-planning stage from primary care departments or were self-referred.

Responses of the patients to the utility assessment varied widely from patients who were emotionally totally unable to deal with their values explicitly to patients who were so pleased with the technique that they returned years later to reconsider their changed utilities with subsequent pregnancies. One couple called to request a repeat application of decision analysis, this time on whether or not to perform myringotomies on the child whose conception had been "too precious" to expose to amniocentesis.

To provide information about diversity of patient attitudes, we present in Table 1 a histogram of these values for both men and women. Recall that a utility of zero implies that the burden of elective abortion is negligible compared to the burden of an affected child and that a utility of one-hundred implies that the burden of an elective abortion is equal to that of having an affected child. In all cases, the disutility assigned to spontaneous abortion after amniocentesis was no greater than the disutility of elective abortion.

Table 1 : Distribution of utilities toward elective abortion

	0-9	10-19	20-29	30-39	40-49	50-59	60-69	70-79	80-89	90-99	100
Women	128	54	65	20	14	59	33	31	11	24	29
Men	141	55	35	15	9	39	17	22	3	19	26

ILLUSTRATIVE CASE EXAMPLES

The following case histories illustrate the range of patients facing the amniocentesis decision.

Case 1 : Prior infertility

Mrs. H.A. (Case #628929) was an 11 week pregnant, 38 year old architect married for 7 years to a 42 year old mathematician at the time of their counseling. After trying for 4 years to conceive, they had succeeded with clomiphene citrate. Since their miscarriage 3 years ago, a paternal cousin gave birth to a Down's child at age 40. Their own risk for having a Trisomy 21 baby at maternal age 39 at the time of delivery was 1/139.

Despite the preciousness of this pregnancy and the unwillingness of this couple to jeopardize a gestation conceived with so much difficulty, they worried about their ability to raise a Down's child while pursuing their active careers.

Utility assessment : They were indifferent between carrying the pregnancy to term and having an elective abortion when their chance of having a child with Down syndrome reached 30 %. Using the decision graph and plotting their burden of therapeutic abortion of 30 on the ordinate and their maternal age of 39 (at the projected delivery) on the abscissa, we were able to advise the potential parents that their values fell within the range where amniocentesis was indicated.

Follow-up : This couple proceeded with an uncomplicated amniocentesis which indicated a normal karyotype. They currently are parents to a fine normal son.

Case 2 : Previous child with Trisomy 21

At age 28, Miss D.U. (Case #453692) worked as a transcriptionist at the local state school for the retarded. By separate fathers she had had 3 miscarriages and a liveborn Trisomy 21 son who was 5 years old. At the time of counseling she was 15 weeks pregnant and faced a 1 % risk for Trisomy 21, although her age-related risk of Down syndrome would have been 0.1 %.

She related that her son's development had been quite good and that he "was a pleasure". His intelligence quotient was estimated at 80, but her exposure at work to more severely affected retarded children and adults had enhanced her anxiety about her recurrence risk. She had planned the current pregnancy which had taken only two months to conceive. She was uncertain about her feeling about elective abortion and the amniocentesis risks.

Utility assessment : The 27 year old father of the pregnancy was not present for the genetic counseling session and the patient did not try to estimate his values. In the process of using the lottery technique and encouraging her to be explicit about her own values, she was able to realize that even if Down syndrome were a virtual certainty in her current pregnancy, she probably would not undergo an elective abortion (utility = 100).

The patient was advised that amniocentesis was not recommended, given her values, even at her recurrence risk. She appeared comfortable with the conclusion of the analysis.

Case 3 : Previous normal child

With a 15 week gestation, Mrs. C.H. (Case #789456) was a 36 year old research psychologist married to a 42 year old economics professor. They had waited 10 months to conceive their second pregnancy. By the time of delivery, her Down syndrome risk would be 0.5 % for this pregnancy. Their 6 year old son was well, bright, and healthy.

These parents stated that they did not want an invasive procedure but they feared the effects of a Down syndrome sibling on their normal son.

Utility assessment : Following routine counseling, the patients requested decision analysis. Mrs. H. said she could not decide between an elective abortion and carrying the pregnancy to term at a risk of Down syndrome of 25 % (utility=25). Her husband's utility was 30, reflecting a slightly higher threshold level before amniocentesis would be indicated.

At Mrs. H's age, however, both utilities fell within the range that indicated the advisability of performing an amniocentesis. This conclusion was shared with the patients.

Case 4 : Professional hyperanxiety

Mrs. S.T. (Case #041282) is typical of many of the patients counselled in that, as a young professional in Boston, she was exposed to many couples in their early 30's who have chosen amniocentesis to detect and prevent as many birth defects as possible. At age 31, she was 13 weeks into her first pregnancy, which was planned with no delay in conception. A counsellor in a developmental evaluation unit, she had been married for 4 years to a 31 year old urban planner.

Although their family history for retardation was negative, Mrs. T. was exposed daily to many learning disabled children. These potential parents were not sure that they could perform an elective abortion, even for Down syndrome.

Although they usually felt facile in dealing with numbers, they were baffled as to how to go about comparing the relative risks of amniocentesis versus a major chromosomal defect when the probabilities were so low.

Utility assessment : Mrs. T. gave a utility of 5, while Mr. T. assessed his utility to be 10. Because Mrs. T. would be age 31 at delivery, it was apparent that an amniocentesis was indicated for them. They agreed that they would "feel better intellectually" if they did indeed have the test.

Case 5 : Perceived divergent attitudes :

Mrs. M.C. (Case #209748), a 34 year old artist, thought her attitudes about having an amniocentesis on her planned pregnancy which took two years to conceive would be very different from those of her 38 year old carpenter husband. He was sure he wanted to take the risk of the test to help assure a normal child. She had kidney stones as did her father, had grown adverse to medical intervention, and was uncertain as to whether she could undergo the test.

This couple assumed an irresolvable dilemma.

Utility assessment : Mr. C. could not choose between elective abortion and carrying the pregnancy to term at a 3 % risk of Down syndrome (utility = 3). When asked the lottery questions, Mrs. C. could fairly quickly and easily indicate that her utility was 5.

Plotting these values against a maternal age of 35 at delivery showed that both parents' utilities fell very securely into the range where amniocentesis was indicated.

Follow-up : These patients were surprised at how close their values actually were and were pleased to have been able to share their thoughts in each others' presence for the first time. They planned to schedule the amniocentesis.

Case 6 : Truly divergent attitudes

At age 39, Mrs. D.O. (Case #762007) had had 4 elective abortions according to the medical record, while her husband, age 42, had spent 11 years in jail. Reunited, they were in the 17th week of a pregnancy which Mr. O. very greatly desired.

A teacher with a family history positive for a developmentally delayed distant cousin, Mrs. O. was willing to have a child, but was thoroughly cognizant of her Down syndrome risk of 1 % by the time of her possible delivery. In her private thoughts, she had assumed having an amniocentesis on any future pregnancy. During the counseling session to which they had been sent by their obstetrician, Mrs. O. stated she was a primigravida.

When asked if they had considered an amniocentesis for the medical indication of advancing maternal age, Mr. O. adamantly stated that testing was "totally out of the question" since elective abortion was impossible "for them". He said he was desperately anxious to have this baby and that he would raise a Down's baby himself if that were the outcome. His wife appeared shocked and drained.

Utility assessment: To better define their positions, the lottery technique was applied. Confirming their diametrically opposed attitudes, Mr. O. gave a utility of an absolute 100 while Mrs. O. felt that a 0.1 % risk of Down syndrome was too high to carry to term (utility less than 0.1). The decision diagram was shared with them. They were advised to schedule a potential amniocentesis due to their advancing gestation, but to return after further private discussion since decision analysis could provide no resolution for them.

Follow-up: Shortly after, their obstetrician appeared saying that Mr. O had threatened her with her life if she performed an amniocentesis on his wife. Meanwhile, Mrs. O. scheduled an amniocentesis with a private physician. Reassured by the normal results which she shared only with her obstetrician, she continued the pregnancy through its normal outcome.

Case 7 : Values change over time

Mr. and Mrs. R.H. (Case #227057) sought genetic counseling about a planned pregnancy when Mr. H. was 27 and Mrs. H. was 28. Her family history was positive for a brother with severe meningomyelocele for whom she was legal guardian. This couple agreed that they desired all available prenatal diagnosis and both gave utilities of 10, indicating the point where they couldn't decide between having a baby with a neural tube defect and electively aborting. They were set to abort if a recurrence of this handicap were prenatally diagnosed.

Eight years later they returned for decision analysis. They were both now managers, one in business, one in medicine. They were enjoying their normal 7 year old twins and had lost their enthusiasm for prenatal diagnosis. Abortion now seemed a much heavier burden, especially since their current pregnancy took two years to conceive. They had begun to use decision analysis in their own work, recalled the model from the previous pregnancy, and requested the technique.

Utility assessment: In fact when we worked through the lottery questions and ascertained the values which they had thought had changed dramatically over time, they both gave revised utilities of 15, as the point of indecision for both neural tube defects and Down syndrome (for which they were now at increased risk). Although their values did indeed change, reflecting the preciousness of this pregnancy and their normal daughters, the change from 10 to 15 is very slight, on a scale of 0 to 100.

Follow-up: The couple proceeded with an amniocentesis. The alpha-fetoprotein and ultrasound were within normal limits and the karyotype and newborn son were normal.

Case 8 : Language difficulties

Mrs. J.G. (Case #152292) was 34 years old when she presented for genetic counseling. She had heard about the availability of prenatal diagnosis for the birth defects she feared, associated with her advancing maternal age. Although Spanish was her native language, she spoke English very well and brought her Boston-born sister to the counseling session to assist in interpretation. They could repeat the given Down syndrome risk of 1/365 at the time of delivery and the given test risks.

Utility assessment : The father of the pregnancy was not involved in decision making. Mrs. G. felt comfortable taking a 50 % risk of carrying a Down syndrome baby to term but at a 90 % risk, she would electively abort. At a 75 % risk (utility=75) she was at the point of indifference. She and her sister agreed that this value represented Mrs. G.'s feelings.

Due to her strict Catholic upbringing and her strong belief that "God will protect me" from an abnormal outcome, she said she felt completely comfortable with the advice based on her own values that an amniocentesis was not indicated for her at that time.

Follow-up : Mrs. G. carried the pregnancy to term without testing and delivered an otherwise healthy daughter with Trisomy 21. Initially, she refused to nurse the baby, bewailed not having had testing, raising the obvious question of whether she had understood the counseling. She was incredulous that this undesired fate had befallen her, despite her faith.

By the time of her next genetics appointment 2 weeks later, she was successfully nursing the baby. She said that she now felt that she had made the right decision about testing given her feelings at that time, but that she truly had believed that "such a thing could never happen to me".

Mrs. G. did not have amniocentesis on her next pregnancy, despite her 1 % recurrence risk, and gave birth to a normal son.

Case 9 : "Too hypothetical"

Mrs. C.O. (Case #1240086) was 38 years old and 12 weeks pregnant when she stated that she "would readily abort a defective fetus". Her husband was age 51, and both prospective parents were writers. Family history was positive for congenital hydrocephaly in four paternal aunts and uncles. This pregnancy had taken longer than they had planned to conceive; 18 months had passed since they had stopped birth control.

They were certain that they wanted maternal serum alpha-fetoprotein testing and ultrasound to rule-out hydrocephaly for which they might have been at a slightly increased risk, but they were undecided about amniocentesis as an invasive procedure. Decision analysis was offered.

Utility assessment : Although they began to participate in the derivation of their utilities via the lottery technique, they broke off sharply saying the questions were "too hypothetical". They said they would electively abort only if the fetus were known to be affected and they refused to accept the possibility of a false positive or negative report.

They became angry at being asked to consider probabilities and the session was terminated.

Follow-up : They chose to have an amniocentesis which showed 46,XX plus a small satellite which was felt to be insignificant. Their daughter was speech delayed at age 3 but was otherwise well with no evidence of hydrocephaly.

Case 10 : Counter-intuitive utilities

Mr. and Mrs. B.R. (Case #889539) were both 35 years old when they conceived their second pregnancy after 3 years of trying. Their normal 5 year old was well known to the genetic counsellor (SPP) who had advised them on the first pregnancy and was the pediatrician for their daughter.

This was a particularly precious pregnancy for the parents who wanted a second child, were not anxious to take the amniocentesis risk, but did not want a Down's child, for which their current risk was 1/365.

Mrs. R., a lawyer, and Mr. R., a hospital administrator, both worked fulltime, but enjoyed sharing in the responsibilities of raising their bright daughter.

Utility assessment : Both parents felt they would continue to carry a baby to term rather than electively abort until the Down's risk was raised to 90 %, at which point they were undecided (utility = 90). The questions were rephrased and the answers were consistent.

Although their utilities and maternal age would place them in the "no amniocentesis" category, this was counter-intuitive to the patients who felt that they had been inclined to have an amniocentesis, despite their aversion to the invasive risk. It was also counter-intuitive to the clinician who felt that they had underestimated the impact of a potential Down's child on both their demanding daughter and on their complex life-style.

The advice was given that the patients reconsider their values and meet with a resource person from the local retarded citizens' group in order to be better informed by actual parents of Down syndrome children as to their experiences and reactions.

Follow-up : This couple opted to avail themselves of amniocentesis after further consideration. The results and their son were normal.

DISCUSSION

It has been our experience that decision analysis has been readily applicable for a wide variety of patients who are candidates for prenatal diagnosis. Using a formal logical model, the technique allows the patients' values to be incorporated into their decision making.

It is important to present outcome risks in both a positive and a negative frame to allow more neutral decision making. For example, saying that a patient has a 3 % chance of having a Down syndrome newborn at maternal age 45 gives a different message to the prospective parents than the converse risk of 97 % that the child will not have Down syndrome. We routinely phrase the risks both ways to minimize the effect of framing on the patients' attitudes.

Assets of the technique

By encouraging patients to be individually explicit about their attitudes toward specific pregnancy outcomes, this decision analytic technique allows some patients to confront their own values for the first time.

It also allows partners to share their values openly, often for the first time. Some couples who thought that they were far apart on their views were surprised to appreciate that their differences were not significant in terms of their final decision. Other couples whose attitudes were far apart often profited from more information about the potential significance of having an affected child. A patient strongly and vocally opposed to abortion who had chosen not to have prenatal testing for neural tube defects despite her husband's wishes and a positive family history was sorry that she had not known more about the required intensity of caring for her newborn spina bifida baby before she set her decision.

Although pregnancy is an emotionally-charged time for many parents, this technique provides a clear logical visual framework for a complex, high-impact, far-reaching decision. Emphasizing the importance of the patient's own values in this process helps the patient to tune out irrelevant input to the decision, e.g., the neighbor's opinion or the experience of a friend.

Application of this formal technique provides documentation in the medical record of the elements of the decision support provided.

Patients who recall the decision analytic process after the time of delivery relate the value of the technique and may return for other significant medical decisions. Patients can refer to their explicitly derived values after the pregnancy in future counseling sessions.

Problems with the technique

The additional questions and explanation of the decision tree and graph add approximately 10 minutes to a routine prenatal diagnosis counseling session. Furthermore, second sessions are occasionally required to be certain that all elements of the counseling have been understood with time for patients' questions and reactions.

Sometimes patients' sense of anxiety is raised when they are encouraged to examine their values about elective abortion and the possible impact of a baby who is not perfect. This can be allayed by explaining that there is comfort in reaching a well-considered decision and this technique can help. Some patients become acutely distressed at the difference between their partner's values and their own. This is a good time to suggest mental health couples' therapy so that they can resolve their feelings prior to the birth or termination.

For many patients, the process of determining their values is the first time that they have confronted their increased risk of the problem, such as having a brother with hemophilia or translocation Down syndrome. The recurrence risk figures take on a new and intense meaning when the patient begins to respond to the lottery questions. Reactions may be strong and need to be anticipated.

When patients become fatigued at the effort to narrow the utility range, the counsellor must be sensitive and try to establish where the utilities fall relative to the threshold of the decision quickly. One can then go back and test the conclusion by rephrasing the question, using the inverse risks.

Some patients refuse to deal with numbers or probability figures. Sometimes it helps to relate the odds to gambling situations or other circumstances with which the patient is more familiar or comfortable. Sometimes all efforts fail, and the technique is simply not applicable to that patient or couple.

CONCLUSIONS

This study has demonstrated the feasibility of deriving individual patients' attitudes and incorporating them into individually-tailored analyses based on current risk. The technique appears to enhance communication between the geneticist and the patient and allows patients to understand their own attitudes better.

Acknowledgement

The authors happily acknowledge Juli Horwitz, M.S., Genetic Associate, who was the next to routinely incorporate this technique into her counseling, and their children, who inspired the model and tolerated their absence during its development.

REFERENCES

Beeson, D. and Golbus, M.S.
Anxiety engendered by amniocentesis.
in : Risk, Communication, and Decision Making in Genetic Counseling (Epstein, C.J., Curry, C.J.R., Packman, S., Sherman, S., Hall, B.D., eds), Part C of Ann Review of Birth Defects, 1978. National Foundation-March of Dimes. Birth Defects Original Article Series XV:5C, Alan R. Liss (New York), pp 191-197, 1979.

Evers-Kiebooms, G., Fryns, J.P. and Van den Berghe, H.
Prenatal diagnosis and genetic counseling in 21 trisomy : impact on family planning.
J. Génét. Hum. 28, 147-159, 1980.

Grobstein, R.
Amniocentesis counseling.
in : Genetic Counseling : Psychological Dimensions (Kessler S, ed), Academic Press (New York), pp107-113, 1979.

McNeil, B.J., Pauker, S.G., Sox, H. and Tversky, A.
On the elicitation of patient preferences for alternative therapies.
New Engl. J. Med. 306, 1259-1262, 1982.

Murphy, E.A. and Chase, G.A.
Principles of Genetic Counseling.
Yearbook (Chicago), 1975.

Pauker, S.P. and Pauker, S.G.
Prenatal diagnosis : a directive approach to genetic counseling using decision analysis.
Yale J. Biol. Med. 50, 275-289, 1977.

Pauker, S.P. and Pauker, S.G.
The amniocentesis decision : an explicit guide for parents.
in : Risk, Communication, and Decision Making in Genetic Counseling (Epstein, C.J., Curry, C.J.R., Packman, S., Sherman, S., Hall, B.D., eds), Part C of Ann review of Birth Defects, 1978. National Foundation-March of

Dimes. Birth Defects Original Article Series XV:5C, Alan R. Liss (New York), pp289-324, 1979.

Pauker, S.G., Pauker, S.P. and McNeil, B.J.
Implications of prospective parents' attitudes on alternative policies regarding prenatal diagnosis.
in : Critical Issues in Medical Technology (McNeil, B.J., Cravalho, E.G., eds), Auburn House (Cambridge, Mass), pp343-357, 1982.

Pauker, S.G., Pauker, S.P. and McNeil, B.J.
The effect of private attitudes on public policy : prenatal screening for neural tube defects as prototype.
Medical Decision Making 1, 103-114, 1981.

Pauker, S.P.
Prenatal genetic diagnosis by amniocentesis : The human problem.
in : Critical Issues in Medical Technology (McNeil, B.J., Cravalho, E.G., eds), Auburn House (Cambridge, Mass), pp317-324, 1982.

Pearn, J.H.
Decision-making and reproductive choice.
in : Counseling in Genetics. (Hsia, Y.E., Hirschhorn, K., Silverberg, R., Godmilow, L., eds) : Alan R. Liss (New York), pp223-228, 1977.

RISK ASSESSMENT, RISK PERCEPTION AND DECISION MAKING ABOUT COURSES OF ACTION INVOLVING GENETIC RISK : AN OVERVIEW OF CONCEPTS AND METHODS

Charles VLEK

Department of Psychology, University of Groningen, Institute for Social and Organisational Psychology, 9718 JP Groningen, The Netherlands.

Abstract

Developments in medical diagnostics and shifts in the ethics of human reproduction increasingly present prospective parents with deliberate choice problems involving possible child deficiencies. An adequate handling of such problems may be supported by explicit methodologies for judging risks and making decisions under uncertainty. The paper gives an overview of concepts, models and methods concerning risk analysis, risk perception and "good" decision making. Several different (stimulus) definitions of risk are presented, and it is shown that "perceived risk" (a response-defined concept) may be operationally measured at different levels of an organism's activity. Disputes on the meaning of probability statements are related to differences in the available information basis which may result from a combination of frequentistic/nonfrequentistic data about, and external/internal determination of possible consequences. After a listing of various notions of "acceptable risk", three different approaches towards making good decisions are discussed. The paper concludes with a summary and some suggestions for the improvement of genetic counseling procedures.

"Vater werden ist nicht schwer,
Vater sein dagegen sehr."
(a German saying).

1. Introduction

For more than one reason, it is difficult to be a prospective parent these

Birth Defects: Original Article Series, Volume 23, Number 2, pages 171–207

days. For some mothers, perhaps the German saying quoted above should be reversed : once you have got a healthy baby, it is not so difficult to be a mother; to become one, however, may require an extensive process of judgment and decision making which may take away the fun of just trying and seeing what comes of it. The developments in medical diagnostic technology and gradual shifts in the ethics of human reproduction are important factors in pushing people towards ever deeper and more-encompassing problem explorations, consequence assessments and value weightings. With it comes a rational-analytic way of decision making which radically differs from the emotional-affective style in which most people have to, and perhaps like to make decisions whose outcomes are personally important to them.

The paper offers a survey of risk assessment, risk perception and decision making under uncertainty in relation to problems involving genetic risks. As you may expect, "risk" will be treated as a psychological concept, not a statistical one. Its underlying components are the uncertainty and the displeasure associated to possible unwanted consequences. The paper is organized in three parts. First, we will consider some essential concepts and methods of risk assessment. Secondly, we will look into the concept of perceived risk and pay some attention to its underlying factors. Third, we will distinguish different kinds of uncertainty associated to specific data bases for probability estimation. Fourth, we will list various different notions of "acceptable risk". And fifth, we will examine rational-analytic as well as psychological perspectives on decision making under uncertainty, and ask ourselves : in what way, or ways, could one arrive at "good decisions"? The paper concludes with a summary and a number of further suggestions.

2. The objectifying assessment of risk

Genetic risk analysis and estimation may be considered to meet with similar conceptual and methodological problems as the assessment of technological risks from industrial activities. Let us, therefore, briefly look into the way risk analysis is defined and what it looks like in connection with problems of industrial safety.

Risk analysis as an engineering discipline developed during the 1970's. It is now an established, although not unambiguous, methodology for the identification and estimation of risks from complex technical systems or processes. In the industrialized countries, almost no large scale technical facility is sited without an accompanying risk analysis. The latter is aimed at spotting hazardous components, suggesting specific measures for increasing safety, and giving quantitative estimates of so-called residual risks that have to be evaluated for their acceptability. Table 1 lists the steps in current risk analysis and reveals that identification, structuring and quantification are the main points of interest.

Table 1 : Steps in technical risk analysis.

I. Identification of possible unwanted events :
- process safety analysis (determining process parameters and safety margins);
- failure mode and effect analysis ("What may go wrong where, with which effect?");
- drawing of event trees, fault trees (structuring events that may follow from a basic initial event, or modeling of possible faults that logically combine into a total system failure).

II. Quantification of consequences and effects of identified unwanted events :
- analysis of damage and effects (e.g., through pressure or vapor cloud dispersion models);
- (evaluation of identified accident effects not emphasized).

III. Quantification of probabilities of unwanted events :
- through use of data banks yielding recorded accident statistics;
- through applying probability combination rules to elements and paths in fault tree;
- through expert (personal) judgment of probabilities of either elementary or compound events.

Risk analysis is customarily used as a policy instrument to explain that the (residual) risks of a carefully designed technical system are extremely small, and that they may be further reduced at certain costs. It is left up to the politicians to weigh these risks against the associated benefits of the project in order to decide whether or not the risks are acceptably low, or at what costs they should, if possible, be further reduced.

Risk analysts used to carry a strong pretense of being able to objectively assess technical risks, as if these were something that existed in reality and could be measured if one used the proper instruments. Increasingly, however, the conceptual basis of risk analysis as a quantitative instrument has come under heavy fire from probability and decision theorists.

Some difficulties with the methodology relate to the impossibility to pay attention to every possible way in which improbable elementary events may combine into an almost but not entirely impossible catastrophe that one wishes to avoid at all costs. Most serious accidents are the result of unfortunated coincidences that few people believed could ever occur. Many of the "technically excluded" ways of letting things go wrong reside in the human operator of a system, who regularly proves to be a rich source of failure probabilities. This contributes to making a valid assessment of accident probabilities highly problematic.

In addition to this it appeared that the evaluation, not the quantitative description, of accidents and their effects poses socio-cultural questions which are no engineer's special responsibility to answer. What is the value of one life lost as compared to the value of 10 people partially handicapped for the rest of their lives? How should immediate, direct harm to the surrounding population be weighted against long-term, creeping health effects that may cause numerous unknown victims in a much larger area?

These and other issues and questions allow us to list a number of shortcomings of both the conceptional framework and the methodology of risk analysis. First of all, the definition of risk is unclear and tends to become more encompassing and less quantitative over the years. One traditional definition of risk is the probability of a negatively valued event. This and other quantitative definitions are given in table 2.

Table 2 : Alternative definitions of risk

1. The probability of a negatively valued event;
2. The product of the probability and the size of a possible loss;
3. The size, or the seriousness, of a possible loss or accident;
4. The variance, or the probability-weighted dispersion of all possible consequences of an activity;
5. The set of points obtained when the probabilities of various possible negative consequences are plotted against the size or seriousness of their effects.

Originally, these and other statistical definitions of risk are stimulus definitions, i.e., they indicate and combine parameters of the external environment so as to quantify the situation's potential for realizing an unwanted event. Risk exists "out there"; it is a measurable quantity; it may be reduced by safety measures; and it can be controlled. These are key phrases often used by adherents of any one stimulus definition of risk. We shall see below (section 3) that response definitions come into play when we consider risk from the standpoint of the beholder. There the emphasis lies on the way a risky activity or situation is represented in the perceiver's mind or behavior.

The second weakness of risk analysis revolves around the possibilities and uses of the probability concept. Formally speaking, probability is an "empty" mathematical concept referring to a number between 0 (representing impossibility) and 1 ("necessity") which has to fulfil certain axioms (like : the probabilities of the elements of a mutually exclusive and exhaustive set of events have to sum to 1). For practical use, however, probability needs an interpretation. Across the past few centuries three interpretations have developed : the frequentistic, the personalistic and the logical points of view.

Traditional risk analysis is mostly connected to the frequentistic interpretation of probability as the limit of a relative frequency of a stochastic event under substantially similar conditions. Practical use of the frequentistic probability concept requires unambiguous definitions of the critical event under consideration, and of the occasions at which it might or might not occur. It also requires that you make a sufficient number of repetitive observations of occasions and critical event occurrences. And, of course, an observed relative frequency cannot be transformed into a probability assigned to a future critical event if one cannot assume the observation conditions to remain essentially the same. These requirements cause the frequentistic probability concept, despites its being the statisticians's ideal, to be of rather limited value in situations which are relatively new or unique.

For perfectly unique probability situations, like the possibility of Prime Minister Margaret Thatcher agreeing to the establishment of economic sanctions against South-Africa (we write July, 1986), one would have to rely on personal (or subjective) probability judgment, which may of course be more or less valid. Expert probability judgment may rely on scenarios the assessor has been able to construct, and which to him or her may give an impression of high probability the more plausible and consistent they look. Clearly enough, personal judgment of probabilities is a basically intractable process the result of which is hard to validate at the time it is made (see Kahneman et al., 1982 for an overview of emperical research).

Complex, unfamiliar systems or processes may often be decomposed into a number of reasonably familiar elementary events. When this is so, one may compose an overall unique system-failure probability from elementary probabilities that could be assessed on either a frequentistic or a personalistic basis. For example, a group of engineers may assemble a collection of valid probability assessments concerning, e.g., pipe leakages, valve ruptures and small operator errors, which may be aggregated into an overall system-failure probability along the lines provided by an appropriate fault tree modeling of the system. This third way of using the probability concept falls under the logical interpretation of probability. An "honest" chance apparatus such as a fair coin or a die would offer opportunities for simple applications.

The frequentistic, personal, and logical interpretations of probability all have their own methodological strengths and weaknesses. The frequentistic interpretation seems the most "objective", but, alas, the conditions required for its valid use are only rarely met in practice. The personalistic interpretation may sound the most honest, but, alas, personal probability assessments are difficult to validate. And the quality of "logical" probability assessments very much depends upon (1) the validity of the fault tree structure used to model the system, and (2) the validity of the elementary probabilities which it is meant to aggregate.

The third problem with risk analysis concerns the assessment of the size and seriousness of possible accidents and their effects. The standard conceptualization of a large-scale accident is in terms of fatalities, number of people wounded and material damage to property and the environment. However, a large-scale accident may have both short and long term effects; it may cause damage and discomfort in the vicinity but also at a more remote distance of the accident site. Loss of life, limb or property may be accompanied by individual emotional suffering as well as by societal disruption and long term losses to the economy. In a somewhat different vein, such considerations also apply to accidents in someone's personal life. What seems to be required is a relatively sophisticated model of what it means to be the victim, either individually or collectively, of an accident, and how its meaning is to be assessed and evaluated.

In sum, due to inherent shortcoming in its operational basis, risk analysis as an objectifying methodology can only be a limited instrument to be used for decision under uncertainty : (1) it remains unclear how the concept of risk could be best defined; (2) the essential notion of probability has a variable interpretation, depending upon the quality of available data and the conditions under which the assessment is to be made, and (3) the personal and/or social significance of a serious accident is not easily modeled and evaluated. These conclusions seem to imply that at least for complex decision situations the "objective" assessment of risks is virtually impossible, so that any risk analysis report is doomed to be the subject of personal scepticism and scientific critique.

Despite these shortcomings one may keep thinking that risk analysis is the only rational framework available for the identification and assessment of risks. If so, one might formulate some conclusions and recommendations for the assessment of genetic risks.

(1) Try to be a good book-keeper : as much as possible attempt to identify and define causes of actual and of possible genetic deficits and record how they develop and what their ultimate outcomes are; this may be of help in making frequentistic probability estimates.

(2) Try to be a genetic system expert who knows how mechanisms and processes work that may bring about genetic disorders; this may help you formulate logical rules for the assessment or calculation of deficit probabilities.

(3) Try to become a fair assessor of personal probabilities in case you have got too little data to go by. It appears difficult to be coherent; it has also appeared to be difficult to assess probabilities independently from the value attached to the event under consideration. The use of explicit methods seems therefore advisable.

(4) Modern engineers are wise enough to define "risk" as some function of the probabilities and sizes of possible accidents, associated with a course of action. For genetic counselors this would mean that they communicate probability assessments as well as descriptions of the personal and social significance of genetic deficits, and to leave evaluative judgments and, of course, accept-reject decisions to the people who are most involved.

3. The subjective judgment of risk

On first sight it might seem as if "perceived risk" simply is the subjective counterpart of the "objective risk" assessed by statistical engineers (or by geneticists for that matter). This is only true, however, to the extent that the possible event considered, the data base for probability assessment and the model for evaluation seriousness of effects are basically similar. A (somewhat artificial) example from the casino would be the risk of losing your stakes when taking a one-shot bet at the first six numbers of a roulette wheel. Here you know exactly how the critical event and the opportunity for it to occur are defined; you might calculate - though not believe - the probability of losing; and the possible loss is evaluated in terms of socio-economic standard : money.

In what ways might your perceived risk differ from the statistically calculated risk? To begin answering this question we should be aware of the fact that perceived risk may be considered at several different levels of psychological measurement (Vlek and Stallen, 1980), see table 3.

Table 3 : Operational levels for measuring perceived risk

1. Physiological : "arousal" or anxiety as expressed in autonomic nervous system activities (glandular secretions, heart beat interval regularity, electrodermal responding);
2. Behavioral : autokinetic patterns interpretable as : adopting a defensive strategy, being frightened (e.g., screaming), turning or fleeing away from the risky situation; denying the risk and getting apathetic;
3. Cognitive : verbalized descriptions of and/or attitudes towards critical event or activity; evaluative comparisons of alternative courses of action; judgmental consequence assessments, etc.

In fact table 3 is underlying of attempts to formulate response definitions of risk, i.e., definitions covering what happens in the human reaction to situations having a potential for generating unwanted events. One such definition, for example, could be in terms of increased irregularity of heart beating, a general sign of emotional stress. Or one could measure perceived riskiness in terms of the effort with which the subject moves away from the threatening situation. And a third possibility would be to define risk as the subjective image of a serious loss or accident.

The importance of distinguishing several different levels at which perceived risk could be defined and measured is that one may gradually learn what stimulus risk "does" to people in terms of psychological response patterns. This eventually may lead to a third type of risk definition, a transactional definition, which delineates the process by which situational risk characteristics and psychological response patterns are interconnected. If well elaborated, a transactional definition of risk would come close to a psychological theory of risk judgment and risk taking. This might be of great help in bridging the communication gap between technical risk analysts and non-technical "risk perceivers".

A conceptual communication gap may also exist between the genetic counselor (a "technical" risk analyst) and his or her non-expert client. The bridge to be built should in fact connect the stimulus and response definitions, respectively, which seem to underly the views and attitudes of either party. It does not seem to make sense to address clients in terms of deficit probabilities when they themselves mainly think in terms of how they could cope with the possible burden.

Looking once more at table 3, an obvious conclusion may be that perceived risk is a multi-faceted concept which is more appropriately measured in terms of an individual's response pattern than in terms of a single variable. This is already true when we try to capture perceived risk at the level of cognitive-verbal representations. As it is problematic to let subjects experience and react to actual risks in a controlled laboratory setting, cognitive-verbal measurements have been used most frequently. Let us consider a few "cognitive" studies and their results.

Payne (1975) had subjects evaluate the riskiness of well defined experimental gambles, and found that when probabilities and sizes of possible loss are well specified, perceived risk is primarily associated to the probability of any loss. But gambling risk appeared to depend on other variables as well. Somewhat desperately, after an extensive laboratory study, Coombs, Donnell and Kirk (1977) conclude that "the several good and bad aspects of lotteries other than expected value are cognitively composed into a one-dimensional variable that mediates preferential choice conditional on expected value. We call this variable risk."

Slovic, Fischhoff and Lichtenstein (1982, 1984) undertook various psychometric studies of perceived riskiness. Their subjects were basically asked to rate a large number of activities, or technologies, with respect to a set of explicit risk characteristics such as, e.g., familiarity of consequences, potential lethality of effects, and voluntariness of exposure. A factor analysis performed on the ratings revealed that three factors were sufficient to explain the observed variance in the subjects' ratings. Factor I was interpreted to be the "catastrophic (or "dread") potential" of an activity. Factor II was labelled "unfamiliarity" or "unknown risk", while factor III could be called "number of people simultaneously exposed". The validity of these factors, of course, depends upon the larger set of risk characteristics used, and upon the collection of activities judged by subjects.

Vlek and Stallen (1981) followed a different strategy in asking many subjects to compare and rank order a set of 26 risky activities - ranging from "storing LPG (liquefied petroleum gas) near petrol stations in cities" and "operating a nuclear power station" to "receiving full anaesthesia before a medical operation" and "riding on a moped in city traffic" - with respect to the "seriousness of their risks and dangers" (disregarding associated benefits). The rank ordering differences among subjects were analyzed using a multidimensional scaling technique. The latter revealed that two dimensions could explain the variety of riskiness orderings. The primary dimension was interpreted to reflect the "size of a potential accident", while the secondary dimension was labelled "degree of organized safety". Interestingly enough, subjects appeared to be quite in agreement in their ordering of the 26 activities following the "size of a potential accident", with "storing LPG at a petrol station" and "operating a nuclear power station" receiving high scores and "receiving full anaesthesia" and "riding on a moped" obtaining low scores. With respect to "organized safety" however, about half of the subjects appeared to associate higher risk with <u>de</u>creased organized safety (so that, e.g., "drunken driving" was judged very risky), whereas the other half saw riskiness increase with <u>in</u>creased organized safety (so that "storing LPG" received a high riskiness rank). Figure 1 presents the full two-dimensional configuration of the 26 activities.

Note that only in the laboratory studies based on well defined gambles did probability of loss come out as a significant variable underlying perceived risk. In the psychometric field studies of Slovic et al. (1984) and Vlek and Stallen (1981) probability of accident turned out to be a subordinate variable. This obviously has to do with the fact that accident probabilities are very hard to come by when one is dealing with realistic risks. In genetic counseling studies, too, it appears that clients are very bad in probabilistic reasoning and find it hard to understand quantitative risk estimates (Leonard, Chase and Childs, 1972; Lippman-Hand and Fraser,

1979; Tijmstra and Huisjes, 1983; Evers-Kiebooms, Vlietinck, Fryns and Van den Berghe, 1984). One explanation is that clients certainly do not think in terms of the data-base and computational formulae used by genetic risk analysts. Another explanation is that, if they did, they would probably find it hard to accept the underlying assumptions and, thus, the resulting risk figures. It is hard to communicate a genetic deficit probability whose validity is already doubted by the communicators, and whose meaning is the subject of a scientific controversy.

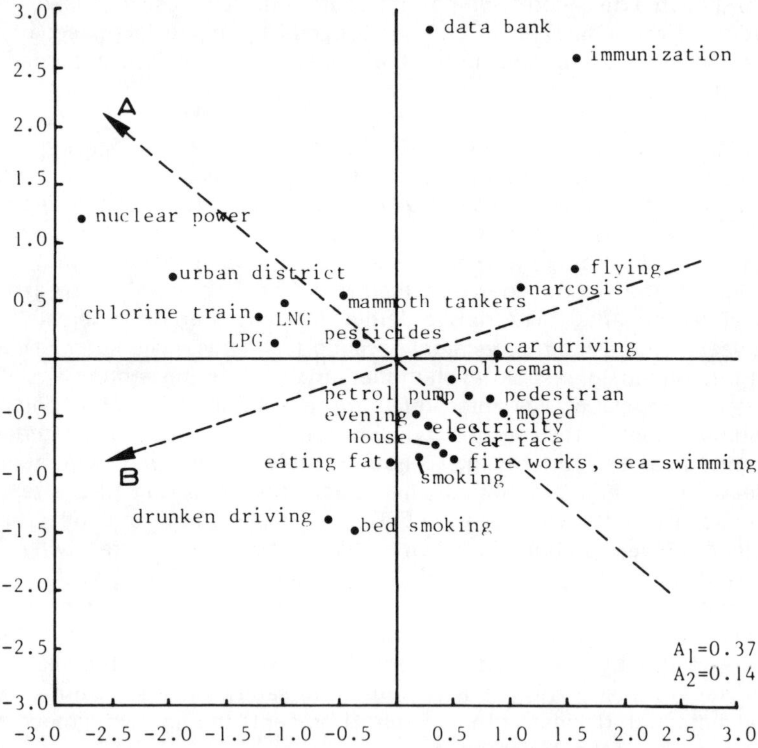

Figure 1 : Two-dimensional configuration of 26 briefly described activities following "seriousness of their risks and dangers", as individually rank ordered by about 450 respondents. From right to left activities were interpreted to increase in "the size of a potential accident"; from bottom to top they were supposed to increase in "degree of organized safety". Lambda 1 and 2 in the bottom-right corner represent the eigen-values of the computed "solution". The dashed arrows labelled A and B represent typical respondents conceiving "riskiness" to be a function of increasing "size of a potential accident" and increasing (A) or decreasing (B) "degree of organized safety", respectively. Source : Vlek and Stallen (1981).

In a summary chapter Kuyper and Vlek (1984) conclude that a major conclusion of this work is that perceived risk is a multidimensional or a multiattributed concept, whose basic dimensions may be differently weighted by different persons. For the variety of industrial or technological activities judged by experimental subjects in recent studies at least five factors appear to be strongly associated to variations in perceived riskiness; notoriously absent among them is the probability of a serious loss or accident (whose place seems to be taken by the controlability variable). The five factors are given in table 4.

Table 4 : Five major factors underlying perceived risk.

1. Potential degree of harm or lethality
2. Controlability through safety and/or rescue measures
3. Number of people simultaneously exposed
4. Familiarity of consequences and effects
5. Degree of voluntariness of exposure

These and other, more physical risk dimensions (see, e.g., Hohenemser, Kates and Slovic, 1983) may be fruitfully used to classify risky activities or situations into basically different categories. The advantage of this would be that for each category of risks one may specify a proper way to deal with the problems posed by that category. For example, one may select particular methods for assessing and representing the risk; specific safety recommendations may be formulated; and an optimal method for evaluating and deciding upon the activity's acceptability may be found. By implication, a particular approach to a risk problem may work well for one category of risks, but it may fail for another category.

I know of no studies aimed at uncovering psychological or physical dimensions of <u>genetic</u> risks. Undertaking these would seem potentially fruitful. It could increase our understanding of the essential difficulties of particular genetic risk problems. And it could help us specify the optimal approach to decide upon them. Comparative thinking about risks (e.g., the risk of dying from cancer compared to the risk of a road accident, or the risk of delivering a child suffering from Down's syndrome as against the added iatrogenic risk of a spontaneous abortion after amniocentesis; see Tijmstra, Huisjes and Ten Kate, 1982; Pauker and Pauker, this volume), is tempting more often than it is logically meaningful. A general rule is that risks should only be compared when they are part of one and the same decision problem (as in the second example just mentioned). A good system for characterizing different risks may help genetic decision makers realize when it makes sense to compare risks and how this could best be done.

In a more fundamental way, the cognitive-psychometric research on perceived risk just discussed may not help us that much in the long run. For indeed, this research is rather atheoretical and it does not, therefore, increase our insight into the psychological processess of judging risks and deciding to take or to reject them. Fortunately, there is some psychological theorizing about how people come to appraise a threatening situation and how they might react to it. Remarkably, the abstract concept of risk plays "low profile" in these models.

The general line of thinking is (see, e.g., Coyne and Lazarus, 1980; Stallen and Thomas, 1985) that a situation, or task environment, may be perceived as threatening, and thus cause stress, to the extent that the functional demands put upon the subject by that situation exceed the subject's abilities to cope with it. Both the functional demands and the person's own abilities are subjectively assessed. Perceived risk, and the resulting stress, are a function of the perceived discrepancies between assessed task demands and subject capabilities. Thus a subject may perceive a difficult examination, or a critical job interview, or a troublesome pregnancy as something hardly manageable and therefore failure-prone, if the subject's coping abilities are judged to be below the required levels. Conversely, these same situations may be experienced as challenging if the subject assessed his or her coping abilities to be (just) above the appraised demands. Figure 2 gives a schematic representation of this model.

The experience of successes and failures add a dynamic character to this model of "coping with risk", success increasing one's feeling of being able to cope with similar risks, while failure obviously reduces one's self-appraisal. Too much success may make a person overconfident and risk-seeking (if only for the sensation of it). Too many failures may gradually turn one into a helpless personality.

In the context of the model two essential components for genetic counseling would seem to be the following. First, the client should be provided with an expert assessment of the future demands that may be put upon her or him if a particular course of action would be selected or allowed to continue. Numerical probability estimates would not likely to be playing a major part in this, although uncertainty would. Secondly, the client should try, and perhaps may be helped, to assess her or his (expected) abilities to deal with the likely consequences of the course of action under consideration. Comparisons among alternative courses of action should be made in similar terms, one course of action being judged as more demanding and less well to cope with than another.

Admittedly, "demand appraisal" and "assessment of coping abilities" are not purely factual tasks; they also involve motivational components. Demands also seem to depend upon what one aspires to make of a situation. Ability to cope also depends upon one's willingness to invest energy and be creative. Such considerations, however, still seem to be far remote from the purely decision-analytic approach of putting the assessed costs, risks and benefits in a pan balance and comparing alternative courses of action with regard to the scales' position.

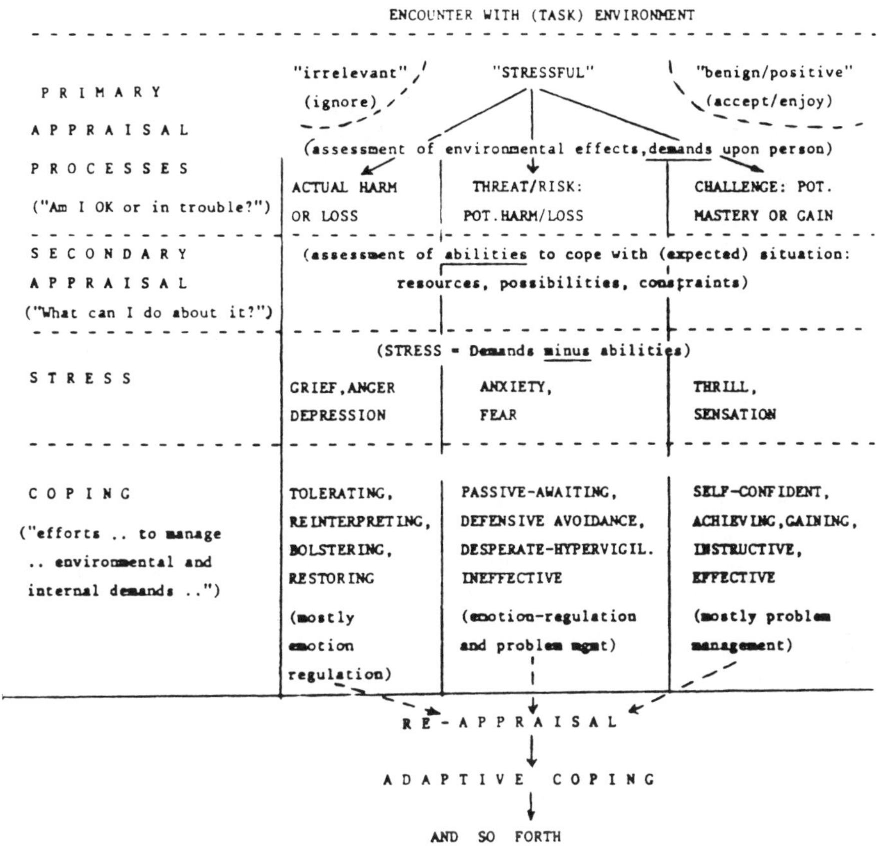

Figure 2 : Transactional model of risk appraisal and coping

There is a final psychological model of risk taking that is worth considering here. In Janis and Mann's (1977) model of emergency decision making it is assumed that more often than not human decision makers are under the stress of problem difficulty, shortage of time, lack of information, social pressure, and the like. These conditions do not allow one to decide in a fully rational manner. Rational decision making is defined by Janis and Mann in terms of seven different criteria which amount to the classical idea of knowing your options, exploring all relevant consequences, being aware of the essential value attributes, adequately processing new information, etc. (see, e.g., Braybrooke and Lindblom, 1970, chapter 3).

According to Janis and Mann's model (see figure 3) a person confronted with a risky situation implicitly poses four successive questions : (1) Are the risks unacceptably high when I don't shift to another course of action? (2) If so, are the risks still unacceptably high when I do take another, available course of action? (3) If so, is there any hope of finding an acceptable course of action? (4) If so, will there be enough time to explore and evaluate the acceptable course of action? Depending upon the sequence of answers to these questions the subject may develop a particular state of stress. Resulting stress states are defined in terms of certain feelings and corresponding quality of decision making behavior. Figure 3 gives a representation of the model.

The implications of Janis and Mann's (1977) theory for decision counseling are that counselors should do everything to help clients become aware of the state of stress they might be in and of its consequences for the quality of their decision making. Also, clients should be provided with the criteria and some methods for good decision making, notably centered around the timely recognition of available courses of action together with an ordered listing of possible consequences. In their practical recipe for improved decision making Janis and Mann (1977, chapter 6) emphasize the need for decision <u>structuring</u> aids rather than the methods for <u>quantifying</u> probabilities and utilities of specified decision consequences.

4. Kinds of uncertainty; different bases for probability estimation

The present treatment of technical risk analysis and of psychological research on the judgment of risk harbors the suggestion that "assessed risk" and "perceived risk" may turn out not to be as different as one might think. What does seem to be of crucial importance for understanding disputes between technical (genetic) risk analysts and their nontechnical discussion partners is the recognition that there are several basically different kinds of uncertainty about possible future outcomes of an activity or situation. Each kind of uncertainty is rooted in a specific data-base for probability estimation.

The logical, frequentistic and personalistic interpretations of probability discussed in section 2 in fact differentially apply to frequentistic and non-frequentistic sources of information about risks. The logical probability concept is ideally associated with a chance apparatus or a stochastic process with known outcome-generating parameters, as in coin throwing or in playing roulette.

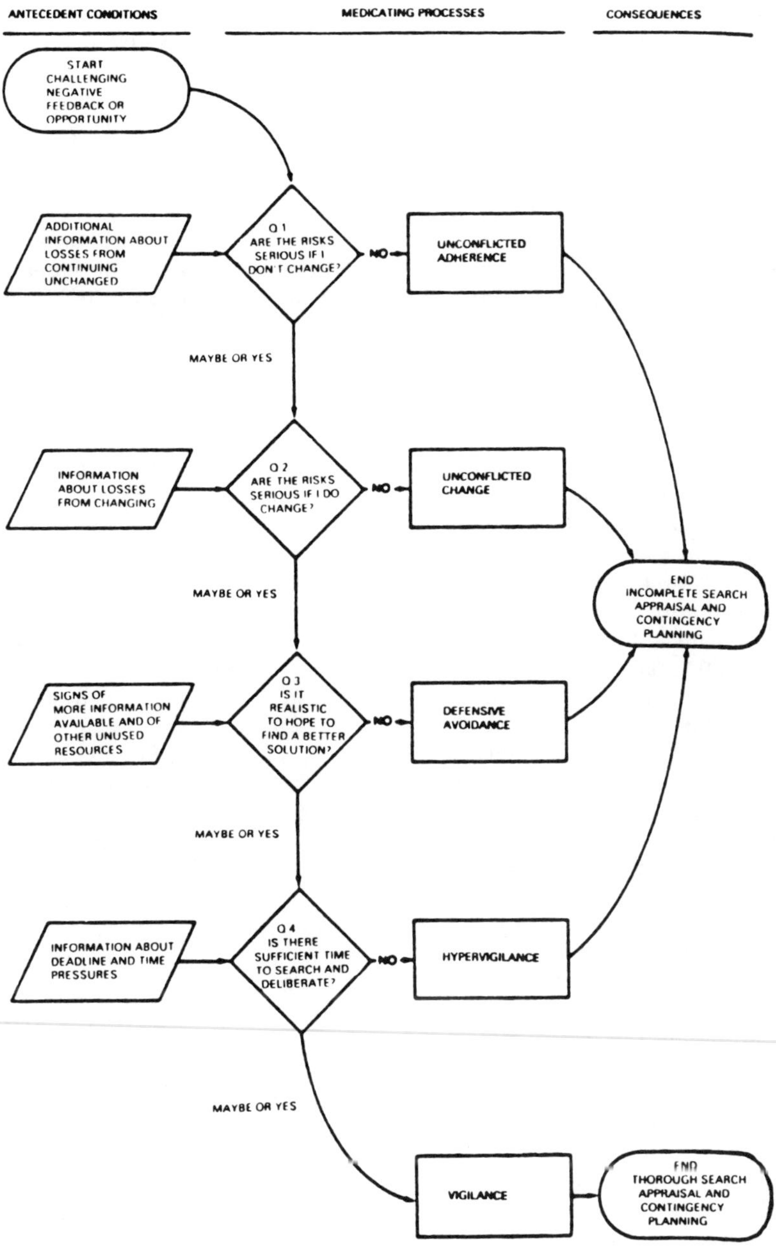

Figure 3: Janis and Mann's (1977; chapter 3) conflict theory model of decision making.

As such the logical interpretation is inherently frequentistic, since a specified set of outcome probabilities may always be validated by means of a long sequence of outcome-generating trials.

The frequentistic probability concept naturally relies on observed relative frequencies of past events occurring under substantially similar conditions, where outcome-generator parameters are in principle unknown. Personalistic probability is basically <u>non</u>frequentistic. Its underlying data base may consist of intuitive beliefs, lines of explicit reasoning, or scenarios about possible future developments of an activity or situation. Thus the availability of a frequentistic versus nonfrequentistic data base constitutes one major variable for the distinction of different kinds of uncertainty.

A second major variable originates in the observation that the occurrence of some probabilistic events (like a house being struck by lightning, or a newborn baby turning out to be a girl) is determined by "external" factors over which the persons concerned have virtually no control. However, other events (like correctly remembering someone else's name, or a spontaneous abortion shortly after an amniocentesis) are largely determined by "internal" factors such as personal knowledge, abilities and competence. The "internal" determination of risks is especially relevant for evaluating activities over which one or more persons can or may exert a considerable amount of control.

Combining the two variable, frequentistic versus nonfrequentistic information and external versus internal determination of risks, leads to the taxonomy of table 5 (see also Howell and Burnett, 1978; Kahneman and Tversky, 1982). Nine different information bases for estimating probabilities are specified as underlying of nine different kinds of uncertainty about the outcome of a given course of events. Naturally, the categories of table 5 are ideal types. In practice the available information base for risk assessment may be a mixture of two or more categories (as in, e.g., estimating the risk of spontaneous abortion after amniocentesis).

The scheme of table 5 may help us realize : (a) that technical risk analysts customarily operate (and like to operate) in the upper left corner, where probabilistic events are externally determined and a frequentistic data base is available, (2) that the psychological dimensions of "controlability" and "familiarity" underlying perceived risk (cf. table 4) can be understood in terms of the relative degree of "internal" determination and the nonfrequentistic data base applying to the risk under consideration, and (3) that the practical use of a formal probability concept may be quite problematic for the quantification of uncertainties identified in the lower right corner of table 5.

The various kinds of uncertainty seem to necessitate different associated methods of decision making under risk. The final sections of this paper are devoted to this problem. A natural transition to these is provided by a brief look at some notions of "acceptable risk".

Table 5 : Nine kinds of uncertainty as rooted in different information bases for probability estimation.

	FREQUENTISTIC		NONFREQUENTISTIC
	known outcome generator	unknown outcome generator	"either it happens or it does not"
EXTERNALLY DETERMINED	parameters of stochastic process (chance apparatus)	observed relative frequencies	scenarios, plans, propensities (of objects, systems)
INTERNALLY DETERMINED (skills)	stable stochastic skill or habit (e.g. running stairs)	observed (calibrated) success/failure rel. frequencies	assessments about feasibility of <u>new</u> performance task (e.g., delivering first child)
INTERNALLY DETERMINED (knowledge)	validated stochastic model of quiz-behavior (nonexistent)	observed (calibrated) rel. frequencies of correct response	argumentative reasoning, or intuitive belief (introspection), about hypothesised fact

5. Defining acceptable risk

Given the difficulties of defining risk itself, various notions of what acceptable risk means have been proposed and are being used. Let us consider some of them (see also Fischhoff, Lichtenstein, Slovic, Derby and Keeney, 1981).

First, a risk may be "acceptable" when the probability of loss or accident stays below a specified level. This definition disregards the size of the loss and it is also insensitive to the expected benefits of an activity.
Secondly, a risk could be judged acceptable when the size of a possible loss remains below a given level, the so-called maximum acceptable loss. Obviously, this definition - which is related to the engineers' 'maximum credible accident' notion - ignores the probability of loss as well as expected benefits.
A third definition rests on the (obvious) combination of probability and size of possible loss. The product rule is most often used for this. "Expected loss" reflects a weighting of probability and size of loss such that "low probability/large loss' risks may be evaluated as equivalent to

"high probability/small loss" risks. Again, this definition does not take account of expected benefits that might be weighed against the risks. Moreover, it is psychologically questionable whether the product rule for combining probability and size of loss, when these two components are given, adequately reflects perceived risk.

A fourth definition is directly inferred from a psychological model of perceiving threats, task demands and coping abilities (figure 2). According to this definition risk is a direct function of the discrepancy between assessed task demands and coping abilities. The greater the discrepancy the larger the risk. An "acceptable risk" situation or activity would be one for which coping abilities just exceed task demands. This definition does not rely on quantified probabilities of any expected outcome pattern of the activity under consideration.

A weighting of risks and benefits comes into play in the fifth and sixth definitions. Both of these imply that, before accepting anything, one should evaluate an activity as a whole, not just the risks of it. The fifth definition stipulates that an acceptable risky activity is characterized by a benefit-against-costs-and-risks balance which just exceeds zero. This necessitates the quantification of benefits, costs and risks on a commensurable set of variables. This would allow trade-offs to be made and aggregation formulas to be applied. However, the definition lets you end up with an "acceptable" course of action, not the most attractive one which may have a better benefit-to-costs-and-risks balance.

The latter idea is captured in the sixth definition which says that risk acceptance in fact amounts to selecting the most attractive course of action from among a set of alternative courses of action all of which have some risk associated to them. This seems to be the fullest definition of acceptable risk. Its practical application, however, is quite demanding of the analytic aptitude and the information processing capacity of the decision maker. Table 6 summarizes the six definitions of acceptable risk.

Table 6 : Possible definitions of "acceptable risk"

1. Probability of loss below specified level.
2. Size of loss below specified level.
3. "Expected loss" (e.g., probability x size of loss) below specified level.
4. Assessed task demands just below assessed coping abilities.
5. Expected benefits just above expected costs and risks.
6. Course of action with highest expected utility.

Note that the first four definitions require you to adopt <u>acceptance standards</u> against which assessed risk levels could be tested. Specified levels of probability (def. 1), size of loss (def. 2), their product (def. 3), or of the subject's coping abilities (def. 4) are needed before a decision can be made. Definitions 5 and 6 introduce the task of making trade-offs between attractive and unattractive aspects of a course of action. This implies that the decision maker should be willing to accept greater risk when the expected benefits (and/or the lower the fixed costs) of a course of action are greater. For some kinds of risk this may be problematic. The sixth definition implies two such requirements. Intending to select the course of action having the highest expected utility seems to presume : (1) that one is willing to consider risk as something to be weighed relative to expected benefits, and (2) that <u>no</u> course of action originally admitted to the evaluation procedure is unacceptable in principle.

The six definitions in table 6 suggest that there are several different approaches towards making a "good" decision about a risky course of action. Let us consider three different perspectives, each of which is best associated to one or more of the definitions in table 6.

First, the fullest and ideal decision approach would seem to be rational decision analysis which best connects to the sixth definition of acceptable risk; in a more limited sense it is also associated to definition 5. A second general approach would be "testing courses of action against pre-determined acceptance standards". This would link up with definitions 1-4 in table 6, all of which seem to imply some absolute notion of acceptable risk. "Testing options against standards" may be seen as a means to standardize the evaluation of recurrent decision alternatives on the basis of accumulated experience.

A third approach reflects a compromise solution between the analytic complexity of full-fledged decision analysis and the intuitive-emotional orientation of most personal decision makers. It derives from the psychological model of risk perception and coping discussed in section 3 and attempts to incorporate definitions 4 and 5 of table 6.

In the final sections of this paper we will briefly outline and discuss the three decision approaches in relation to the earlier sections on risk assessment and the subjective judgment of risk.

6. Three different approaches towards making "good" decisions.

6.1. What constitutes "a good decision"?

Before presenting any decision approach one might wish to consider the concept of "a good decision". In attempting to do this, however, we would immediately become aware of the need to define "decision making" itself. Insofar there exists agreement among philosophers, psychologists and management scientists on the notion of decision making, it is concerned with the great variety of ways in which people do, and could make decisions. Important contenders are instinct, habit and intuition on the one hand and formal rules and explicit analyses on the other. Each way of decision making has its own implicit or explicit criteria for evaluating decision goodness and some very general notions seem required to compare alternative conceptions of good decision making amongst one another. Two issues may help us here.

First, it is generally acknowledged among decision theorists that any single decision under uncertainty should not be evaluated by its own consequences. For the subject could have been lucky or not, and the uncontrollable factors in the decision problem may have co-determined what comes out. One notion of good decision, however, is built upon the value or worth of the decision maker's long run average <u>outcome</u>, considered across a sequence of more or less similar decisions. This could be called the <u>frequentistic</u> perspective on good decision making since it requires you to deep records of past decision consequences and tally the positive and negative ones.

On the other hand there is a <u>personalistic</u> perspective which emphasizes the quality of the decision <u>procedure.</u> This notion especially applies to relatively unique decision problems or to problems occurring under specific circumstances. In such cases statistical records on past decision maker performance are unavailable or relatively meaningless. This seems to apply to many personal decision problems involving genetic risks.

The second relevant issue for evaluating the quality of decision making is the concept of rationality. Most of us have learned that good decisions are rational and that we may blame decision makers who are partly or wholly irrational. But what does this mean?
Upon further scrutiny the concept of rationality is not as clear an ideal as we might wish. It seems useful to distinguish four kinds of rationality :

1. Representational rationality (knowing what you talk about);
2. Goal-value rationality (knowing what you want);
3. Methodical rationality (using coherent assessment methods);
4. Balancing synthetic and analytic rationality.

The first two kinds of rationality may be called substantive; maximizing these implies that you obtain a full representation of your decision problem, including your own desires and values. The third and fourth kinds of rationality may be called procedural-supportive. Methodical rationality, for example, may require you to use axiomatic methods for assessing probabilities and utilities of decision consequences.

Note that the first three kinds of rationality may be maximized; taken together this would imply that you maximize <u>analytic</u> rationality. This may create the problem of your never making any choice at all because you keep going on analyzing your problem in ever greater detail and precision. Therefore it seems indispensable to invoke a certain amount of synthetic rationality which amounts to trusting your intuition and making shortcuts in assessing consequences and evaluating them. The art of good decision making, then, seems to require that - for the problem at hand - you strike the correct balance between analytic and synthetic rationality. How this is done is unclear, let alone how it should optimally be done. But the fourth kind of rationality certainly is the source of a number of enduring feelings of scepticism and unease over the usefulness of different recommended decision methods.

Let us now consider the three different decision approaches in a little more detail, starting with what many theorists consider to be the ideal approach.

6.2. Rational decision analysis

This methodology - also called "Bayesian decision analysis" (see Lindley, 1985; Weinstein and Fineberg, 1980; Keeney, 1982, for more extensive overviews) is aimed at clearly laying out the elements of your decision problem, and at evaluating feasible courses of action in order to identify the one which is most attractive or most goal-effective. Roughly, five steps may be distinguished :

1. Delineating and structuring the problem;
2. Uncertainty analysis : assessment of probabilities;
3. Analysis and assessment of goals, values and/or utilities;
4. Optimization analysis : identification of the "best" course of action;
5. Sensitivity analysis : testing the nature of the final decision against variations in the results of steps 2 and 3.

We shall briefly consider each step in turn.

<u>Delineating and structuring the problem</u> requires you to be able to tell yourself after a while : these are my feasible options; for each option these are the relevant uncertain factors with their possible outcomes; and these, therefore, are the final consequences considered relevant at the time horizon adopted. Thus I will not look at other courses of action than the ones I have listed, I do not consider additional uncertain factors relevant, and I therefore do not expect any other consequences to be pertinent for the eventual identification of the best alternative. Pauker and Pauker (1979; see also this volume) provide an excellent example of decision tree modeling in connection with the amniocentesis decision.

<u>Uncertainty analysis</u> implies that you attempt to transform your feeling of uncertainty into quantitative probability estimates assigned to the possible outcomes of uncertain factors. This may lead you to consider the

collection of additional information (at a cost) which should sharpen your probability distributions over specific sets of uncertain outcomes. The optimal revision of probabilities in the light of new information is done under the guidance of Bayes' theorem (e.g, Edwards, Lindman and Savage, 1961; see also Lindley, 1985).

Analysis of goals, values and/or utilities is a job in itself. Given a defined problem structure the ultimate task here would be to assess the relative attractiveness or seriousness (or utility-disutility) of specific final consequences of the various courses of action. This is best done by using values on a so-called interval scale of utility (having arbitrary unit and zero point), which is defined between the most attractive and the least attractive consequence, respectively, of your total set of relevant consequences. The interval scaling of utilities is sufficient to determine the relative attractiveness differences between the various courses of action, and that is enough to determine which course of action is best.

Specific utility or value-judgments, however, are not easily given from the top of one's head. It certainly helps if they are considered as part of a more encompassing goal hierarchy . The latter results from a hierarchical goal analysis starting with very general or "super" goals at the top which are differentiated and specified in a stepwise process. The process ends when the analyst feels that the formulation of utility attributes is sufficiently specific for valid utility judgments to be made. Obviously, the goal-hierarchy as a whole promotes the clarity, completeness and consistency of the value judgments that are to be carried further in completing the decision analysis.

Optimalization analysis is aimed at the identification of the "best" course of action from among the options incorporated in your decision problem. This necessitates the computation of "expected utilities", i.e., the average expected utility of the consequences following from a chance node.

Sensitivity analyses are indispensable to learn which probability and/or utility assessments are crucial and which allow for a wide-margin estimate. Thus one may learn that the assessment of the probability distribution at a particular chance node is crucial for determining which course of action is best in terms of the expected utility of its consequences. Similarly, changes in assessed utilities may carry through to the initial decision point so as to either enlarge or reduce the attractiveness difference between options, or even to shift their rank order of attractiveness.

To complete this utterly short tutorial on Bayesian decision analysis it should be stressed that well-defined, axiomatic methods are available for the assessment of probabilities of uncertain outcomes, and of utilities of specific decision consequences (see the references mentioned earlier). These methods exist for quite a while, they have been tested both in the laboratory and in practice, and they significantly contribute to what nowadays is called the practical toolkit of decision analysis.

If fully dressed up, decision analysis really looks impressive and it is hard to get around the convincing power of its advocates (e.g., Keeney and Raiffa, 1976, chapter 1). There are, however, several basic shortcomings of rational decision theory, that may make prospective decision makers wary of its applied results and recommendations.

First of all, decision analysis can be rationally applied only to well-defined decision problems; no optimizing procedures are available for getting your options fully listed and their relevant consequences fully explored. The quantitative methodology starts from an a priori "edited" decision problem; how the "editing" is done and whether or where it falls short is no concern of the decision theorist; it often does of course, seriously bother the practising analyst.

Secondly, decision analysis is directed at maximizing what we could call "analytic rationality". One of four fundamental problems, however, is to strike the correct balance between analysis and synthesis, between ever greater decomposition and explication on the one hand, and aggregate judgment and evaluation on the other. Decision theory holds no recipe for determining what that balance between analytic and synthetic information processing should be for a particular type of decision problem.

The third major problem of decision analysis is that it may get you into an infinite regress into ever more detailed justifications of original preferences and expectations. At the simplest level the argument for using decision analysis may be that it is too difficult for you to directly state your relative preferences for the set of available courses of action. You would rather calculate these from component probabilities and utilities which you have assessed after the decision problem has been decomposed. The next step might be that you feel unable to directly assess the overall utility of a particular, reasonably complex decision consequence; you would rather decompose it in terms of underlying utility attributes, assess attribute-wise utility functions and let some utility aggregation rule (e.g., weighted addition across attributes) determine the value to be assigned to the consequence as a whole. But one may start wondering how valid the attribute-wise utility functions are, and whether they perhaps had no better be decomposed further in order to get at a level that the subject is really able to manage.

Decision analysts operate on the assumption that the subject is unable to directly report his or her preferences, but that he or she can do so validly

at a decomposed level where things look much simpler. This strategy may easily become the subject of cartoonists, and it already has, who may ridicule the idea that crucial decisions are construed from answers to extremely simplified preference questions.
Taken together, decision analysis, although well developed and good looking, may not be that convincing to someone contemplating to decide on matters of life and death. If applied wisely and with restraint, it may be of some assistance. If used overenthusiastically, you may no longer know what you are doing, or you may even get stuck.

6.3. Testing separate courses of action against acceptance standards

The second approach towards making good decisions is called "testing options against acceptance standards". This is a suitable decision approach when standards have been set on relevant decision variables, and when you can afford to pay little attention to alternative options than the one currently under consideration. Also, setting standards and subsequently using them is appropriate when a general policy is to be followed which should be applicable to a series of future individual cases. For example, any diagnostic equipment purchase considered that exceeds a price of Dfl 50,000 needs an approval stamp of the hospital budget office director. Or : no expecting mother over 35 years of age and with a prior history of obstetric complications should be advised to deliver her child at home. Thus, testing options against standards amounts to applying one or more if-then rules for arriving at accept-reject decisions.

Depending upon the number and relative importance of criterion variables and upon their way of combination, "standards testing" may be done under several different decision models. Most of these play important roles in the methodology of personnel selection and student counseling, a popular topic of psychological research. For convenience, let us refer to the example of giving genetic advise to parents while discussing three well-known models.

(1) In the <u>conjunctive model</u> critical values on two or more variables or aspects <u>all</u> have to be met before a tested course of action is judged acceptable. For example, prospective parents are advised not to engage in a pregnancy when there is a greater than 10 % chance of their getting a baby suffering from Duchenne's muscular dystrophy, they already have at least one child, and they can make it convincingly clear that they could not handle an affected child satisfactorily in the future.

(2) In the <u>compensatory-weighting model</u> the same variables - probability of Duchenne's muscular dystrophy, having at least one child, and insufficient expected coping - may be relevant, but they may be differently

weighted, and high scores on one variable may compensate for low scores on another. For instance, if the probability of the child having the disease is relatively large, but there is no earlier child in the family and the mother's expecting coping ability is judged high, then the parents may judge it to be acceptable to engage in the pregnancy.

(3) In the lexicographic model the decision variables dominate each other in a particular order of importance. Therefore, the most important variable is considered first and a given option is accepted when its score on that variable exceeds the pre-set standard. Only if the option fails to meet the acceptance standard on the very first variable does one move on to the variable that is second in importance, and the process is repeated.

For example, probability of Duchenne's muscular dystrophy may override both the existence of an earlier child and the mother's coping ability. If that probability is lower than a critical value, say 5 %, the pregnancy option is accepted. If the probability is higher than 5 %, the pregnancy option is only accepted if there is no earlier child in the family. If there are both a high probability and an earlier child, then the pregnancy plan is only accepted when the parents' coping ability is judged sufficiently high. Otherwise the pregnancy is rejected.

Note that "standards testing" is simplest under the conjunctive model requiring that all relevant standards be met for an accept-decision to be made. More complicated but perhaps more realistic is the compensatory weighting model which in fact amounts to an acceptance formula rather than a set of acceptance standards.

There are several fundamental problems inherent to the decision approach of testing a course of action against pre-determined acceptability standards. The first is that you have got to have standards which are sufficiently clear and accepted by themselves; the set of standards applying to a particular case should also be complete. Ambiguous standards may lead to endless discussions about their specific meaning in separate cases. Insufficiently accepted standards may give rise to controversies among experts, and between experts and clients. And an incomplete set of standards would not allow you to arrive at a singular decision.

The second problem with accept-reject standards is that the cases which they are meant to handle may not be similar enough. This means that the standards are too general, which may render them factually invalid for the solution of individual decision problems. Only too well known, I presume, is the argument that "our standards would prescribe the choice of action A, but in this particular case we believe it would be justified to choose B". The reverse side of this coin is the possibility of doing injustice to the individual case, when anyone recommending an alternative to the chosen course of action meets with the rebuttal that "we are sorry, but according to our standards we are bound to take this action now". Thus, existing standards may not help you enough because they are too general; or they may help you too much when the implied policy is too rigid.

A third problem with any standards testing approach is that it in principle does not allow the decision maker to make ad hoc weightings of positive and negative aspects of a decision alternative (according to a predetermined formula this is done in the compensatory-weighting model). Thus standards testing seems suitable for distinguishing between acceptable and unacceptable courses of action, but it does not help you get an idea about how acceptable an option is, let alone which would be the best of the acceptable options. A standard testing approach helps you identify a satisfactory solution, not an optimal one.

Notwithstanding the above weaknesses and shortcomings, testing options against standards may be a highly goal-effective, efficient approach that relieves decision makers of the burden of exploring each separate decision problem in depth and preparing a specific problem representation. However, to be convincing, and to remain so, as instruments for good decision making, adopted standards and their combination rules have to be validated and open to intermittent revision. This seems only possible on the basis of a sequence of regularly occurring similar decision problems which allow you to keep statistics of their actual outcomes. Thus standard testing seems to be intimately connected to a frequentistic notion of good decision making (see section 6.1).

6.4. Deciding on the basis of task demands, coping abilities and desirable scenarios

The third perspective on good decision making is psychological rather than statistical-utilitarian. It capitalizes on the notion of "internal" uncertainties (cf. section 4), and it is based on the psychological models for risk perception and coping discussed in section 3. It also supposedly meets with several of the shortcomings and difficulties inherent in the two approaches discussed above. Perhaps the most general shortcoming of formal decision models is that they are best applicable to static decision problems. Such problems allow you to take a snapshot and freeze the picture obtained in order to decompose it at your leisure and make the assessments required for identifying the optimal course of action. Indeed, there do not exist tractable models for dynamic decision making in a continually changing environment over which the subject may exert a certain amount of control.

A psychological decision approach presumes that people are limited-capacity information processors who adaptively strive to attain a set of flexible goals in a continually changing environment. Given these conditions rationality itself becomes a concept of relative significance - as we have seen (section 6.1). Behaving as if one were the carrier of fixed sets of outcome probabilities and consequence utilities would make a caricature of what human survival actually means.
Therefore, we had better forget about decision methods that claim to provide us with the optimal course of action. What we should, and can only aspire for is to make acceptable decisions in a way that connects our common modes of information processing, respects the limits of our cognitive system, and helps us recognize the essential components of our "real" problems. This approach combines the need to evaluate a course of action by its possible consequences with the need to look into its demands and one's ability to cope with these.

Figure 4 represents the four basic components of evaluating a single course of ("stressful") action for its acceptability : desirable as well as undesirable scenarios forming part of a future course of action-under-uncertainty, a profile of assessed "task demands" upon the decision maker, and a profile of subjective coping abilities (cf. the model of figure 2). Assessing and evaluating these four components would allow the decision maker to make two aggregate judgments. One is made in a decision-analytic vein and concerns the expected desirability of the course of action under consideration. This is based on both the positively and negatively valued possible future developments ("scenarios") whose uncertainties are restricted to a number of factors outside the decision maker's control (as in playing roulette).
The second aggregate judgment pertains to the expected level of stress caused by the course of action considered. This is a function of the discrepancy between assessed functional task demands and the subject's assessed coping abilities. The size and sign of this discrepancy is determinant of different patterns of stress and different coping strategies as explained in figure 2.
To arrive at an overall decision, the subject has to weigh the "expected desirability" and "expected stress" of a given option against one another. Presumably, this is best done in an educated-intuitive fashion, after the subject has become aware of the several underlying components of this overall evaluation.

Figure 4 also suggests that the essential components underlying the overall acceptability judgment may be decomposed further as one moves away from the center. In fact this is what happens in attempts to analyze a complex decision problem. The continued decomposition towards the periphery of figure 4 allows one to structure the problem in greater detail.

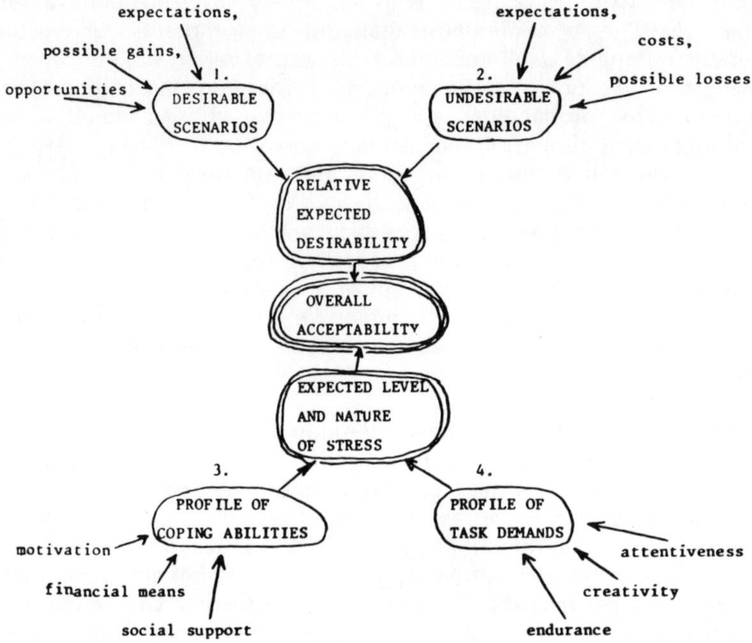

Figure 4 : Structural model for evaluating the acceptability of a stressful course of action.

At the same time, however, the question arises how one is to aggregate the judgments made on all decomposed elements back into the more-encompassing components closer to the central acceptability judgment. Figure 4 thus gives an impression of the dilemma between analytic and synthetic rationality. It pictures the temptation to get away from the center first and analyze your problem into its basic elements. It also is suggestive of the difficulties of finding aggregation rules that help you get back from the periphery to the center.

Considered in pairs, the four pivotal components of figure 4 are indicative of the main psychological factors underlying acceptability judgments. Components 1 and 2 both reflect that what may happen to you is partly dependent upon environmental uncertainties that are outside your personal control; you can only wait and see what the outcome shall be. In contrast, components 3 and 4 indicate that what would happen also depends to some extent on your own ability to deal with external task demands. Thus you may exert control over the outcomes of your decision.

Components 1 and 3 together present the desirable and "achieving" sides of the course of action; some valuable outcomes may occur, and this may be stimulated by your efforts. Components 2 and 4, on the other hand, make you realize that things may also turn out badly and that this may be strengthened by the demands put upon you by the situation you will engage in.

A basically three-step decision procedure inspired by figure 4 could be formulated as follows. In step 1, for each course of action to be evaluated you consider and list the desirable and undesirable scenarios making up that course of action. For example, a 38-year old pregnant woman considering amniocentesis may list the possibility that this may proceed favorable, that it may provide her with the information that the foetus may develop a mild form of Down's syndrome, whereupon she may decide to carry the baby to full delivery and that it (later) happens to be mildly retarded.
These and other scenarios describing a particular development of the course of action considered, are first rank ordered, then rated on some interval scale with respect to their relative value. Formally, a scenario could well be conceived as a path (one path) in a decision tree. Uncertain factors in a scenario could be captured by probability estimates and these could be used to discount on the "certain" evaluation of a scenario, much like in an expected utility calculation. Step 1 of the procedure would be concluded by a joint consideration of desirable and undesirable scenarios in an attempt to assess the relative expected desirability of the course of action considered as a whole.

Step 2 of the decision procedure is directed at components 3 and 4 of figure 4. Here the decision maker attempts to identify and judge the functional task demands which are expected to be posed upon her or him. And (s)he assesses the various abilities (resources, options, skills) that (s)he would have available to cope with the extended demands. For example, delivering and rearing a mildly retarded girl when you already have a normal son may be judged to require your constant initial availability, financial resources for letting the child later on go to a day-care center, an enduring willingness to protect the child from both over- and underattention from its brother and other children, and a continued effort to maintain your own self-confidence and self-esteem as a mother. With respect to his profile of task demands one could subsequently assess one's means and abilities to cope with this scenario.
Step 2 of the procedure would be concluded by the subject making up the balance of coping abilities and task demands in an attempt to determine whether the expected stress from the course of action considered would constitute a threat, or a challenge that could be met. Obviously, task demands and corresponding coping abilities connected to improbable scenarios should be discounted in the overall aggregate judgment of

expected stress.

In step 3 of the procedure the expected desirability of the course of action is weighted against its expected stress level. This means that the decision maker considers the extent to which (s)he likes the possible outcomes of this course of action in relation to her or his relative ability to cope with the required task demands. In doing this, a strongly preferred course of action may turn out to be fairly stressful. But the subject may accept this upon the assumption that (s)he will be especially motivated to keep things under control and make the best of it. Alternatively, an appreciably lower level of expected stress may nonetheless deter the subject, when it is associated to a course of action which is only weakly preferred.
If the weighing of expected desirability against expected level of stress would be done on an interval scale rather than in an ordinal manner, the procedure might be extended to allow the decision maker to make comparative judgments about the acceptability of alternative courses of action. This, however, would be a "quantitative escalation" that this approach essentially wishes to avoid.

As derived from figure 4, the procedure just outlined is mainly directed at helping the decision maker to become aware of the essential components (and some of their underlying determinants) of an overall acceptability judgment to be assigned to a given course of action. The procedure also may help the subject (and the counselor) realize the dangers of either conducting too extensive an analysis, or of cutting things short and relying too much on intuitive judgment.
The scheme of figure 4 could be taken as a basis for elaborating various quantitative models and rules for aggregating decomposed judgment at the periphery into overall judgments required in the centre of figure 4. Such quantification, however, may be a risky venture in itself, as it reflects a tendency to "analyze out and formalize" subjective feelings, emotions and beliefs. Quantification thus may be <u>deceptively</u> helpful, whereas in fact it withdraws the decision process from the subject's comprehension.

7. Summary, conclusions and suggestions

In the earlier sections of this paper an overview has been given of the basic concepts and some methods of (technical) risk analysis, risk perception research and decision making under uncertainty. The ordering of these topics reflects the development-over-time of a critical debate about the analysis and evaluation of technological risks, and about adequate ways to decide on their acceptability. Much of this debate is directly relevant for understanding and structuring discussions on <u>genetic</u> risks, their evaluation and the judgment of their acceptability.
It appears that a statistical-engineering approach to risk requires a

sufficient frequentistic data base and/or valid causal models for estimating risks, as well as a proper multifaceted modeling of the personal and social significance of possible serious losses. This approach, therefore, cannot easily handle nonfrequentistic and "internal" uncertainties (see section 4, table 5), nor does it adequately take account of dynamic changes in, and/or adaptations to the risky activity or situation.

"Perceived risk" has been shown to be a multidimensional concept, whose basic dimensions - "size of a possible accident", "controlability of consequences", "voluntariness of exposure", etc. - may be differently weighed by different individuals. In several studies "probability of loss" proved to be a variable of secondary importance, and a problematic one at that. "Perceived risk" does not seem to be primarily based on statistical considerations. Rather it is reflective of a relative lack of personal control over a demanding course of events, which may be defined as a discrepancy between a set of expected task requirements and a profile of coping abilities. Thus, perceived risk is mainly rooted in other kinds of uncertainty (cf. table 5) than are relied upon in technical risk analyses.
Given the ambiguities of objectifying risk analysis and the multidimensionality of perceived risk, one should not be surprised that comparisons between "objective risk" and "subjective risk" are meaningless more often than that they make sense. One may speculate that this is particularly true when it comes to judging genetic risks whose objectifying assessment is wrought with various kinds of uncertainty. Unfortunately, there is little or no research on lay persons' judgments and evaluations of different kinds of genetic risk.
"Acceptability of risk" as a concept may be defined in various ways (see table 6) which can be related to different approaches towards making "good" decisions on problems involving risk. Three different perspectives on good decision making were presented. The first is rational (or Bayesian) decision analysis, an analytical ideal which is rather demanding of the decision maker's information processing capacities. Pauker and Pauker (1979; also this volume) give an account of their extensive decision-analytic practice concerning problems of genetic risk taking. Decision analysis may be criticized for its reliance on well-defined problems, its lack of a "stopping-rule", and its risk of getting you into an infinite regress in justifying your preferences and expectations. Decision analysis, too, is not easily applicable to highly dynamic kinds of problems.

The second perspective is "testing separate courses of action against predetermined acceptance standards". This approach is simpler and may be highly effective, but it requires the prior availability of an unambiguous and complete set of acceptance standards and a rule for combining them. The approach is directed at evaluating the degree to which an available course of action is satisfactory rather than optimal, and it seems to be best applicable to relatively simple, repetitive decision problems that allow you to keep statistical records of their actual consequences. For "difficult" decision problems, however, the formulation, validation and intermittent revision of sets of operational acceptance standards may be problematic.

In a third decision approach - weighing desirability against expected stress - an attempt is made to incorporate both the expected utility notion of decision analysis and some basic ideas from a psychological model of perceiving risks, task demands and personal coping abilities (figure 2). This approach deliberately shuns quantitative assessments of elementary variables. Instead, it capitalizes on the explicit structuring of someone's decision problem in terms of four basic components. These are the desirable and the undesirable scenarios making up a particular course of action, and the assessed profiles of task demands and of coping abilities, respectively. The model - see figure 4 - illustrates the dilemma of analytical versus synthetic rationality and it explicitly acknowledges the importance of dynamic decision making behavior. It stands in considerable contrast to what would be done under a full-fledged decision analysis.

From the present treatment of risk analysis, risk perception and "good" decision making several conclusions concerning the design of genetic counseling (or, more generally : decision counseling) procedures may be inferred. First, communication about possible consequences, especially risks, of feasible courses of action is difficult when it takes place between parties having totally different views, expectations and stakes in regard to what seems to be one particular problem involving genetic risk. Some mutual agreement and understanding of different possible definitions and psychological dimensions of risk seem essential for effective exchanges between clients, counselor and (other) experts.

Secondly, given that genetic risk is not easily dealt with in the form of a single quantitative variable, the major task of the genetic counselor may be to help the client structure the decision situation in terms of possible courses of action, initial and later decision points, and likely and unlikely (but crucial) consequences. This would reveal "external" and "internal" sources of uncertainty and it would indicate the assessments to be made (and the information needed to make those assessments) while one attempts to identify an acceptable or even the optimal course of action to be undertaken. Humphreys and Berkeley (this volume) present a deliberate view of how this structuring and assessment process could be organized. It may be useful to realize that the geneticists's technical information and assessments form only part of the total package of relevant considerations.

Third, "good" decision making may be achieved in different ways. Neither "untouched intuition" nor far-fetched decision analysis carries the guarantee that one arrives at an optimal course of action. Compromise approaches aim at cutting short on the depth and breadth of analysis by standardizing assessment variables and sets of acceptance criteria. Or they provide a mixture of expected utility assessment and an appraisal of the degree to which the decision maker will be able to cope with future task demands. The latter approach hedges away from a precise quantitative assessment of elementary decision variables, and it does so under the assumption that one could not (and should not) "analyze out" intuitive beliefs and basic emotions. This is well in line with the ideas and conclusions of, among others, Lippman-Hand and Fraser (1979) and it takes account of the difficulties most clients of genetic counselors have in probabilistic reasoning and expected utility analysis referred to in section 3 above. In the field of genetic counseling there seems to be little practical experience with explicit judgment and decision methods other than decision analysis. A concerted research effort may provide us with some very helpful insights on this point.

How could genetic counseling procedures be evaluated? On what grounds should the need for their revision be assessed? The answer to these questions is best formulated in terms of a model of "good" decision making. If that model follows the lines of rational decision analysis (section 5.2) one might look into a subject's understanding for and retention of information about the possible consequences of feasible courses of action and their evaluations in terms of probabilities and utilities.

A more psychologically oriented approach (section 5.4) would suggest that the genetic counseling procedure be judged in terms of understanding for and valuation of desirable and undesirable scenarios, and of the person's appraisals of expected task demands and his or her abilities (resources, skills etc.) to cope with them.

A general set of variables for evaluating genetic counseling relates to "client satisfaction". This, however, could be defined in terms of different ideas about what would make for a "satisfied client". A client may wish to be "happy with the result" of the procedure (measured immediately or after several years..?). Or the client may wish to establish that his or her fundamental beliefs and emotions have been given acknowledged roles in the procedure which otherwise is designed to pull the subject <u>beyond</u> the intuitive emotional level by the compelling force of its internal logic and (maybe) its empirical validity. Given the basic unpredictability of someone's future, the recommended point of view is that the client should judge and decide upon his or her genetic risk problem in a way that (s)he understands, feels comfortable with, and is able to control, and which is seen as appropriate for the situation at hand. From the point of view taken in this paper, people facing difficult decisions seem to be best helped when they are taken through a careful judgment and decision procedure to which they subscribe beforehand. Which conceptual framework and which methods are most suitable for which kind of people and in which situation, is a matter of theoretical and empirical research.

Acknowledgments

Ms. Magda Bootsma of the author's institute deserves gratitude for her careful typing of the manuscript.

8. References

Braybrooke, D. and Lindblom, C.E.
A strategy of decision; policy evaluation as a social process.
New York/London : The Free Press/Collier McMillan (Second edition; First edition, 1963) 1970.

Coombs, C.H., Donnell, M.L. and Kirk, D.B.
An experimental study of risk preferences in lotteries.
Michigan Mathematical Psychology Program MMPP 77-6, University of Michigan, 1977.

Coyne, J.S. and Lazarus, R.S.
Cognitive style, stress perception and coping.
In I.L. Kutsh, L.B. Schlesinger and Associates (Eds) : Handbook on stress and anxiety. San Francisco : Jossey-Bass, 1980.

Edwards, W., Lindman, H. and Savage, L.J.
Bayesian statistical inference for psychological research.
Psychol. Rev. 70, 193-242, 1961.

Evers-Kiebooms, G. , Vlietinck, R., Fryns, J.P. and Van den Berghe, H.
Impact on family planning of the birth of a child with 21 trisomy; the effect of genetic counseling.
In J.M. Berg (Ed.) : Perspectives and progress in mental retardation. Volume II : Biomedical aspects. I.A.S.S.M.D., 1984.

Fischhoff, B., Lichtenstein, S., Slovic, P., Derby, S.L. and Keeney, R.L.
Acceptable risk.
Cambridge : Cambridge University Press, 1981.

Hohenemser, C., Kates, R.W. and Slovic, P.
The nature of technological hazard.
Science 220, 378-384, 1983.

Howell, W.C. and Burnett, S.A.
Uncertainty measurement : a cognitive taxonomy.
Organizational behavior and human performance 22, 45-68, 1978.

Janis, I.L. and Mann, L.
Decision making; a psychological analysis of conflict, choice and commitment.
New York : The Free Press, 1977.

Kahneman, D., Slovic, P. and Tversky, A.
Judgment under uncertainty : heuristics and biases.
Cambridge : Cambridge University Press, 1982

Kahneman, D. and Tversky, A.
Variants of uncertainty.
Cognition 11, 143-157, 1982.

Keeney, R.L.
Decision analysis : an overview.
Operations Research 30, 803-838, 1982.

Keeney, R.L. and Raiffa, H.
Decisions with multiple objectives; preferences and value trade-offs.
New York : Wiley, 1976.

Kuyper, H. and Vlek, C.A.J.
Psychologisch onderzoek over de beoordeling van activiteiten met gevaarlijke stoffen, in het bijzonder vloeibaar autogas (LPG). (Psychological study on the judgment of activities concerning hazardous materials, especially LPG).
Part III of Report No. 3, Division of Energy and Environmental Studies, University of Groningen, December 1984.

Leonard, C.O., Chase, G.A. and Childs, B.
Genetic counseling : a consumer's view.
New Engl. J. Med. 287, 433-439, 1972.

Lindley, D.V.
Making decisions.
New York : Wiley (Second Edition; first edition, 1971), 1985.

Lippman-Hand, A. and Fraser, F.C.
Genetic counseling : parents' responses to uncertainty.
In C.J. Epstein et al. (Eds) : Risk, communication and decision making in genetic counseling : Annual review of birth defects (1978), Volume XV,

number 5c, 1979.

Pauker, S.P. and Pauker, S.G.
The amniocentesis decision : an explicit guide for parents.
In C.J. Epstein et al (Eds): Risk, communication and decision making in genetic counseling : Annual review of birth defects (1978), Volume XV, number 5c, 1979,

Payne, J.W.
Relation of perceived risk to preferences among gambles.
Journal of Experimental Psychology : (Human Perception and Performance) 104, 86-94, 1975.

Slovic, P., Fischhoff, B. and Lichtenstein, S.
Why study risk perception?
Risk analysis 2, 83-93, 1982.

Slovic, P., Fischhoff, B. and Lichtenstein, S.
Decision theory perspectives on risk and safety.
In K. Borcherding, B. Brehmer, Ch. Vlek and W.A. Wagenaar (Eds) : Research perspectives on decision making unde r uncertainty. Amsterdam : North-Holland, 1984.

Stallen, P.J. and Thomas, A.
Public concern about industrial hazards.
Paper presented at the Annual Meeting of the Society for Risk Analysis, Washington D.C. Internal Report of TNO Centre for Technology and Policy, Apeldoorn (Netherlands), 1985.

Tijmstra, Tj. and Huisjes, H.J.
Over het slagen van voorlichting aan zwangeren omtrent alpha-fetoproteïnebepaling in het bloed ter opsporing van een defect van de neurale buis bij de vrucht. (On the success of counseling pregnant women about alpha-fetoprotein determination to detect possible defects of the fetus' neural tube).
Nederlands Tijdschrift voor de Geneeskunde 127 (13), 541-545, 1983.

Tijmstra, Tj., Huisjes, H.J. and Ten Kate, L.P.
Vruchtwateronderzoek wanneer? Informatie-en beslissingsprocessen bij prenatale diagnostiek op leeftijdsindicatie (Amniocentesis : When? Information processing and decision making around age-indicated prenatal diagnostics).
Medisch Contact 26, 2 juli, 1982.

Vlek, Ch. and Stallen, P.J.
Rational and personal aspects of risk.

Acta Psychol. 45, 273-300, 1980.

Vlek, Ch. and Stallen, P.J.
Judging risks and benefits in the small and in the large.
Organizational Behavior and Human Performance 28, 235-271, 1981.

Weinstein, M.C. and Fineberg, H.V.
Clinical decision analysis.
Philadelphia : Saunders, 1980.

EXPERIMENTS ON GENETIC RISK PERCEPTION AND DECISION MAKING : EXPLORATIVE STUDIES

Géry d'YDEWALLE and Gerry EVERS-KIEBOOMS

Laboratory of Experimental Psychology
Center for Human Genetics
K.U. Leuven, B-3000 Leuven, Belgium.

ABSTRACT

In cognitive psychology, considerable attention has recently been given to studies on risk perception and decision making under uncertainty. The attempt to apply the cognitive frameworks to the genetic counseling setting is a major challenge.

After reviewing the relevant literature in cognitive psychology, the aim of our first study was to understand how people process and memorize genetic information about Huntington's disease. Although we did not obtain clear-cut data about the mental representation of this genetic information in our subjects, the context in which the information was given was a surprisingly strong variable affecting its memorability.

Pauker and Pauker (1979) developed a tree model helping the prospective parents to use the probabilities as well as the costs of different outcomes to decide on having an amniocentesis performed. Specific attention was paid to the estimation of the costs of the outcomes. While repeating the same experiment, the goal of our second study was to investigate whether the subjects agree with the advice given by the model and whether their final decision was affected by using the technique or not.

In a third experiment, we scrutinized the joint decision process of two persons as compared with the decision process of people not discussing together. They all received genetic information, either about Hemophilia or about Down syndrome. The joint decision process was completely different for the two genetic diseases. As the two diseases have highly different risk probabilities, we had to unravel the influence of the importance of the risk and the burden of the disease on the ongoing decision of two persons.

The set of findings at least suggests that the existing models in the literature have overlooked the importance of the context in providing the

Birth Defects: Original Article Series, Volume 23, Number 2, pages 209–225

information and the complexities of the decision process when two people have to agree. Moreover, the serious problems in carrying out an experiment when a decision tree is imposed upon the subjects, reveal the potential inadequacy of the assumed total rationality of the decision maker.

INTRODUCTION

During the last decade, a number of studies at the Center for Human Genetics in Leuven have been carried out to evaluate the impact of genetic counseling in families facing a genetic risk. The studies revealed that many individuals have problems to grasp the meaning of probability figures and difficulties to use probabilistic information for decision making. Against this background, a collaboration was initiated between the Center for Human Genetics and the Laboratory of Experimental Psychology. It was our purpose to explore whether cognitive psychology may contribute to a better understanding of perceiving risk probabilities and of decision making within the genetic counseling context.

Experimental psychology is basically process-oriented, while the whole field of risk perception and decision making is mainly characterized by descriptive and prescriptive models. It was considered as a major challenge to bridge the gap between basic research in (experimental) psychology and the applied field of human genetics, keeping in mind the processes involved in the situations of counseling. Besides the basic work of Tversky, Kahneman, Slovic and Fischhoff (we refer to Kahneman, Slovic and Tversky, 1982 for a collection of reviews and previously published articles on judgment and inference) risk perception and decision making studies have a distinguishing European output, as evidenced in Borcherding, Brehmer, Vlek and Wagenaar (1984) and Brehmer, Jungermann, Lourens and Sevon (1986). A European research flavor makes it more attractive in terms of conceptual frameworks and exchanges of research ideas.

In Billen, Evers-Kiebooms and d'Ydewalle (in press), we reviewed the following major issues on risk perception : the most important heuristic inference processes, the impact of problem representation upon the perception of risk, the differences between the concepts of risk and uncertainty, and the impact of motivational and emotional factors in risk assessment. It became clear progressively that the existing literature does not allow us to apply the findings in the context of risk perception in genetic counseling directly. Most studies were carried out with "very simple risky situations" which were verbally presented, mostly to university students. In the studies which will be presented in this paper, we also used volunteering students, and the problems were presented verbally. Still, by presenting a problem situation concerning "genetic risk", we do hope to unravel some of the processes involved in risk perception and decision making in the context of genetic counseling. It should be well understood that the studies presented in this paper are our first explorative studies which must allow us to embark in the future on a larger research project with clinical applications.

EXPERIMENT 1

Purpose of the experiment

In genetic counseling (we refer to the paper of Swerts in the present volume for a definition of genetic counseling) prospective parents are often provided with information concerning risk probabilities. It is important for an optimal decision to remember and to have available the risk probability. As we know that risk probability is not well recalled (Evers-Kiebooms and Van den Berghe, 1979; Evers-Kiebooms et al., 1984), a first research goal could be to define the critical elements in the context which may help to understand and remember this probability. The information is always given within a context which may have strong emotional consequences either for the patient or for the parents. What is the impact of the context on recalling the risk probability ?

Procedure

Subjects were 335 students from two colleges, with a higher proportion of female volunteers. They all saw a Canadian movie entitled 'Living with Huntington's disease' which was produced by the Alberta Educational Communications Corporation in collaboration with the Canadian Huntington Association. The movie was subtitled in the Dutch language (presenting foreign movies with subtitles in the local language is a quite common practice in Belgium).

The movie was composed of four well-defined parts. One part was on the medical background of the disease, together with information about its genetic risk probability (.50 if one of the parents is affected). The concept of the .50 risk probability is richly documented with many examples and illustrations. A second part is about the emotional consequences for the affected person, for the partner and for their children who have a 50% risk to carry the mutant gene and to develop the disease. Part 3 discussed the problems Huntington families are facing concerning the decision to have children. In the final part, prospects about future treatment of the disease symptoms and about presymptomatically diagnosing the disease for at risk family members are described (it should be noted that the movie was made before the availability in the near future of a predictive test was announced). The four parts of the movie were about equally long, and it was easy to separate the four parts.

To assess the importance of the context in which the information about risk is embedded for remembering the risk probability, a factorial design was used. All subjects received Part 1 of the movie, with the medical background of the Huntington's disease and with the 'objective' risk probability. The presence of the three other parts was orthogonally manipulated as to provide 2 x 2 x 2 conditions. Figure 1 gives the outline of the factorial design involving the eight conditions.

Half of the subjects in each condition received a preliminary questionnaire, with two parts. One part was requesting some objective information about the sex of the subject, his/her age and the socio-economic status of the family, while the second part included questions on the attitudes towards having children and towards genetic diseases in general. A preliminary questionnaire can make the subjects more sensitive to the issue and this can have an impact on their recollection of the risk probability. Therefore, it was considered as a fourth factor in the design.

After watching the movie, a new questionnaire was given to all subjects. The questions were all on the information provided in Part 1 of the movie which was given to all subjects. Part of the questions could be answered directly from memory, while the answers to other questions implied an inference process based on the memory of the genetic information provided.

Results

The analyses were limited to nine questions which could be coded as either correct or incorrect (the questions are given in the appendix). A multivariate analysis of variance was carried out on the coded answers in the questionnaire following the movie. After a significant multivariate effect was obtained, appropriate univariate analyses were performed on the answers of separate questions. We only report here the significant values from the multivariate and univariate analyses. Throughout the paper, the significance value was set at at least $p<.05$.

For a number of questions, Part 3 has a main effect on the correctness of the answers (multivariate F value $=13.06$, $p<.0001$). Looking at a discussion about the opportunity for potential carriers of the disease to have children affects negatively the memory of risk (Question 1, $F=3.99$, $p<.05$; and Question 7, $F=4.93$, $p<.05$), except when the question involves a query whether the emergence of the disease may be stopped in the future (Question 2, $F=107.45$, $p<.0001$).

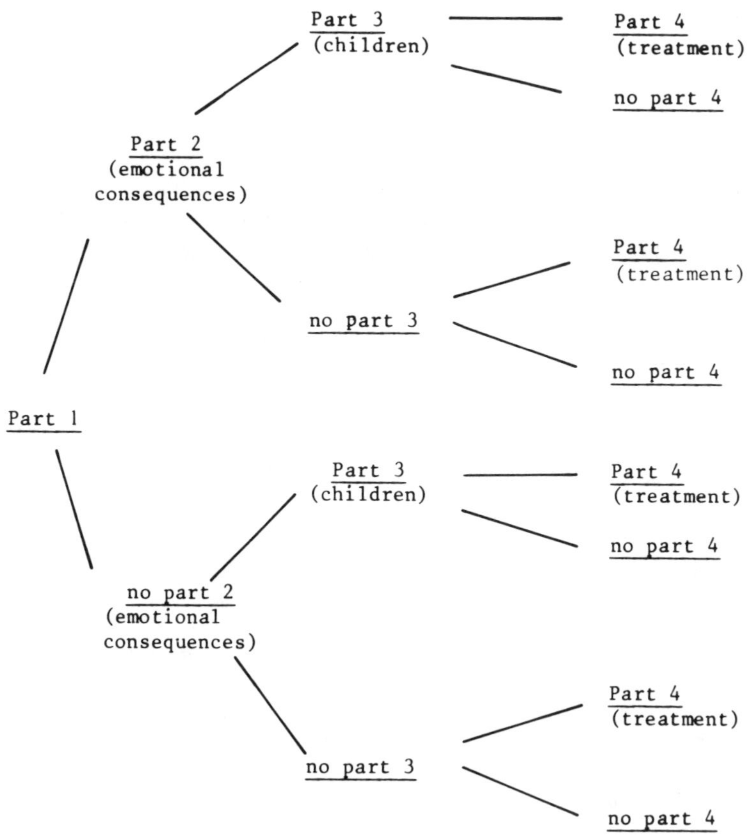

Figure 1: Factorial design of Experiment 1.

However, the presence vs. absence of Part 3 also interacts significantly with the presence vs. absence of other parts. Table 1 gives the average proportion of correct answers as a function of the significant interactions. The headings give a summarizing formulation of the question in the questionnaire as involved in the significant interaction.

Summarizing the main findings is a difficult task when so many significant interactions are involved. However, it must be clear from Table 1 that providing or not Part 3 (Children) has a major impact on the correct answers of the subjects, as all interactions involve the presence vs.

absence of Part 3. Those interactions may be divided into three sets as a function of the pattern of findings.

One set shows that the preliminary questionnaire together with the presence of Part 3 is detrimental (multivariate $F=3.04$, $p<.005$). This is especially clear with Question 8 ($F=10.39$, $p<.005$), although also evident in Question 9 ($F=4.37$, $p<.05$). Does the combination of one's attitude (which is activated by the preliminary questionnaire) with information about facing problems with prospective children (Part 3) complicate the task of assimilating information about risk probability ?

A second set of interactions suggests that it is detrimental to provide either Part 3 without Part 4 or Part 4 without Part 3 (multivariate $F=1.94$, $p<.05$). This can be seen in Table 1 with the data of Question 3 ($F=11.99$, $p<.001$), Question 6 ($F=13.36$, $p<.0005$), and Question 9 ($F=14.57$, $p<.0005$). We have no idea how to explain this set of findings.

More understandable is the final set which involves the interaction between Part 2 and Part 3 (multivariate $F=1.94$, $p<.05$), which is only due to the data from Question 2. Presenting Part 3 and Part 2 on the emotional consequences together boosts the proportion of correct answers how to stop the disease (.67) because the information of both parts unequivocally reinforces the dramatic side of the disease. Without Part 3 and Part 2, the proportion of correct answers is only .11 (see Table 1).

Conclusion

From the large number of unpredicted interactions, we must conclude that our knowledge of how genetic information is encoded and influenced by context is in its infancy. General models of information processing and human memory don't provide us with clear guidelines to understand the performance of our subjects. Two general but conflicting predictions could have been formulated. Providing more context may overload the subjects' memory of the information provided in Part 1 on the risk probability. The first prediction must be rejected because the best performance did not occur in the absence of Parts 2, 3 and 4. The second prediction -that the context may help to reinforce the memory trace- was at the core of the experiment when it was designed. Unmistakingly, context was important as revealed by the large number of interactions. However, the pattern of findings could not be explained easily. Providing Part 3 (the discussion about the children) is critical but its impact varies as a function of the presence of the other parts. Our failure to explain its impact is likely to be due to our ignorance about what is remembered. We have assumed that the probability is stored as such in memory. It is possible, however, that the subjects' correct performance was based on a completely different memory representation.

Table 1: Proportion of Correct Answers Experiment 1.

Question 2 : Is it possible that Huntington's disease will no longer occur in the future?

With Part 3 (Children)	With Part 2 (Emotion)	.67
	Without Part 2	.41
Without Part 3	With Part 2	.09
	Without Part 2	.11

Question 3 : Suppose the father of five children has Huntington's disease. Is it possible for all of this children to be affected?

With Part 3 (Children)	With Part 4 (Treatment)	.97
	Without Part 4	.86
Without Part 3	With Part 4	.87
	Without Part 4	.97

Question 6 : Consider a family with one son and one daughter. Father as well as son are affected. What is the risk for the daughter to develop the disease?

With Part 3 (Children)	With Part 4 (Treatment)	.89
	Without Part 4	.78
Without Part 3	With Part 4	.84
	Without Part 4	.95

Question 8 : Has a person affected with Huntington's disease the same risk of passing on the disease as an at-risk individual of this disease?

With Part 3 (Children)	With Preliminary Questionnaire	.47
	Without Preliminary Questionnaire	.73
Without Part 3	With Preliminary Questionnaire	.70
	Without Preliminary Questionnaire	.60

Question 9 : What is the risk for a child to inherit Huntington's disease of his affected father or mother?

With Part 3 (Children)	With Preliminary Questionnaire	.79
	Without Preliminary Questionnaire	.93
Without Part 3	With Preliminary Questionnaire	.92
	Without Preliminary Questionnaire	.88

With Part 3 (Children)	With Part 4 (Treatment)	.94
	Without Part 4	.78
Without Part 3	With Part 4	.84
	Without Part 4	.95

EXPERIMENT 2

Introduction

In order to help future parents to come to a decision about having an amniocentesis performed, Pauker and Pauker (1979, but see also in this volume) developed a technique to determine the relative costs associated with different potential outcomes in a decision tree (see Figure 2). The different outcomes correspond with the different branches of the decision tree. Pauker and Pauker (1979) used this decision tree to help consultants to make a decision about either having an amniocentesis performed or not for the detection of Down syndrome in couples with advanced maternal age.

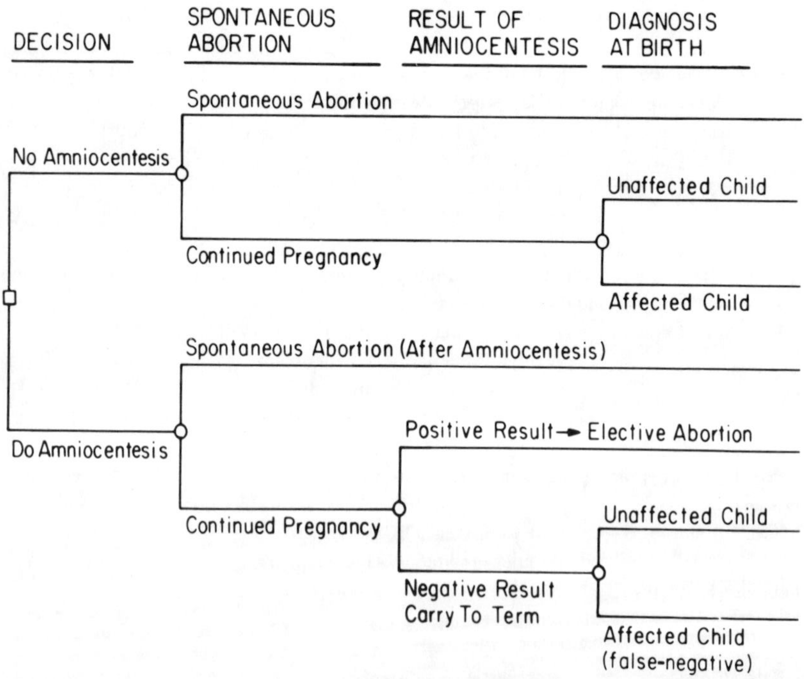

Figure 2 : Decision tree from Pauker and Pauker (1979)

In order to help them, two critical questions are presented : the future parents are asked to specify the risk probability of having an affected child whereby the burden of continued pregnancy would exactly balance the burden of elective abortion (Question 1) or spontaneous abortion (Question 2). We refer to figure 2 in S.P. Pauker's paper in the present volume for an illustration of the question on these balance "probabilities". With those two probabilities, it is possible to define the relative psychological cost of elective abortion and spontaneous abortion, assuming that the cost of an affected child is 100 and that of a normal child being zero.

Purpose

The central question of Experiment 2 is whether it is possible for young adults to specify the above mentioned balance of hypothetical risk probabilities. The Pauker and Pauker (1979) model can only provide advice when such a balance can be achieved. We also intended to check whether the subjects agree with the advice given by the model, and whether their final decision was affected by using the technique or not.

Procedure

In order to answer the central question of Experiment 2, we followed more or less closely the procedure as published in Pauker and Pauker (1979). We presented general information about Down syndrome. They all received the information about the probabilities of spontaneous abortion with and without amniocentesis, respectively. They were asked to imagine that they (or their wife) were 38 years old and pregnant, and they were informed that the objective probability of having an affected child at that age is 1 to 183 or .055. This information was presented to the group as a whole but also on an individual sheet to each subject.
It should be noted that we needed to go through several pilot studies before starting the experiment. Although we followed as closely as possible the procedure as published in Pauker and Pauker (1979), our subjects had serious problems in understanding the two critical questions. We had to change the wordings of the questions a few times before embarking with the experiment. One of the potential reasons may be that we used volunteering students (69 subjects) who had to imagine they were pregnant (or having a pregnant wife) at the age of 38.

In Condition 1, the subjects immediately received the two critical questions of Pauker and Pauker (1979) to determine the psychological cost of elective abortion and the cost of spontaneous abortion. Then they went through the formula leading to an advice about amniocentesis. In a final set of questions, they had to decide about amniocentesis, thus expressing their (dis)agreement with the provided advice.
In Condition 2, they first had to decide about amniocentesis -completely independent of the procedure- before going through the two critical questions bringing them to an advice which may or may not be compatible

with their former decision.

Results

Although all our subjects had at least a high school level, it still (considering the changes we already had to introduce after some pilot studies) was very difficult for most subjects, and even next to impossible for some subjects, to understand the instructions and to specify the probability to have an affected child, whereby the burden of continued pregnancy would balance the burden of elective abortion (in Question 1) or spontaneous abortion (in Question 2).

In terms of the final decision, there is a significant difference between the two conditions (chi-square = 4.33, $p<.05$). If the subjects go through the two critical questions first (Condition 1), 66% of the subjects decide in favor of amniocentesis, and 34% against. In Condition 2 (deciding first, before answering the two questions), only 41% are in favor (with 59% against). It pinpoints to the fact that the spontaneous decisions may be quite different from the decisions following the Pauker and Pauker (1979) model.

There is no significant difference between the two conditions in terms of the agreement of the subjects with the advice as provided by the formula. However, there is a significant difference ($t=2.06$, $p<.05$) between the two conditions looking at the differences between the costs of elective and spontaneous abortion. The cost of elective abortion was considered to be only slightly more important than the cost of spontaneous abortion in Condition 1 (with a t-test at the borderline of significance, $p=.07$) but the cost of elective abortion was definitely larger than the cost of spontaneous abortion in Condition 2 ($t=3.88$, $p<.0005$). The difference could be an artefact resulting from the prior decision which was rather against amniocentesis (59% of the subjects; see above) in Condition 2. A larger difference between the two types of costs justifies a negative decision. The several rating scales about the certainty of their answers did not produce a difference between the two conditions.

It is worthwhile to report that there are subjects who find that the costs of spontaneous abortion either equal or exceed the costs of elective abortion. Although 58% of the subjects find the costs of elective abortion higher than the costs of spontaneous abortion, still 28% find them equal and 14% consider the costs of spontaneous abortion higher than the costs of elective abortion.

Conclusion

After following the Pauker and Pauker (1979) model (Condition 1), subjects clearly come to another decision than without the advice according to the model (Condition 2). Our findings suggest that working through the model may lead to a more positive attitude towards amniocentesis. Besides the importance of ethical issues involved there is the theoretical problem "how" people arrive to a decision in such a situation.

EXPERIMENT 3

Purpose

The decision making about a pregnancy, in principle, involves two people. If there is an increased genetic risk, they will have to assess and evaluate (explicitly or at least implicitly) individually and together the importance of the risk. The central question of Experiment 3 is how the individual and common assessments combine together into a decision within the context of a prospective pregnancy. Moreover, the decision may be made either with or without a preceding discussion between the two persons involved, about the importance of the risk. Moreover, it can be predicted that the (individual and/or common) assessment, leading to the decision, may vary as a function of the 'objective' risk probability.

Procedure

Subjects were 48 male and 130 female volunteering university students. Small groups of subjects were invited together. About half of the groups received approximately a one-page description of Hemophilia, describing the genetic disease and the 'objective' risk probability of .50 to have an affected son when the mother is a carrier of this X-linked disease. The other groups of subjects received a similar description about Down syndrome, with the 'objective' risk probability of .01 to have another child with Down syndrome in young parents who already have an affected child and who themselves have a normal karyotype.

In Part 1 of the Experiment, all subjects had to assess individually the importance of the risk and their affective evaluation of the disease on a seven-point scale. The rating was carried out immediately after reading the text. After that, they all received a personality questionnaire. While the subjects were answering the questionnaire, the experimenter checked their rating. She tried to form groups of two subjects on the following basis. The assessment ratings of the importance of the risk should differ as much as possible, and the two should be from a different sex as far as the unequal proportion of the two sexes in our sample made it possible.

In Part 2 of the experiment, the two subjects (the couples) were introduced to each other and they had to go together in smaller rooms, one room for each couple. The couples were now divided into two experimental conditions. In Condition 1, the couples had to discuss together the importance of the risk, and to provide jointly a new assessment rating. After the rating, they had to decide jointly about a pregnancy. The couples in Condition 2 had not to discuss together about the importance of the risk; they only had to decide jointly about the pregnancy.

Results

The importance ratings of the two genetic risks (Hemophilia vs. Down syndrome) were significantly different, as could be expected because the two 'objective' risk probabilities were quite different ($F=35.97$, $p<.0001$). The affective evaluation of the disease, however, did not differ significantly. For both diseases, female subjects rated the importance of the risk significantly higher than male subjects ($F=5.02$, $p<.05$). While there was a significant correlation between the two ratings in the case of Hemophilia ($r=0.36$, $p<.01$), the correlation disappeared completely in the case of Down syndrome.

In Part 2, only in Condition 1 (with a discussion among the two about the importance of the risk) subjects had to make a joint importance rating of the risk. A critical question is what is the nature of the shift of the joint rating of two persons as compared with the initial rating of the individual subjects in Part 1 of the experiment. From the individual ratings we derived a "predicted joint rating" of the two persons (the average). After that, the average of the two individual ratings was subtracted from the joint rating and this difference was weighted against the absolute difference between the two individual ratings. The "deviation score" of couples receiving the text about Down syndrome did not differ significantly from zero. The other group with the Hemophilia text (with a higher 'objective' risk probability) did change (although only marginally significant, $t=1.76$, $p=.09$) : after a joint discussion, they lowered the assessment of the importance of the risk.

The final question in Part 2 was about the decision to have a pregnancy. In the group receiving information concerning Hemophilia, there was a marked difference between the two conditions ($F=4.84$, $p<.05$). When a joint discussion about the importance of the risk and a joint rating preceded the question (Condition 1), subjects were more willing to accept a pregnancy than subjects without a discussion about the importance of the risk (Condition 2). Subjects receiving the genetic risk probability of Down syndrome did not differ in their decision in the two conditions. This pattern of findings fits well with the joint rating of the importance of the risk. Only in the case of Hemophilia there was a decrease of the importance rating; accordingly, those subjects were more in favor of a pregnancy.

In the case of Down syndrome, couples of different sexes were also more willing to decide in favor of pregnancy than couples with only female subjects ($F=4.70$, $p<.05$); this pattern of findings did not emerge with Hemophilia.
In terms of a decision to have a pregnancy, the two diseases led to a completely different pattern. In the case of Hemophilia, 24 couples are in favor and 23 couples are against, with only two couples undecided; in the case of Down syndrome 12 couples are undecided (with 19 couples in favor, and 9 against). The larger number of undecided couples in the case of Down syndrome is striking.

The correlation between the joint rating of the risk importance and the decision for a pregnancy in Part 2 was significant for both diseases (Down syndrome, $r=-.35$, and Hemophilia, $r=-.32$; in both cases, $p<.05$). When the risk importance rating is higher, subjects are less inclined to have a pregnancy.

Conclusion

We presented two completely different genetic diseases (Hemophilia and Down syndrome) with very different "objective" risk probabilities. As could be expected the importance ratings of these two genetic risks were significantly different. Obviously, the impact of a joint discussion of the importance of the risk (and the fact that a joint rating had to be given) greatly differs as a function of the two probabilities. In the case of Hemophilia, a disease with a high risk, subjects, after discussion, reassessed the importance of the risk downwards. Accordingly they were more in favor toward a pregnancy than subjects who did not discuss the importance of the risk. It remains an open question whether this pattern as a function of the 'objective' risk probability is a general one, or is also linked with the specific type of genetic disease involved.

Although we used students in Experiment 3, it is worthwhile to notice that the experiment was carried out smoothly. The reactions of the subjects during the experiment revealed that they felt highly involved in the experimental setting. This is obviously in contrast with Experiment 2.

GENERAL DISCUSSION

We presented our first three explorative studies in the field of genetic risk perception and decision making involving genetic risk. The first goal was to explore the field. The studies were not designed to investigate thoroughly one or other psychological process involved in genetic counseling. We wanted to know in what direction a systematic and extensive empirical approach could be initiated.

We outline the main results of our explorative studies.
It is clear that the context shapes the memory encoding and availability of provided genetic information (Experiment 1). The use of a decision aiding technique was explored in Experiment 2. After following the Pauker and Pauker (1979) model subjects clearly come to another decision than subjects who come to a decision without the advice according to the model. Reassessing jointly the importance of a high risk influences the decision about a pregnancy (Experiment 3). Generally speaking, we had difficulties in explaining the obtained differences. The failure to explain the findings is partially due to the fact that the available frameworks in cognitive psychology (but also in social psychology, see especially Experiment 3) are difficult to apply in this field. Obviously, more theoretical and empirical work will be needed to unravel the processes involved. While the findings are encouraging in continuing to design the experiments more or less in a similar way, in the next step we will have to focus on the obtained but unexplained differences.

We like to emphasize that more work will have to be carried out on the mental representations the subjects construct about provided risk information. There are some indications in Experiment 1 that many subjects don't store numbers : risk probabilities are remembered in a different 'mental' format.

Two final cautionary notes must be given. First, only students with a higher educational background were participating in our experiments. This may severely restrict the external validity of our studies, and we must acknowledge the problem. Still, a number of issues addressed in the present paper could be independent from the investigated group of subjects. The problem of the mental representation of risk probabilities, the effect of the context, the influence of a joint reassessment of risk probabilities and working with a decision tree are problems of very general nature, and could be studied, independently of the genetic counseling situation.
A second problem concerns the nature of the dependent variables in the three studies : they were all either answers or ratings on verbal questions. The final behavior of prospective parents may be quite different. This problem can be generalized for almost all studies on risk perception and decision making in cognitive psychology. Cognitive psychology has recently addressed the link between verbal 'protocol' and instrumental behavior within models of information processing (see, for example, Ericsson and Simon, 1980, 1984). Moreover, social psychology has investigated the problem, mainly by looking at the mediating variable of attitude (see especially Fishbein and Ajzen, 1975). While a decade ago most investigators were quite sceptical about a direct link, now a growing consensus seems to emerge that the gap is not that large as to discredit completely the value of verbal reports.

Acknowledgements

We greatly acknowledge the contribution of A. Van de Casteele (Experiment 1), S. Ceuppens (Experiment 2), and D. Kronenberger (Experiment 3) in carrying out the experiments in partial fulfillment of their licence degree at the University of Leuven.

REFERENCES

Billen, A., Evers-Kiebooms, G. and d'Ydewalle, G.
Risico perceptie en erfelijkheid: een bijdrage vanuit de cognitieve psychologie. (Risk perception and heredity : a contribution from the perspective of cognitive psychology)
Lisse, the Netherlands, Swets and Zeitlinger, in press.

Borcherding, K., Brehmer, B., Vlek, C. and Wagenaar, W. A.
Research perspectives on decision making under uncertainty: Basic theory, methodology, risk and applications.
Amsterdam, North-Holland, 1984.

Brehmer, B., Jungermann, H., Lourens, P. and Sevon, G.
New directions in research on decision making.
Amsterdam, North-Holland, 1986.

Ericsson, K. A. and Simon, H. A.
Verbal reports as data.
Psychol. Rev. 87, 215-251, 1980.

Ericsson, K.A. and Simon, H. A.
Protocol analysis: Verbal reports as data.
Cambridge, Mass., MIT Press, 1984.

Evers-Kiebooms, G. and Van den Berghe, H.
The impact of genetic counseling : a review of published follow-up studies.
Clin. Genet. 15, 465-474, 1979.

Evers-Kiebooms, G., Vlietinck, R., Fryns, J. P. and Van den Berghe, H.
Impact on family planning of the birth of a child with 21 trisomy.
In J. Berg (Ed.), The effect of genetic counseling : Perspectives and progress in mental retardation vol II, 323-333, University Park Press, Baltimore, 1984.

Fishbein, M. and Ajzen, I.
Belief, attitude, intention and behavior : An introduction to theory and

research.
Reading, Mass., Addison-Wesley, 1975.

Kahneman, D., Slovic, P. and Tversky, A.
Judgment uncertainty : heuristics and biases.
Cambridge, Mass., Cambridge University Press, 1982.

Pauker, S. P. and Pauker, S. G.
The amniocentesis decision : an explicit guide for parents.
In C. J. Epstein, C. J. R. Curry, S. Packman, S. Sherman, and B.D. Hall (Eds), Risk, communication and decision making in genetic counseling (pp.289-324). Washington: National Foundation, 1979.

Appendix : Questionnaire from Experiment 1

Question 1 : Suppose somebody's mother died of Huntington's disease and he and his partner are both healthy. What is the risk for their child to get this disease?

Question 2 : Is it possible that Huntington's disease will no longer occur in the future?

Question 3 : Suppose the father of five children has Huntington's disease. Is it possible for all of his children to be affected?

Question 4 : Is it possible for Huntington's disease to skip a generation?

Question 5 : Suppose somebody's father and brother are affected with Huntington's disease and he and his partner are healthy. What is the risk for his son to develop the disease?

Question 6 : Consider a family with one son and one daughter. Father as well as son are affected. What is the risk for the daughter to develop the disease?

Question 7 : Is it possible for someone to be a carrier of the gene that causes Huntington's disease without ever developing the disease?

Question 8 : Has a person affected with Huntington's disease the same risk of passing on the disease as an at-risk individual of this disease?
Mark the right answer :
An at-risk individual has
- more chance to pass on the disease
- the same chance to pass on the disease
- less chance to pass on the disease.

Question 9 : What is the risk for a child to inherit Huntington's disease of his affected father or mother?

REPRESENTING RISKS : SUPPORTING GENETIC COUNSELING

Patrick HUMPHREYS and Dina BERKELEY

Department of Social Psychology

London School of Economics and Political Science, London

Abstract

This paper discusses issues involved in decisions to bear a child given the knowledge that the child may be subjected to a genetic risk. It argues that the problem of whether to take the risk or not is predicated on the way the prospective parents have conceptualised this risk and its effects. Five levels of abstraction are described at which this risk can be represented and the implications of conceptualising the problem at each of these levels are outlined. Recommendations are made about how to explore the way - or different ways - parents conceptualise the problems involved and how to go about helping them make the decision which they will be least likely to regret subsequently, whatever the actual outcome.

Introduction

Genetic risk taking, unlike other personal decisions involving risk, is taken under the knowledge that an undesirable outcome of one's own decision will primarily affect another person. While, if the feared outcome of a pregnancy were to materialise, one would have to live with the consequences of such a decision, one's offspring is the person who would be primarily affected.

Furthermore, it is a decision which is invested with uncertainty : uncertainty about outcomes and how one would feel about them, uncertainty about the likelihood of any one outcome materialising, uncertainty about current and future development of science to deal with a particular condition which may only develop in later life, and in some cases (e.g., Huntington's chorea) even uncertainty about one's own health is involved.

Birth Defects: Original Article Series, Volume 23, Number 2, pages 227–250

Moreover, the results of this decision may not be immediately obvious, so that the decision maker will know for certain whether the child is symptom-free and will remain so. For example, Duchenne's muscular dystrophy sets in at about 3 years of age and kills by the early teens. In some cases, one does not even know whether any future offsprings will have to run the same risk : having one symptom-free child does not necessarily imply that any later children will be symptom-free. One may also be running the danger of passing the decision onto one's children as, for example, in the case of amaurotic idiocy (Auerbach, 1969).

It is also a decision which in some instances cannot be reversed. Diagnosis of foetal abnormalities through ultrasound scan or amniocentesis is usually possible only around the 16th to 20th week of a pregnancy, by which time the pregnancy cannot easily be terminated. Even if the pregnancy were to be terminated, the physical and emotional consequences of carrying out the operation necessitated by the advanced pregnancy can be very unpleasant. Conversely, a decision not to have children under the high genetic risk involved may not subsequently be open to change if the woman has by then passed child bearing age.

In cases where the decision has been made to conceive a child who will run a genetic risk, the long waiting period of pregnancy will continually offer to the prospective parents the possibility to reconsider their initial decision. Nine months is a long time to live under the uncertainty of not knowing the outcome of their decision (of course, it is much longer in the case of disease which only appears later in life). Even in cases where tests exist enabling one to determine whether the foetus is affected or not, the reliability of these tests is not always 100 % certain : false positives and false negatives can have dramatic effects (Rakusen and Davidson, 1982). For sex-linked genetic risks (such as haemophilia or muscular dystrophy) it is possible to determine the sex of the foetus with certainty. In such cases, one will know for certain that a female child is symptom-free and further investigations can indicate whether a male child is affected by the disease or not (here again, however, the reliability of tests is brought into question).

These are some of the issues that make decision making concerning child bearing under conditions of genetic risk especially hard, both for the prospective parents and for any professional counsellor who may inform and advise them. Any regret arising from taking the wrong decision will have to be coped with both in the case where the child develops the feared symptoms and in the case where pregnancy was actively avoided or aborted, the latter as a phantasy of the attractions of being the parent of a living symptom-free child (Parkes, 1971). It is this regret that will concern us here (rather than the satisfaction of giving birth to a symptom-free child) : how can one prepare and support parents in taking and implementing the decision they take and in helping them live with its consequences.

Issues involved in child bearing decisions with genetic risk

In a seminal work on birth planning decision making, Beach et al. (1976) developed and tested a decision aiding tool (the Optional Parenthood Questionnaire; Beach et al., 1978) to help prospective parents reach a decision concerning whether or not to have children. The key categories of this questionnaire concern three main areas of consideration for the prospective parents :

(a) Self and partner - as persons, as parents and as family
(b) Children - in the family and their well being
(c) Other people - relatives, friends and society.

We refer to this study here as a starting reference point for the range of issues one should consider when faced with a family planning decision. (We will discuss its use as a decision aid later on). In this questionnaire, the issue of how one would cope with the possibility of having a child with an inherited defect is raised in regard to its impact on the feelings about oneself and partner as persons, on their relationship as parents of such a child, and on the effects of having such a child on their already existing children. Having the opportunity to consider this issue while planning a family is different, however, to having to consider this issue for the first time when one is already pregnant.

At the outset, one can differentiate between decisions involving genetic risk which are taken <u>during</u> the planning stage of a pregnancy and decisions taken <u>after</u> the pregnancy has been confirmed. In the former case, we are dealing with prospective parents who have to face the possibility that their offspring may be subjected to a genetic risk. In the latter case, the prospective parents may or may not have known that there existed such a possibility prior to conception, and would have found out about it only as a result of the routine medical investigations carried out after the woman was diagnosed as pregnant (e.g., testing for Down's syndrome). During these investigations, one can also find out about other chromosomal abnormalities (such as XXX or XYY), which lead to even more difficulties in deciding as they indicate the presence of <u>borderline</u> types of foetal "abnormality". Information about the presence of this type of abnormality can make the decision, whether to continue with the pregnancy, very complicated. The child, if born, could well be expected to live a relatively long and happy life but not the one parents may have previously phantasised for their child.

In the case where parents know of the risk of genetic abnormality prior to

conception, the options within the decision making process will be either
(a) not to take the risk at this time and opt for a life without (further) children (avoiding choosing the option now may involve a repetition of the decision making process at a later stage), or
(b) to try to conceive a child and, if successful, decide on the fate of the particular pregnancy later on.
Option (b) involves gambling on the risk of the birth of an abnormal child if one is not prepared to consider a termination of pregnancy or if there are no reliable tests to depict the suspected genetic abnormality in the foetus. One also has to consider what a termination of pregnancy entails and the possible adverse effects which may result from this (e.g., Berkeley et al, 1984).

When prospective parents did not know before conceiving a child that they were facing a genetic risk but they have become aware now (i.e., during the pregnancy) that the expected child may be affected, we are dealing with a decision where the undesirable outcome has a much higher probability of materialising : the only uncertainty concerning the odds is based on the possible unreliability of the particular test which depicted the condition and any possible lack of any further tests to cross validate the results of the original test.
Although parents facing the decision for the first time during pregnancy will have much more severe psychological problems with which to cope, such as the loss of the particular expected child and its attendant problems (e.g., Marris, 1974), and the significant modification in their "sense of coherence" as prospective parents (Antonovsky, 1980), in terms of how the prospective parents will need to think about the particular problem they are facing (which is the vital issue to consider in genetic counselling and in any attempt to provide support for them), the issues are much the same as when the decision is faced before embarking on a pregnancy. As we shall show below, any decision problem involving genetic risk (whether known for certain or envisaged as a possibility) may be represented at five levels of abstraction which define qualitatively different kinds of cognitive operations the decision maker has to perform on the material available to him or her in order to reach a decision.

In earlier papers (Humphreys and Berkeley, 1983; 1985; in press), we have argued that it is important to understand how the decision problem has been represented at each level if we are to be able to account for differences between different individuals considering similar problems and if we are to provide support to their decision making activities. In the case of genetic counselling, this is particularly important, given that issues not properly resolved at each level may have severe repercussions for the well-being of all persons involved. Thus, in this case, we would argue, it is vital that, when attempting to provide help, the counsellor finds out the level at which prospective parents are encountering difficulties or will have to negotiate differences with each other in conceptualising their decision problem.

Levels of conceptualisation of decision problems involving genetic risk

A major difficulty for people facing a decision about whether to bear a child, in the knowledge that there is evidence for genetic risk, is to know how to think about the problem. This is something which they have to work out for themselves insofar as they will have to live with the consequences of the decision and any regret that unanticipated sequelae may engender ("I wish I had thought then about the problem the way I do now"). Severe problems can arise when the two prospective parents conceptualise the problem in different ways, and so cannot understand each other's account of the basis for their preferred course of action. A counsellor may form a clear picture of the risks associated with the various courses of action he or she conceptualises as open to the prospective parents, but then find that attempts to explain the probabilities and value trade-offs involved are met with incomprehension, rejection or frustration by the clients, who seem to have quite a different preoccupation with the problem. We discuss below possibilities and methods aiding the resolution of such difficulties, based upon the thesis that these types of misunderstanding and incomprehension often stem from a failure to apprehend the level at which difference in or difficulty in conceptualisation occurs.

Our discussion of methods is organised within a five level scheme, which when applied sequentially within any particular genetic counselling situation, will give an indication of the level at which the process of displaying and resolving differences or difficulties in problem conceptualisation should start. The scheme, when taken as a whole, is characterised by the following key formal properties : (1) what is qualitatively different at each level are the <u>cognitive operations carried out</u> in thinking about the problem at that level; and, (2) the results of the operations carried out on a particular level constrain the ways operations are carried out at all lower levels. We shall present the scheme in descending order from level 5 to level 1, since property (2) implies that in order for risk presentation or decision aiding activities at any level to be successful, differences or difficulties must first have been resolved at all higher levels.

Level 5 : Exploring the boundary of the "small world" within which the problem is located

Decision problems, whether concerning genetic risk or some other aspect of a person's life, are located within a "small world" which defines the bounds of the material which the person is prepared to retrieve from memory and attempt to structure in handling the decision problem (c.f. Toda, 1976; Humphreys and Berkeley, 1983; 1985; in press).

However, small worlds, complete with contents, do not exist as complete entities pigeonholed away in a person's mind ready to be retrieved intact. From the outside we infer the contents of the small world the person is using by looking at what he or she explores, and guessing its bounds or possible "holes" within it by what he or she leaves out. We are left with uncertainty of the bounds of this structure, in the same way cartographers of the physical world in the middle ages experienced uncertainty about where to draw bounds when they had access only to explorers' reports and guesswork to fill in the gaps.

From the standpoint of this analogy, though, the person facing the decision problem is not the cartographer, but the explorer. He or she can only establish the bounds by backwards and forwards processing (Jungermann, 1983; 1984), exploring alternative futures in a territory for which there are no maps and there may be considerable uncertainty not only about where the boundary is but also what unforeseen rewards - or terrors - lie there, or along the route.

Traditionally, risk assessment has been characterised as the process of determining the probability of a worst case scenario, whose subjective expected (dis-)utility can then be set against that of other, more attractive scenarios in determining the overall attractiveness of a risky option. However, attempts to explore "worst case scenarios" with real world, habitual gamblers usually lead to a denial that they "are taking much of a risk". The worst case scenarios they volunteer are usually bounded in that they claim to have contingency plans which would enable them to cope with the outcomes envisaged in them (Wagenaar et al., 1984).

However, experience of risk is suddenly magnified when a person, having reached a particular outcome in a worst case scenario, says "I just don't know what I would do if this occurs". Why this is so has been discussed by Sandler and Sandler (1978) in terms of a "background of safety" built up through play; that is, structured and guided exploration of ways of setting bounds or having bounds provided by one's parents or others for one's "worst case" phantasies. When a person, exploring within the small world of a decision problem, finds a "gap" in the boundary of the background of safety (that is, where no contingency plans exist for handling the situation), then the negative utility associated with the scenario is unbounded, and considerable fear can result. Janis and Mann (1977) describe how the anticipation of even the lowest possibility of going beyond the background of safety will often induce stress, leading to defensive avoidance of such exploration.

In the case of genetic risk, this "background of safety" may be provided by a belief that medical science will progress and the feared condition will be treatable in the future and so a contingency plan could be developed in that, should the starting condition for the worst case scenario materialise (i.e., one's offspring is diagnosed as actually having a genetic defect), medical science will be able to help. Alternatively, the background of safety can be maintained prior to conception of a child potentially at risk through the belief that a contingency plan will always be available in case of conception : e.g., a reliable test could be carried out to determine whether the expected child is affected by the feared condition. Conversely, a potential genetic risk condition of which one has no experience may become extremely fearful if one does not know about, or has no access to information which could restore the background of safety through allowing one to explore realistic contingency plans.

Facilitating the representation of genetic risk at level 5

Difficulties in providing an adequate representation of risk at this level may stem from defensive avoidance of exploring the implications and possibilities which may well have to be faced in the future, or through an unwillingness of one prospective parent to explore his or her partner's ideas about possible contingency plans for handling worst case scenarios, as they lie outside his or her own background of safety. In the latter case, genuine constructive or creative opportunities for handling the genetic risk problem may be lost through fear and defense on the part of one partner, and frustration or disillusionment on the part of the other concerning the possibility of even being able to negotiate or realise his or her contingency plan. How could one alleviate these difficulties, thus facilitating the representation of the genetic risks that need to be considered? Should a counsellor endeavour to <u>extend</u> or <u>restrict</u> the range of considerations explored by the prospective parents?

<u>Extending the range of considerations</u> would by necessity lead to a wider exploration of issues that may impinge on the outcome of a pregnancy, thus increasing the chance of encountering consequences which for one or both of the prospective parents involve unbounded worst case scenarios. For example, undiscriminate screening for the level of alpha-foetoprotein in the mother's blood (the AFP test which can determinate neural tube defects) can have far-reaching emotional effects through the introduction of a simple blood test, "particularly if careful attention is not paid to the way it is given and to its meaning generally" (Rakusen and Davidson, 1982, p. 78).

Moving to the other extreme, <u>restricting</u> rather than extending what one should think about in family planning decisions in the hope that scenarios in certain areas will not be explored (thus unduly scaring some prospective parents), is likely to be counter-productive as it would simply throw such exploration into the realm of taboo or "the occult", wherein phenomena excluded from consideration, rather than being neutralised, are experienced as having special agency and potency (c.f. Leach, 1964; Douglas, 1966; Douglas and Wildavsky, 1982).

We would suggest that an alternative and more promising method of facilitating the representation of risks at this level would be to consider ways of extending the background of safety, helping people develop and bound scenarios in areas where, at present, they "don't know how to think about what would happen". This strategy will enable them to feel safe in the knowledge of what options are open to them were any unexpected consequence to materialise. Janis and Mann (1977) describe a way of solving this through outcome psychodrama, where the client is asked to suppose that he or she had decided on a particular option, and then to imagine, one year in the future, having a "heart-to-heart talk with a friend", "at a time of a crisis when things were going very badly, worse than you thought they would" (Janis and Mann, 1977, p.381). The aim of this procedure is to combat defensive avoidance, with the reassuring presence of the counsellor as the audience for the heart-to-heart talk providing a temporary background of safety so that the client can explore in directions from which he or she would otherwise have shied away. During the ensuing "outcome psychodrama", the client is encouraged not only to explore worst case consequences further, but also to "work out ways of reassuring himself", and the counselor supports the client's efforts to arrive at effective reassuring beliefs by "supplying him with accurate new information about how potential setbacks (uncovered during scenario exploration) can be handled or their effects mitigated" (Janis and Mann, 1977, p.395).

In this way, the background of safety remains extended in the mind of the client, ways of bounding previously avoided and unbounded aspects of worst case scenarios have been discovered, and stored in memory for future use if and when required. Thus, at this level, one is not interested so much in aiding the client to assess the probabilities of the risks involved, but to characterise what such probabilities might refer to, and to anticipate and evaluate realistic ways of coping with feared outcomes.

Level 4 : Problem expressing language

The manner in which a prospective parent explores within the boundaries of the small world comprising genetic risk scenarios effectively sets the constraints within which he or she will express issues that need to be structured and assessed in order to arrive at a decision. The simplest way of expressing the problem is to define a single frame within which options may be conceptualised : for example, a "multiattribute frame", where the problem is structured through identifying those criteria (attributes) which are important for the person in distinguishing between alternative consequences. For example, a prospective parent knowing that she faces the risk that any future offspring may have Down's syndrome, may express the problem simply as how to characterise the positive and negative attributes of the consequences "remain childless", "bear a normal child" and "bear a child with Down's syndrome", and as how to make trade-offs between these attributes as a basis for choice between the options of whether or not to try to conceive a child.

Humphreys and Berkeley (1985) describe how decision theory in its current state of development, provides a technology for developing structure within four different types of frames in representing the types of uncertainty which may have to be faced in decision making under risk. The multiattribute frame is one of these four, and is focussed on resolving expressed uncertainty about how to evaluate the benefits and drawbacks of consequences. The other three frames aid the resolution of uncertainty about subsequent events concerning (i) the impact of what has preceded them in an act-event sequence in a forward moving scenario, (ii) the impact of influencing events extraneous to the forward moving scenario, and (iii) the impact of prior beliefs or historical information in determining the likelihood of particular events.

These four decision analytic frames are distinguished in <u>analytical terms</u> , that is, concerning the resolution of particular types of uncertainty irrespective of the substance of the problem expressed. There is, however, no automatic requirement that the frames identified within a person's problem expressing language should belong to an analytic, rather than a substantive taxonomy. On the contrary, von Winterfeldt (1980) has described how, in handling real problems, decision analysts prefer to distinguish frames according to their <u>substantive</u>, rather than analytical features, and Beach et al. (1984) have described how intuitive decision makers (students), faced with a set of ten decision making tasks commonly used in psychological experiments, always chose to classify them into frames based on substantive features (e.g., "problems about people", "maths problems", and so on).

In fact, there can be no fixed definition of what is a "right" or "wrong" frame for use in problem expressing language. Operating at level 4, a stakeholder in a decision problem involving genetic risk is able to exercise his or her discretion on the selection and utilisation of frames through the use of problem expressing language. Each prospective parent, and any genetic counsellor they consult about their options, is in some sense a "problem owner" (Checkland, 1984), but the problems they own are not necessarily the same, even if they are located within the same, agreed small world. The counsellor may seek to express the problem in terms of frames which reduce uncertainty about medical investigative and diagnostic procedures during pregnancy, about the typical nature and progress of disability associated with a particular genetic syndrome, and about the support procedures (community, institutional, therapeutic) available should the disability manifest itself in the client's offspring. A prospective mother, hoping to resume her career after childbirth might, equally legitimately, wish to express the problem in terms of frames which characterise her role in caring at home for a mongol child, in order to evaluate the change of lifestyle which would then be imposed on her, and whether she would have to give up that part of her identity which she found in her "career world" (Parkes, 1971; 1975). The prospective father, never considering an interruption in his career, might be especially concerned with expressing the effects on his lifestyle and relationship with his partner which would result from their both becoming parents of (i) a normal child, or (ii) an abnormal child.

In the above example, and in general, the problem owners' idiosyncratic choice of frames may lead to a successful handling of his or her own problem, provided that structure can be developed within the frame in an appropriate way to handle the aspect of the problem delegated for consideration within each frame selected. For example, it is little use deciding that part of the problem should be handled within a frame identified as "effects on relationship with partner" if one has no idea of how to characterise and structure such "effects" within the frame.

The problem expressing language which stakeholders are likely to want to use in representing genetic risks, and the consequences entailed by decisions involving such risks, usually involves more than each stakeholder matching a problem to a particular frame that he or she wishes to employ. Rather, it can be understood as a way of generating and linking together the various frames which a person may wish to use. Even when a pair of prospective parents locate their genetic risk decision problem within the same small world, they can still find each other's problem expressing language incomprehensible because they are each using it to link different frames in different ways. This problem is quite commonly encountered in doctor-patient interactions (Robinson, 1978; Katon and Kleinman, 1981; Zola, 1981; Berkeley, 1985). It also causes difficulties in negotiations between prospective parents, particularly where they anticipate different roles in coping with possible consequences of the decision that they will make (Haley, 1976).

Analysing problem expressing language

Within the interview, discussion and argumentation of situations which typically characterise sharing views between stakeholders to a decision involving genetic risk, problem expressing language can be considered as directed natural language discourse. Methods for analysing discourse usually identify propositions as the fundamental structural units of interest (Anderson, 1976; van Dijk and Kintsch, 1983). However, if propositions are viewed simply as syntactically organised sets of words (i.e., phrases) then we are left with the problem of how to "fix the meaning" of these words in a denotational sense. Structural representations based on selection and linking words with clear denotational referents (in terms of acts and events in the world of implementation of the problem solution) involve the development of highly complex patterns of linkages. The alternative strategy of keeping the structural linkage simple by using language to construct what are in effect "cognitive maps" (Axelrod, 1976; Eden et al., 1980) often requires the use of words or phrases with complex signification (e.g., "child has Down's syndrome") as semantic primitives. Direct "fixing" of denotational meaning is difficult in these cases, which is one reason why cognitive maps have rarely been found to provide an effective guide to reasoned action in supporting decision making under risk.

An approach which we prefer is to analyse knowledge representations present in problem expressing language in terms of the frames which are being proposed by the speaker for exploration, development, or use in representing risks and arriving at a decision. (The denotational meaning expressed within each frame can subsequently be investigated separately through operations developing structure within that frame). Thus, cognitive operations at level 4 are viewed as setting the agenda for problem structuring in a way that can transform desires and fears into action, but the analysis of the problem structuring process is completed piecemeal (within each frame identified) at level 3 in ways we shall outline later.

One way of displaying differences between stakeholders at level 4 is simply to list the frames that each person identifies as relevant in handling the decision. However, two other types of priorities are important in analysing the problem expressing language of those parties to a decision who know that other stakeholders may hold different views, and hence need to be argued with, or persuaded about the issues which need to be taken into account. Hogberg (1984) and Vari et al. (1986) have identified these as <u>warrants</u> and <u>backing</u> , following Toulmin's (1958) argumentation theory. For example, a prospective parent may suggest to his partner "I think that, rather than making a final choice now, we should explore the option to have an amniocentesis later on at sixteen to twenty weeks, after conception, and then consider the possibility of an abortion if the results of the test indicate foetal abnormalities. Doctor X says that the results are very reliable, and he promises that, in the case of an abnormality being indicated, there would be no difficulty or embarrassment involved in obtaining an abortion."

The first sentence quoted above expresses a frame within which the person would like an aspect of the decision problem to be structured. The second sentence provides the warrant for including the frame in the representation of the genetic risk decision problem (exploring issues involving amniocentesis and abortion are (i) likely to reduce uncertainty about the genetic risk, and (ii) not likely to complicate the decision situation significantly). It also contains the backing ("Doctor X says..." implying medical expertise and experience).

Differences between the types of frames identified in stakeholders' problem expressing language may not be obstructive when the way the decision problem is to be structured is negotiated amongst themselves, with each stakeholder employing warrants and backing which are accepted by the others. In this way a "requisite" decision structure can evolve (Rowbottom, 1977; Phillips, 1984) which each party recognises as a legitimate basis for a group decision making process on a genetic risk problem. However, difficulties arise when warrants and backing are not accepted. For instance, the suggestion made in the above example may be rejected by the stakeholder to whom it is addressed (the proposer's partner) because, (i) on moral grounds she does not want to even consider an abortion, however medically justified or straightforward the procedure might be (rejection of warrant), (ii) she does not trust doctors (rejection of backing).

In cases where frames are not shared across stakeholders and warrants and/or backing for their inclusion in the problem representation are rejected by one or more parties to the decision, these differences must first be resolved at the level 4 through negotiating problem expressing language, before developing structure at level 3 within frames whose legitimacy in representing risks would otherwise be disputed.

Level 3 : Developing structure within a particular frame

Operations represented at level 3 are concerned exclusively with developing structure within a particular frame identified within whatever knowledge representation was developed (or selected on the basis of "received wisdom") to characterise a genetic risk problem through the use of problem expressing language at level 4. For example, if a selected frame has the function of providing an evaluation of (multiattributed) consequences, then, within this frame, development of structure implies eliciting and re-defining the set of attributes to be included in a multi-attribute utility structure (Humphreys and McFadden, 1980; Edwards and Newman, 1982; Berkeley and Humphreys, 1982).

Structuring risks within a particular frame : an example

Beach et al. (1976) have described in detail how such structuring was performed in the pilot studies which led to the development of their Optional Parenthood Questionnaire (Beach et al., 1978). The introduction to the questionnaire explains the use that it "may help you to decide whether or not to have (another) child at this time in your life. It will help you explore your attitudes about parenthood and to rationally consider the pros and cons of the many issues involved." The questionnaire is structured within a single multiattribute utility frame (i.e., a decomposed and structured value frame). Beach et al. (1976, p.103) give the following warrant for this frame being important, indeed dominant, in this type of decision problem.
"A recently developing subsection of the birth planning literature has focussed on the kinds of values (utilities) that children seem to satisfy for parents and, implicitly or explicitly, assumes that birth planning decisions are rationally related to the satisfaction of these values (e.g., Fawcett and Arnold, 1973; Hoffman and Hoffman, 1973)".
This warrant, which indicates the existence of a body of research rather than a universal preoccupation of prospective parents, does not guarantee that the frame of the Optional Parenthood Questionnaire will automatically be welcomed by all stakeholders in a decision of whether or not to attempt to conceive a child. For instance, in the example given in the previous section, where amniocentesis was expressed as an issue for consideration, and the two prospective parents disagreed over the frame to be used in handling that aspect of their decision problem, neither of them expressed the desire to use a value-based frame.

While this implies that decision aiding procedures based within single frames should be offered as panaceas within counselling on genetic risk decision problems, the strength of the warrant still indicates that the Optional Parenthood Questionnaire might well deserve a place within a library of (single-frame) decision problem structuring and aiding tools (Humphreys, 1984) each of which can be selected for use in cases where the frames on which it is predicated is expressed by a stakeholder as relevant in handling his or her problem.
Working within a multiattribute frame, Beach et al. (1976) describe how they developed the structure of their questionnaire, starting from a list of values that children apparently fulfill for parents which they gleaned from the literature. This list was structured into a provisional value hierarchy, provisional in the sense that the list was considered too vague. The provisional structure was refined through interviews with seven married couples, aimed at identifying value-laden outcomes. The descriptions of these outcomes were copied onto "outcome cards", and subsequently sorted by the couples into hierarchically ordered classes, which they could revise and develop during the sorting process. The value hierarchy

developed by each couple was thus a composite of "received wisdom" (the hierarchy offered to them at the start of the sorting process) and their own value-structuring operations.

Representing differences in structures developed within a frame

If the various stakeholders in a decision can agree on the components of the structure developed within a particular frame, then differences between them can be represented at level 3 in terms of the differences of emphasis they place on each of the components in the structure. If we can resolve these differences, we can treat the structures as fixed and proceed to the two lower levels in the multilevel scheme for representing risks. In the example described above, Beach et al. (1976) appointed one of their research team to "retire with all the outcome decks and hierarchies to try to coalesce all of the material into a representative final outcome deck and a final hierarchy". They then used two large groups of subjects to test whether the result was meaningful to persons other than those who had participated in the development. Given reasonable indications of acceptability, this "final" hierarchy was then employed to provide the fixed structure within which prospective parents could indicate the values and relative importances they each attributed to its various components through completing the Optional Parenthood Questionnaire.

This approach, relying on the acceptability of a generic structure of (presumed) fixed denotation to all parties to a decision, is common in the literature on perception of environmental risks (e.g., Slovic et al., 1979; Vlek and Stallen, 1980; Humphreys and Berkeley, in press), where the assumption of the acceptability of use of the generic structure is rarely questioned. However, investigations of stakeholders' acceptance of an a priori-defined structure in real-life social decision making (Linnerooth, 1984) and counselling situations (Wooler, 1985) has indicated that it is generally preferable to negotiate a "requisite" structure between stakeholders, acceptable to all parties, rather than impose a generic one which may fail to represent key components of risks experienced by one or more stakeholders as governing their decision (Katon and Kleinman, 1981; Berkeley and Humphreys, 1982; Humphreys and Berkeley, 1985). It is possible to provide decision aids which support this negotiation process, but they are usually computer based, as they must possess interactive re-structuring capability at level 3 (Humphreys and Berkeley, 1985).

Level 2 : Exploring "what if" questions

The result of the operations carried out at level 3 is a decision problem representation whose structure is now conditionally fixed : all the syntax is in place. At level 2, there is no longer any discretion over, say, which attributes are to be considered in a multi-attribute utility structure, but sensitivity analysis may be used to explore "what-if" questions about the impact of changing values at nodes or reference points within the structure developed at level 3. An example would be changing the probability of a particular subsequent event (e.g., "the amniocentesis indicates abnormality") to see what effects are propagated throughout the decision tree structure in which that event is embedded. Hence, at level 2, the content manipulated within the structure is not "facts" (where the decision maker is expected to exercise discretion over their true value) but hypotheses (opinions, views, etc.). At this level it is explicitly recognised, for example, that probabilities can vary according to prospective parents' varying views on future states of the world and that their utilities may vary in reflecting the range of stakeholders' roles, interests and preferences within the various options considered in facing the genetic risk problem.

Explaining differences at level 2

The advantage of exploring the dynamic properties of different stakeholders' problem representations at level 2 within a fixed frame is that the resulting sensitivity analysis may indicate nodes of crucial interest within the structure where change of values makes very little impact (e.g., that defining a choice between immediate courses of action like "try to conceive a child" and "take precautions to avoid conception"), or where views of the stakeholders conflict (e.g., concerning the desirability of a therapeutic abortion).

If differences in stakeholders' opinions are found to impact on crucial points in the decision process, then they can be discussed in a focussed way, so that the compromise which is reached limits the regret experienced by a stakeholder who accepts a decision which goes against his or her own assessment of the best course of action at a particular point. This is because he or she is now able to identify exactly those issues in the representation of risks where a compromise has been made, and can be reassured that the rest of the decision making process fully accords with his or her beliefs and values.

Level 1 : Making best assessments

At level 1, the only degree of discretion left for the decision maker is to decide on how to make a "best assessment" of the value to be assigned to each node in the knowledge representation whose structure has now been completely fixed through the operations carried out at the higher levels. Making best assessments is necessary in order to determine the tradeoffs between the various courses of action structured within the problem representation, so that one can choose what to do. An example of a case where a person is accorded discretion only in representing the problem at level 1 would be a self-assessment "genetic risk preference questionnaire" in which each question is prespecified and the person is only allowed to check a box indicating his or her answer (from a pre-defined set), or provide a response on a predefined scale.

In general, the freedom accorded to a person operating at level 1 is to decide the assessment of the value to be assigned to each node in the knowledge representation whose structure has now been completely fixed through the operations carried out at the higher levels. This implies deciding what the appropriate referent would be for the assessment. For example, should a prospective parent use his or her own subjective assessment or consider the opinion of an expert (e.g., physician, consultant, counsellor), or other stakeholders (e.g., sponsors, parents) in forming the assessment?

Once the representation of risks has been completed by making best assessments at level 1, prescriptions for action can be made through "rolling back" the decomposed information about risks distributed throughout the fixed frames negotiated as requisite for expressing the problem within a shared small world (Raiffa, 1968). The result is an estimate of the relative attraction and riskiness of each course of action under consideration for the person whose assessments are modelled at level 1, conditional on how the constraints were set at all higher levels.
If the result is not acceptable to one or more stakeholders in the decision it is then necessary to re-examine how the various higher-level constraints were set, and thus discover the level at which adjustment or negotiation is necessary as a precursor for displaying differences or for setting the constraints on how risks are represented in a new way which will better reflect the interests of the parties to the decision.

Aiding the representation of genetic risks : received wisdom versus taking responsibility for cognitive operations

So far, we have discussed the general form of the cognitive operations involved in representing risks at each of five levels of abstraction and have hinted that sometimes the results of these operations may be inherited as "received wisdom" by some, or all, of the stakeholders in a decision problem. Sometimes a stakeholder may wish to take the responsibility for carrying out the appropriate cognitive operations at a particular level for himself or herself, thus ensuring that the problem representation developed at that level really is his or her own , and therefore can act as a secure basis for rationalising any regret subsequently associated with whatever outcome actually occurs (Parkes, 1971; Janis and Mann, 1977;

Jungermann, 1980).
This does not, however, imply that we should strive to ensure that all parties to a decision take responsibility for the cognitive operations they use in handling the problem at all levels, since they may well have no experience, or confidence in their capabilities to do this, particularly at the higher levels of abstraction. It is no use insisting on the use of a multilevel scheme which involves cognitive operations which the actual participants in the decision process are unable or unwilling to carry out in practice.

Thus, it is necessary to appreciate that any decision aiding programme which aims to support participants in their use of cognitive operations at progressive levels of abstraction must build on their process of cognitive development. Moving upwards through the levels our scheme starts at the level of cognitive development that Piaget (1972; 1977) calls concrete operational (level 1) the entry points for any theory of cognitive decision making. In order to move to the second level (equivalent to Piaget's formal operational level), a person must be fully conversant with the operations used at the first level, so that patterns of principles underlying these operations (the form at level 1) can itself be used as an operator at the next level. Lack of experience of, or appropriate feedback from, problem structuring operations at one level effectively prohibits a decision maker's progress to the next level.

A prospective parent, aware of the presence of genetic risks but who is willing to take responsibility for operations located <u>only</u> at level 1, will tend to view the decision problem as a purely medical problem, and the assistance any genetic counsellor may offer as equivalent to the assistance a physician may offer to a patient (Berkeley, 1985). This reasoning goes as follows : "One has a problem and one's responsibility lies only in describing one's condition and feelings as well as one possibly can to the doctor/counsellor through answering his or her questions. It is the doctor/counsellor's responsibility to diagnose the problem and propose the best solution. If the solution is unacceptable, then perhaps the fault lies with the doctor/counsellor as he or she may not be skilled or knowledgeable enough to handle the problem, or not sympathetic enough, and thus assistance should be sought elsewhere". This level 1 approach amounts in fact to seeking a magical solution : risks are not represented (as handling them is the responsibility of the person who tells the person what to do); contingency plans are not appreciated ("under the counsellor's guidance I'll cross my bridges when I come to them") and, in the event of an outcome which causes regret, the person will blame himself or herself, blame the counsellor, or anyone else who gave advice which was taken, without any real understanding of the basis for the regret, the risks that were run, or how to cope with the outcome.

For these reasons it is desirable for genetic counsellors to seek to establish a dialogue with their clients at level 2 at least. Here the client will still rely on the counsellor to define the frame(s) which are relevant in handling the problem and fix the structure within the frame, but the client will wish to explore alternative pathways, and their implementations, and be interested in the implications of differences between his or her own point of view, as represented within the structure, and those of other stakeholders in the decision problem. He or she would be likely to appreciate the chance to complete Beach et al's (1978) Optional Parenthood Questionnaire or other pre-structured decision aids addressing currently salient frames, and would find these kind of activity useful in deciding upon choice of action and anticipation of the degree of risks involved; and in making contingency plans to cope with such risks (Pauker and Pauker, this volume).

Difficulties occur at this level when the decision maker feels uneasy about the structures which are being offered as constraints within which to frame his or her problem, as somehow not really appropriate for capturing his or her anxieties and uncertainties about the risks involved, or hopes for possible compensations. Such difficulties can only be resolved through the use of cognitive operations at level 3, where the decision maker takes responsibility for developing a requisite structure for handling the problem within each frame selected. Only a few decision aids currently exist which have the capability for supporting the development of structure in personal decision making (Humphreys, 1984; Wooler, 1985) but aiding clients to operate at this level is a major goal of psychodynamically inclined therapists who may view the essence of a client's problem as inappropriate (or unrealistic) structuring of problem frames, thus trapping themselves in a web of anticipated regret and frustration, and an inability to uncover "silver linings" for themselves : that is, ways of understanding or creating the options which can offer hope and fulfillment when facing the need to cope with the fears associated with an awareness that genetic risks impact on their plans for the future (Haley, 1976; Janis and Mann, 1977).

Few people wish to take responsibility for cognitive operations required to develop (rather than use) problem expressing language at level 4. Conscious setting of bounds at level 5 is an impossibility as it is equivalent to having conscious control of what is in fact the whole of one's unconscious (Lacan, 1977) : a person who could do this would be able to change his real (rather than assumed) identities at will.

Thus, at level 4 a person usually considers his or her own problem expressing language simply to be his or her natural language, without awareness that there is a history to why this language seems "natural" in the particular context, and that the received wisdom that comprises this history may have been generated within motivated social and cultural structures within which the decision maker is positioned according to his or her sex, class, religion and so forth (Barthes, 1972; Douglas and Wildavsky, 1982). Dealing with the difficulties such positioning generates for constructive decision making in the face of genetic risk, however, requires an analysis which goes beyond the representation of risks (i.e., the scope of this paper), addressing and investigating the cultural and social structures which underly stakeholders' conceptualisations of what genetic risks are actually about.

References

Anderson, J.R.
Language, thought and memory.
Hillsdale, New Jersey : Erlbaum, 1976.

Antonovsky, A.
Health, stress and coping.
San Francisco : Jossey-Bass, 1980.

Auerbach, C.
The science of genetics.
London : Hutchinson, 1969.

Axelrod, R.
The analysis of cognitive maps.
In : R. Axelrod (ed), Structure of decision, Princeton, New Jersey : Princeton University Press, 1976.

Barthes, R.
Mythologies.
St. Albans : Paladin, 1972.

Beach, L.R., Christensen-Szalanski, J.J.J. and Barnes, V.
On the quality of judgement : Bad News or Bad Press?
Paper presented at the Fourth International Symposium on Forecasting, London, 1984.

Beach, L.R., Townes, B.D., Campbell, F.L. and Keating, G.W.
Developing and testing a decision aid for birth planning decisions.
Organizational Behavior and Human Performance 15, 99-116, 1976.

Beach, L.R., Townes, B.D. and Campbell, F.L.
The Optional Parenthood Questionnaire : a guide to decision making about parenthood.
Baltimore, Maryland : National Organization for Nonparents, 1978.

Berkeley, D.
Negotiating personal reality : a systems' study of people referred to a hospital outpatient psychotherapy department.
Unpublished PhD dissertation. London : University of London, 1985.

Berkeley, D. and Humphreys, P.C.
Structuring decision problems and the "bias heuristic".
Acta Psychol. 50, 201-252, 1982.

Berkeley, D., Humphreys, P.C. and Davidson, D.
Demands made on the general practice by women before and after an abortion.
Journal of Royal College of General Practitioners 34, 310-315, 1984.

Checkland, P.
Systems thinking, systems practice.
Chicester : Wiley (2nd edition), 1984.

Douglas, M.
Purity and danger.
London : Routledge and Kegan Paul, 1966.

Douglas, M. and Wildavsky, A.
Risk and culture.
London : Sage, 1982.

Eden, C., Jones, S. and Sims, C.
Thinking in organizations.
London : Macmillan, 1980.

Edwards, W. and Newman, J.R.
Multiattribute evaluation.
Sage University Paper Series on Quantitative Applications in the Social Sciences 07-026. Beverley Hills and London : Sage, 1982.

Fawcett, J.T. and Arnold, F.S.
The value of children : theory and method.
Representative Research in Social Psychology 4, 53-65, 1973.

Haley, J.
Problem-solving therapy : new strategies for effective family therapy.
San Francisco : Jossey-Bass, 1976.

Hoffman, C.W. and Hoffman, M.L.
The value of children to parents.
In : J.T. Fawcett (ed), Psychological perspectives on population. New

York : Basic Books, 1973.

Hogberg, O.
Argumentation : a case study of the Swedish Energy Debate.
Department of Business Administration. Stockholm University, 1984.

Humphreys, P.C.
Levels of representation of decision problems.
Journal of Applied Systems Analysis 11, 3-22, 1984.

Humphreys, P.C. and Berkeley, D.
Problem structuring calculi and levels of knowledge representation in decision making.
In : R.W. Scholz (ed), Decision making under uncertainty. Amsterdam : North Holland, 1983.

Humphreys, P.C. and Berkeley, D.
Handling uncertainty : levels of analysis of decision problems.
In : G.N. Wright (ed), Behavioral decision making. New York : Plenum, 1985.

Humphreys, P.C. and Berkeley, D.
How to avoid misjudging judgement.
Social Behaviour, 1, (in press).

Humphreys, P.C. and McFadden, W.
Experiences with MAUD : aiding decision structuring versus bootstrapping the decision maker.
Acta Psychol. 45, 51-69, 1980.

Janis, I.L. and Mann, L.
Decision making. New York : The Free Press, 1977.

Jungermann, H.
Speculations about decision theoretic aids for personal decision making.
Acta Psychol. 45, 7-34, 1980.

Jungermann, H.
Psychological aspects of scenarios.
In : V. Corello et al (eds), Technology assessment, environmental impact assessment and risk analysis. Berlin : Springer Verlag, 1983.

Jungermann, H.
Construction and evaluation of scenarios from a psychological perspective.
Paper presented at the Fourth International Symposium on Forecasting,

London, 1984.

Katon, W. and Kleinman, A.
Doctor-patient negotiation and other social science strategies in patient care.
In : L. Eisenberg and A. Kleinman (eds), The relevance of social science for medicine. Dordrecht, Holland : Reidel, 1981.

Lacan, J.
The agency of the letter in the unconscious.
In : J. Lacan, Ecrits. London : Tavistock, 1977.

Leach, E.R.
Anthropological aspects of language : animal categories and verbal abuse.
In : E.H. Lenneberg (ed), New directions in the study of language. Cambridge, Mass. : M.I.T. Press, 1964.

Linnerooth, J.
The political processing of uncertainty.
Acta Psychol. 56, 219-232, 1984.

Marris, P.
Loss and change.
New York : Pantheon, 1974.

Parkes, C.M.
Psycho-social transitions : a field for study.
Soc. Sci. Med. 5, 101, 1971.

Parkes, C.M.
What becomes of redundant world-models? A contribution to the study of adaptation.
Brit. J. Med. Psychol. 48, 131, 1975.

Phillips, L.D.
A theory of requisite decision models.
Acta Psychol. 56, 29-48, 1984.

Piaget, J.
The principles of genetic epistemology.
London : Routledge and Kegan Paul, 1972.

Piaget, J.
The development of thought : equilibration of cognitive structures.
Oxford : Blackwell, 1977.

Raiffa, H.
Decision analysis : introductory lectures on choices under uncertainty.
Reading, Mass. : Addison Wesley, 1968.

Rakusen, J. and Davidson, N.
Out of our hands : what technology does to pregnancy. London : Pan Books, 1982.

Rowbottom, R.
Social analysis.
London : Heineman, 1977.

Robinson, D.
Patients, practitioners and medical care : aspects of medical sociology.
London : Heineman Medical Books (2nd edition), 1978.

Sandler, J. and Sandler, A.M.
On the development of object relations and affects.
Intern. J. Psychoanal. 59, 285-296, 1978.

Slovic, P., Fischhoff, B. and Lichtenstein, S.
Rating the risks.
Environment 21, 14-20 and 36-39, 1979.

Toda, M.
The decision process : a perspective.
Intern. J. Gen. Systems 3, 79-88, 1976.

Toulmin, S.
The uses of argument.
Cambridge : Cambridge University Press, 1958.

van Dijk, T.A. and Kintsch, W.
Strategies of discourse comprehension.
New York : Academic Press, 1983.

Vari, A., Vescenyi, J. and Paprika, Z.
Supporting problem structuring in high-level decisions.
In : B. Brehmer, H. Jungermann, P. Lourens and G. Sevon (eds), New Directions in Research on Decision Making. Amsterdam :North Holland, 1986.

Vlek, C.A.J. and Stallen, P.J.M.
Rational and personal aspects of risk.
Acta Psychol. 45, 273-300, 1980.

von Winterfeldt, D.
Structuring decision problems for decision analysis.
Acta Psychol. 45, 71-94, 1980.

Wagenaar, W.A., Keren, G. and Pleit-Kuiper, A.
The multiple objectives of gamblers.
Acta Psychol. 56, 167-178, 1984.

Wooler, S.
Let the decision maker decide : a case against assuming common occupational value structure.
J. Occupational Psychol. 58, 217-227, 1985.

Zola, I.K.
Structural constraints in the doctor-patient relationship : the case of non-compliance.
In : L. Eisenberg and A. Kleinman (eds), The relevance of social science for medicine. Dordrecht, Holland : Reidel, 1981.

EVALUATING DECISION AIDING TECHNOLOGIES FOR GENETIC COUNSELING

Gordon F. PITZ

Southern Illinois University, Carbondale, Illinois 62901, USA

In a review of research on judgment and decision making (Pitz and Sachs, 1984), I suggested that a measure of our understanding of human decision making is the ability to use current research and theory to help people make decisions. A technology for aiding decision making has emerged recently, based on psychological research and on developments in mathematical decision theory. Much of this technology has been devoted to decisions made in an organizational context (see Keeney, 1982). There are as yet only a few examples of decision aids devoted to personal decision making (career choice, for example; see Wooler and Wishuda, 1985). Pauker and Pauker (this volume) discuss the use of decision aids in making decisions about amniocentesis. The potential for using such aids has been recognized for some time (Jungermann, 1980), and their use is likely to increase. In this paper I explore some implications of decision aiding technology for the counseling of people who must make decisions in the face of genetic risks.

There are many difficult decisions that a person faces as a consequence of genetic disorders. It is reasonable to suppose that an understanding of judgment and decision making might help people deal with these problems. One must beware, however, of over-selling the technology. The usefulness of decision aiding procedures, especially for helping a person with a very difficult personal decision, is yet to be adequately documented. Only extensive research will determine whether the promise that seems to be offered by the technology can be fulfilled.

Decisions and other problems

I begin by summarizing some fundamental ideas and defining some basic terms. A <u>decision</u> is a problem in which some person (the decision maker)

Birth Defects: Original Article Series, Volume 23, Number 2, pages 251–278

is faced with a choice between at least two options, or alternative courses of actions. One assumes that the need to make a decision has been recognized by the decision maker. It is assumed also that the person's choice will be based on deliberations concerning the advantages and disadvantages of each option. I do not assume, of course, that the deliberation is careful or complete. Describing the decision maker's thought processes, explaining why they might not be as thorough as they should be, and suggesting techniques for helping a person with the deliberations, are basic problems for the psychologist who studies decision processes.

One can distinguish deliberative decision making from other, non-deliberative behavior. Much that is called "decision making" in non-technical discussions does not fit the definition given here, and one cannot expect theories of decision making to account for such behavior. This is especially true of habitual or impulsive reactions. For example, Natalie Sachs and I (Sachs and Pitz, 1981) studied women's decisions about contraception. We are often asked to explain why women "choose not to use birth control". The answer is that usually they do not so choose; there is no deliberation involved, and therein lies the problem.

One can also separate the problem of choosing an option from the problem of implementing the choice. The theoretical treatment of decision making usually ends once a choice has been made; translating the choice into action is a motivational concern that demands a different theoretical approach. Nevertheless, while the theoretical analysis may change, the problems of choice and implementation are not separate ones for the decision maker.

These points illustrate a major difficulty that arises when we use psychological theory and research to address important problems. Theories come in neatly packaged compartments; society's problems do not, and solutions to the problems demand approaches that cross disciplinary boundaries. Theoreticians usually prefer boundaries; they provide structure and definition in a complex world. A decision theorist has useful things to say about the decision making process when a person wants to make a careful and deliberate choice among several options. There will often be other concerns involved, however, that make the contributions of the decision theorist incomplete or irrelevant.

In discussing recent studies of decision making, I have in mind a prototypical problem that involves genetic risk. At several points I use the problem for illustrative purposes. In this hypothetical example it has been determined that there is, say, a probability .4 that a woman is a carrier for Duchenne Muscular Dystrophy. She is pregnant, and is wondering whether to abort the fetus. She is appalled by the prospects of giving birth to a son who will suffer from DMD, but has serious religious and moral objections to abortions. We have in this scenario all of the features of a classic problem studied by decision theorists : two or more options, uncertainty about the consequences of some of the options, well-defined probabilities for these outcomes, and conflicts among two or more values that the decision maker holds. A psychologist who studies decision making should be able to say something helpful to the woman or her counselor or physician.

By way of contrast to this hypothetical case, let me describe a real case. In one with which I am familiar, a woman was referred for diagnosis of a possible genetic disorder. She had two sons who had become deaf early in childhood, three normal children by a different father, and was pregnant again. She was only nineteen years old. For the health authorities, the problem has been defined as diagnosing possible genetic factors in the deafness and giving a prognosis for the new infant. For the patient, the problem was how to escape from an intolerable life style; she wanted to know how she could make arrangements for sterilization. There was no contribution that an expert on decision making could make, for by my definition there was no decision problem.

Normative and descriptive approaches to decision making

The next definitional issue I need to discuss, concerns the distinction between normative and descriptive theories of decision making. Briefly, a theory is normative if it purports to prescribe a person's decisions, i.e., to state which choice ought to be made. It is descriptive if it sets out to explain why or how a person made a particular choice. A normative theory would attempt to show that a particular choice was correct for the woman in the hypothetical example I gave earlier; a descriptive theory would attempt to explain her eventual decision.

The distinction is helpful in reminding us that theorists have approached decision making from different directions, and that there are different questions we might ask about decision problems. It is important to recognize, however, that the distinction is not as clear as at first it appears.

First, descriptive studies of decision making cannot avoid the problem of explaining rational behavior. Normative theories provide systematic treatments of rationality that have useful descriptive properties, so it is appropriate to ask to what degree the normative theory is also descriptive. Several descriptive theories have been derived from adaptations of normative theory; the best known of such approaches is Expected Utility (EU) theory. Based on the normative theories of Von Neumann and Morgenstern (1947), EU theory has been employed by many authors as a descriptive model (e.g., Edwards, 1954). The success of such attempts to describe behavior is still a matter of debate. Whatever the status of EU theory as a descriptive model, however, it is clear that uncertainty and value are important concepts when dealing with decisions. Both descriptive and normative theories must deal with these concepts in some way.

In the same way that descriptive theories must attend to normative considerations, normative theories cannot avoid descriptive issues. Normative models of decision making take as their starting point an axiomatic treatment of the decision maker's beliefs and values. The axioms include various independence assumptions, i.e., assumptions that the person's values and beliefs are stable and consistent in certain well-defined ways. In addition the normative theory assumes that beliefs and values can be expressed through statements of preference or by means of numerical judgments. In other words, normative theories are conditional; they prescribe a person's behavior given that certain assumptions are correct, and given certain expressions of belief or preference. The theories are prescriptions for consistent behavior; they cannot indicate that a certain choice is necessarily best, only that the choice is consistent with a person's other stated preferences. If a normative theory is to be effective, it must begin with an adequate description of those preferences, and there must be evidence that the underlying independence assumptions are correct.

The impossibility of separating normative and descriptive concerns is perhaps best seen in the development of multi-attribute forms of expected utility theory. The usefulness of EU theory is limited as long as utility is treated as a unitary construct. Significant problems involve many attributes of value, and often require the decision maker to resolve conflicts among values. When EU theory is expanded to recognize such conflicts explicitly, it becomes more useful. The best known extension is multi-attribute utility theory (MAUT), as developed by Keeney and Raiffa (1976). This approach to normative theory makes it clear that a normative solution to a problem depends on a descriptive analysis of the decision maker's concerns. It is this interaction of normative and descriptive theory that has led to the successful development of decision aiding technologies.

Decision analysis and decision aiding

In its broadest sense, a "decision aid" is any tool or technique that helps a person make a decision. It might include such diverse approaches as computerized spreadsheets, data base management systems, or so-called expert systems. I shall not address here the most general issues of decision aiding, although there are important psychological concerns in the design of such systems, and it might be interesting to explore their potential value in dealing with genetic disorders. In this paper, however, I am concerned only with those systems that help a decision maker deal with uncertainty and value conflicts. The term "decision analysis" refers to an approach to decision aiding that is based on a combination of normative and descriptive decision theory, and which generally uses some form of MAUT as its normative basis. A broader survey of decision aiding techniques, with primary emphasis on decision analysis approaches, is given by Wishuda (1985). Humphreys and Berkeley (1985) offer a more general perspective, in which decision analysis is presented as part of a hierarchical approach to the representation of decision problems.

Decision analysis can be defined as a set of formal procedures for helping a person arrive at an optimal decision. Keeney (1982) has described decision analysis as "a formalization of common sense for decision problems which are too complex for informal use of common sense." This definition captures the idea that the analysis helps decision makers arrive at their own choice, rather than imposing any prescriptions on them.

Keeney (1982) lists four characteristics of complex problems that make decision analysis appropriate : high stakes involved in choosing among options, a complicated structure for the problem, an absence of experts who can identify the best option, and a need to justify the decision to others. While he discusses these characteristics from the point of view of managerial decision making, it is apparent that they characterize genetic decisions also. The high stakes are obvious, for the quality of a person's life is affected by the outcome of a decision. The problems are made complex by the conflicting values and the emotional depth with which they are held. The need for justification may be less obvious. In a managerial context justification involves explaining a decision to another person; in a genetic counseling context it may involve justifying the decision to oneself (so that one can accept the decision and live with its consequences), or to members of one's family who have an interest in the final outcome.

Formal methods of decision making often elicit objections from both patients and counselors when used to guide highly emotional personal decisions. Some of these objections will be addressed later, but it may be helpful to explain why on a priori grounds a formal analysis should help a person make a decision.

Decision analysis procedures are sometimes justified by asserting that human judgment and decision making is seriously flawed, even irrational, if left unaided. The literature on heuristics and biases (Kahneman et al., 1982) is sometimes taken as evidence that one cannot trust decisions that a person makes intuitively. This literature is now widely known, and can be seen quoted in recent textbooks on, among other things, genetic counseling (Schild and Black, 1984). Unfortunately, it is not as widely known that there is still disagreement over the interpretation of the experimental results. It is premature to conclude that humans are "cognitive cripples", or that intuitive judgments are inherently irrational (see, e.g., Cohen, 1981; Hogarth, 1981).

It is better to think of decision analysis as a form of information processing assistance that is available when the quantity or complexity of relevant information creates difficulties for the decision maker. Formal decision making procedures can serve a need that is recognized by the decision maker, and they do not necessarily replace the decision maker. Consider the electronic calculator as an analogy. Calculators are accepted as useful aids to computation without assuming that people are incapable of performing arithmetic calculations. Simple arithmetic problems are solved faster without using a calculator, but as the problem grows more complex we recognize the need to rely on the speed and accuracy of a machine. There is a similar role that mechanical assistance can play in decision making. Simple judgments and decisions are best made without any mechanical assistance; more complex ones are made more easily if information processing help is available.

In a description of decision analysis techniques, Pitz and McKillip (1984) justify the use of decision analysis by the "principle of decomposition". This is the assumption that judgments are more reliable and more sensitive to relevant information when they are made with respect to simple events than when they concern complex events. Several experimental studies (reviewed by Pitz and McKillip) document the validity of this assumption. The principle provides a strong argument for using methods of analysis that decompose a problem into simpler elements. A decision analysis guarantees that the final decision will be consistent with the decision maker's judgments concerning the elements of the decomposition.

The evidence reviewed by Pitz and McKillip suggests that decision makers have difficulty in identifying the option that best matches their beliefs and values. When making decisions about complex, emotionally disturbing problems, a person is likely to make choices that are inconsistent with her stated preferences. Sachs (1984) examined the effects on behavior of inconsistency between choice and preference. She studied people's use of birth control methods, and compared the reliability of their use of contraception with the degree to which their chosen method of birth control was inconsistent with their expressed preferences. The latter were measured as they would be in a decision analysis. Those who exhibited the greatest inconsistency in their choices were most likely to use birth control unreliably. The lack of reliability presumably indicates dissatisfaction with the chosen method of birth control. The finding provides a strong justification for using formal decision analysis methods. It implies that the decision maker is more likely to accept a decision that is reached using such an analysis. One might predict that those whose decisions concerning genetic risk are guided by a formal analysis will be better able to live with those decisions later.

Decisions in genetic counseling

I turn to the problems that might be faced by a patient who is at risk of suffering from, or giving birth to children who suffer from, genetic disorders. To clarify the potential use of decision analysis with such problems, I quote Schild and Black's (1984) statement of the guiding principles of genetic counseling for social workers. There are perspectives on genetic counseling other than that of the clinical social worker. I quote these principles, however, because they make several points that should be considered by a physician or counselor who looks to judgment and decision theory for help, and by a decision theorist who hopes to provide that help. They offer a point of view that is not always recognized by those who take a formal approach to the analysis of decisions.

> 1. Clinical assessment is based on the biopsychosocial aspects of the person, the environment, and the interrelatedness between the two, including the nature of the resources in both.
>
> 2. Intervention, planning, and goal setting are based upon clinical assessment, relevant theory, and client agreement, addressed to the client's unique situation and not limited by professional preference or expertise of the worker.

Principle 1 provides a statement of the context in which decision analysis might be used. In particular, it illustrates my earlier point that the analysis of a decision cannot be carried out independently of other concerns and problems. Principle 2 suggests how and where a formal analysis of decisions might be helpful. As I shall show, the technology of decision analysis is fully consistent with the spirit of this principle.

> 3. Clinical assessment is an ongoing process that may result in alteration of goals, or the treatment made, and of services of assistance.

Principle 3 points out that a patient's problem can rarely be analyzed as a single decision. This is a perspective that needs to be recognized more explicitly by decision theorists. While in practice a decision analyst may recognize that real problems are dynamic, and develop gradually, typical textbook presentations of decision analysis do not always convey that impression. Connolly (1986) has discussed similar concerns that arise in managerial decision making. He contrasts the "tree felling" approach of traditional decision theory (decide which tree to chop down, then do it) with the "hedge-clipping" nature of most problems (trim a little, step back, evaluate the results, then trim a little more). The same principle applies to many significant decision problems, including those one finds in a genetic counseling context.

> 4. Evaluation of the effectiveness of the helping process is required.

This principle also deserves more concern by decision analysts. It is one to which every decision analyst subscribes in theory, but which is then often ignored in practice. Fischhoff (1980) has expounded at length on the need for evaluating decision analysis. One goal of this paper is to provide some overall evaluation of the effectiveness of decision analysis.

> 5. Clinical social work has the responsibility of documenting deficiencies in resources or harmful conditions for clients and initiating change by making these conditions known to professional and institutional systems. (page 75)

Principle 5 is one that differentiates clinical social work from many other disciplines. It is unlikely that decision analysts would readily consider themselves to be instruments for social change. Nevertheless, the possibility of acting in such a role, perhaps inadvertently, is one that needs to be discussed. The principle suggests some ethical dilemmas that decision analysts might have to confront.

The formal analysis of decisions

I provide here a simplified description of a typical decision analysis. The description hides several complications that are important. I return to many of the complications later, especially as they apply to problems of genetic counseling. Note also that the procedures described here should normally be preceded by less formal methods of the sort described by Humphreys and Berkeley (this volume). In their terminology, the analysis described here deals with uncertainties at level 3 and below, and assumes that uncertainties at higher levels have been satisfactorily resolved.

Earlier in this paper I described a prototypical decision problem involving issues of genetic risk. It is possible to construct a general framework within which to describe any such problem (see Figure 1). This framework consists of two intersecting tree structures. The outline shown in Figure 1 needs to be filled out with the exact details for any given problem.

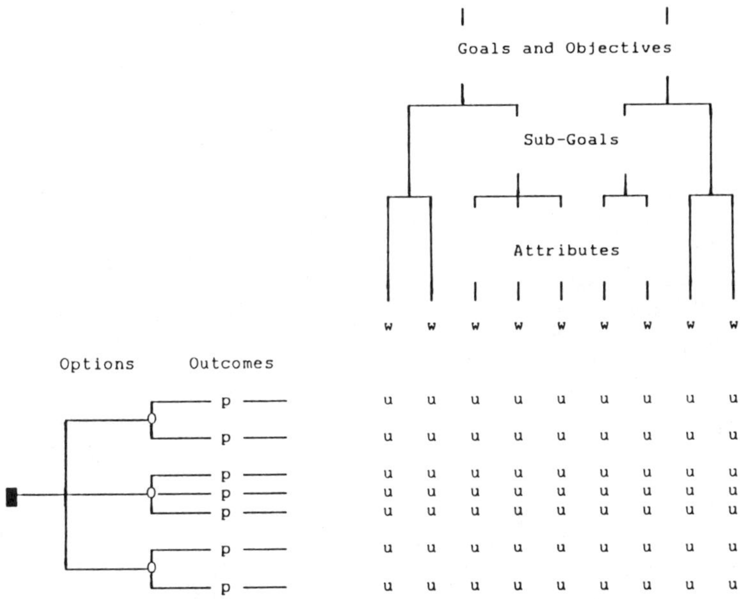

Figure 1 : Representation of a MAUT-based decision analysis.
A decision tree shows (from left to right) the sequence of options and probabilistic outcomes. A value tree represents (from top to bottom) the decision maker's goals and objectives. Three sets of quantities are included : probabilities (p) for each outcome, weights (w) for each attribute, and single-attribute utilities (u) for each cell of the matrix defined by the intersection of the two trees.

One tree structure describes the sequence of events that might unfold over time, and is usally referred to as a decision tree. The far left of this tree represents the present moment. The first set of branches represents the options available to the decision maker; the set might include aborting the fetus, conducting an amniocentesis and aborting only if the fetus is male, or going ahead with the planned childbirth. The chosen option may be followed by one of a number of probabilistic outcomes. If the pregnancy is not terminated, then the child will be either male or female; if male, it will or will not turn out to be affected by DMD, and so on. In a complex problem, each outcome may be followed by further decisions that have to be made, which are followed by further outcomes, and so on. A given sequence of decisions and outcomes traced out along the decision tree will be called a scenario. For complex, dynamic decisions the tree can grow very bushy, and extend into the indefinite future, unless simplifying assumptions are made. In many cases, however, the tree can be sharply abbreviated, only the immediate options being described explicitly. Concerns about the consequences of these options are then considered implicitly when evaluating the options.

The second tree structure represents the decision maker's value system (and so is called a value tree). At the top level the tree branches into a set of major goals or objectives that describe the decision maker's concerns: to enjoy having children of her own, to avoid the pain and suffering of disease, and so on. Top level goals are typically described in very broad, vague terms. For this reason they are further defined in terms of subgoals, which may be decomposed still further. Eventually one arrives at a set of attributes, which are more-or-less measurable properties that can be used to evaluate each scenario represented in the decision tree.

The intersection of the two trees creates a matrix; each cell of the matrix represents the decision maker's evaluation of a single scenario in terms of a single attribute. Eventually the quantities shown in Figure 1 need to be given numerical values. Briefly, one assigns probabilities (p) to the uncertain outcomes in the decision tree to indicate the likelihood of their occurrence, weights (w) to each branch of the value tree to indicate the impact of each attribute, and utilities (u) that represent the attractiveness of each cell of the scenario-attribute matrix. These quantities should reflect the beliefs and preferences of the decision maker.

Once a decision problem has been described in this way, it is possible to use the mathematical rules of EU theory and of MAUT to select an "optimal" choice for the decision maker. An aggregation rule can be used to calculate a utility or expected utility for each available option. The optimal choice is the one with maximum aggregate utility or expected utility. (The description here is intentionally terse; see, e. g., Keeney and Raiffa, 1976, or Pitz and McKillip, 1984, for all the mathematical and calculational details. They are not important for present purposes).

In principle, an analysis of this sort, based on the theoretical assumptions that underlie MAUT, provides a solution to the decision maker's problem. In practice, of course, it is not that simple. At every stage of the analysis there are potential difficulties to be overcome. These complications can be categorized in terms of the three major stages involved in a decision analysis. These are :

1. Problem modeling, in which the decision tree and value tree are created.
2. Quantification, in which the probabilities, weights, and utilities are assigned.
3. Synthesis, in which the appropriate aggregation rule is used to derive a solution to the problem, and the effect of changes in the

analysis are observed.

I review these stages in turn, particularly as they might apply to a problem of genetic risk.

Defining the problem

In the first stage of the analysis the problem has to be defined according to the format required for a formal analysis. The decision maker must decompose her problem into its separate elements, using the tree structures outlined in the previous section. The elements to be defined are the options, outcomes, goals and attributes. There appears to be general agreement that this problem definition stage can be beneficial for the decision maker (e.g., Humphreys and McFadden, 1980; Jungermann, 1980). The process of identifying the options, defining possible consequences of each option, and specifying the goals or objectives, can help the person better understand the problem. Many decision aids offer assistance to the decision maker in creating a structure for the analysis. Such assistance is essential, for, as I point out below, there are many sources of difficulty that confront a decision maker who is asked to define his or her problem, and the analysis cannot be effective unless the problem definition is adequate.

The first step in defining the problem is to identify the decision maker. While in some cases this a trivial exercise, it is sometimes necessary to give the issue some thought. A problem may involve many people - the patient, the counselor, members of the patient's family, the patient's physician, and perhaps others. Each of these individuals may be faced with a decision that he or she must make. It is important to recognize that the decision problem is not the same for all of these people. A description of the options, for example, will depend on the identity of the decision maker. The patient's options might be to abort or not; the counselor's options might be to intervene in this decision or not. The decisions interact, and methods for describing these interactions must be developed, but confusion results when one decision maker proceeds as if his or her options were someone else's.

The identification of the decision maker is also important when considering goals and objectives. The counselor and the patients may hold different sets of values, and these values affect their decision in different ways. Schild and Black (1984) describe the problems that arise when the counselor's values conflict with the patient's. Only by making it explicit that different decision makers face different problems can one effect any resolution of the conflict. It is essential, therefore, to determine the "owner" of a particular problem (a term suggested by Checkland, 1981). In some cases there are multiple decision makers - the patient and the family, the patient and the counselor - who jointly own a problem. Pitz and McKillip (1984) discuss a number of procedures that can be used when several people share ownership in a problem. They introduce the concept of an "audience" to a decision : the patient is an audience to the counselor's decision, the counselor to the patient's. The goals of members of the audience are relevant to the decision maker, but not directly as goals for the decision maker. Consider the possible role of family members in an analysis of the patient's decision. The patient's parents may have a desire for grandchildren - that is one of their goals. Pleasing the parents may be a goal for the patient. The patient's evaluation of an option in terms of her own goal should reflect her knowledge of the parent' goal, but the two goals are not equivalent.

Once a clear understanding has been achieved of whose decision problem is to be addressed, further difficulties arise when the decision maker is asked to describe the important elements of the problem. A patient may not be able to recognize all of the available options, especially if she is under severe emotional duress. Helping a person recognize new options is one of the most valuable contributions that a counselor can make. Procedures for suggesting new options have been discussed and validated by Pitz, Sachs, and Heerboth (1980). The methods involve using the value tree component of the problem description as a device for helping the decision maker develop the decision tree. Pitz, Sachs and Brown (1980) have shown that these procedures can sometimes be more effective than traditional counseling approaches.

It is equally important that the decision maker include all the significant consequences of each option. There is a tendency to view the future in terms of deterministic scenarios that then affect the interpretation of options and outcomes. It is not easy to persuade people to think about the uncertainties that are associated with options. Failure to assess the consequences of a decision realistically is especially troublesome when considering undesirable outcomes. Consider the studies of fault trees reported by Fischhoff, Slovic, and Lichtenstein (1978). When people are asked to identify ways in which an undesirable outcome can occur, they often fail to include entire categories of events. The result may be a serious misjudgment of the desirability of an option. Unless a decision maker has considered all consequences of the chosen option, it is unlikely that he or she will find the choice to be satisfactory later on.

Defining the value tree to be used in an analysis may be even more difficult than defining the options and outcomes that make up the decision tree. Goals, objectives, and attributes are usually not concepts that are well understood by a decision maker who is unfamiliar with formal methods of analysis. When eliciting a description of a person's values, one is asking that person to use a vocabulary and an abstract structure that is unfamiliar and may be incompatible with her own representation of the problem (Pitz and Reidel, 1984). Adelman, Sticha, and Donnell (1986) show that the form of the value tree depends on the procedure that is used to elicit the decision maker's values. The best procedure, then, is one that employs several approaches, and seeks convergence among the different results that might be obtained. Pitz, Sachs and Brown (1980) have described procedures that are effective in helping a person identify his or her goals and objectives. Like the suggested methods for eliciting options, they depend on using one part of the problem structure to suggest others. More recent research in my laboratory has extended this work. We have shown that when decision makers are asked to think about one of the tree structures used to define a problem (the decision tree or the value tree), they are better able to define the elements in the other.

One approach that avoids the difficulty people experience in creating their own structure is to use a pre-defined description of the problem. Either the decision tree or the value tree or both may be created by some "expert". The decision maker's role can then be restricted to eliminating those elements that are irrelevant for his or her particular situation. The analysis is simplified if a complete description of the problem can be provided initially. Sachs and Pitz (1981), for example, developed an aid for contraceptive decision making in which the options and attributes were clearly defined for the decision maker. The approach was very successful, since the problem is very similar for everyone who has to choose a method of contraception. Most genetic counseling problems are not of this sort, and capturing the individual features of the problem is an important step in the analysis. Wooler and Wishuda (1985) discussed the problem of defining the attributes to be used in a decision aid used for career counseling. They suggested using a combination of pre-specified attributes and user-generated attributes, perhaps employing an "expert systems" technology to help decision makers identify relevant attributes. This combined use of a pre-defined structure and a structure provided by the decision maker might be advantageous for some frequently recurring genetic problems.

When decisions concern such value-laden issues as genetic disease, abortion, and sterilization, it is not easy for the decision maker to think about the problem in the analytic form demanded by a formal analysis. The issues are what Janis and Mann (1977) call "hot" problems, in which intellectualized approaches of the kind described here are more difficult to use than they are for the "cold" problems one normally associates with formal analysis. Decomposed descriptions of hot problems seem to some people to violate important intuitions about the problem, intuitions that cannot be captured in the structure and vocabulary of decision analysis. Nevertheless, the justification for using a decomposed description of the problem is strong enough that it is worth some effort to help people define their problem in this way.

If a decision maker finds it difficult to define the fundamental elements of her problem, it may be helpful to use practice problems that deal with other, less emotional problems. There is evidence from a recently completed study in my own laboratory that people can learn to decompose complex problems into options and goals. One of the results of this study was that teaching people heuristic rules to use in decomposing a problem was just as effective as a more traditional feedback procedure. That is, people can learn how to decompose a problem without being told the "correct" decomposition. This is important when dealing with problems for which no correct representation exists outside the private experience of the decision maker. We do not yet know if this procedure can help a person accept a formal analysis of a hot problem after suitable learning has occurred with cold ones, but it is a prospect that is worth investigating.

Phillips (1984) has discussed the process of defining decision problems as part of a decision analysis. He argues that the process is successful if the decision maker, and any others who are involved in the analysis, arrive at a new and satisfactory understanding of the problem. This understanding is achieved by creating a simplified model of the problem, one in which the essential features are retained and unnecessary details are ignored. The model is considered suitable if it captures accurately all of the relevant intuitions that the decision maker has concerning the problem. The end result is a "requisite model", one that enables the decision maker to understand the problem clearly enough to be able to reach a solution. If the process works as Phillips suggests, then it will overcome the objections raised by those who find a decision analysis to be too intellectual and destructive of important features of the problem.

The quantitative analysis of a problem

The next step in a formal analysis involves the specification of probabilities, weights, and utilities. Numerical values must be placed on a person's beliefs and values, which is something that few people find easy to do. Like the decomposition process described in the previous section, quantification is aversive to those who find it inappropriate to make numerical judgments about feelings. In this section I review the quantification process briefly, point out some of the difficulties that arise, and suggest possible solutions.

I begin with a discussion of probabilities. Some treatments of MAUT suggest that the explicit introduction of probabilities is not necessary, and that it unduly complicates the analysis (Edwards and Newman 1982). It is true that a simple decision tree restricted to a list of options is often sufficient to describe a problem (see Pitz and McKillip, 1984, for ways of handling uncertainty without using probabilities explicitly). Nevertheless, with many genetic problems the probabilities are so salient that they should be included in the analysis directly. Otherwise one runs the risk of ignoring critical determinants of the utility of each option.

These salient probabilities will usually be defined very precisely by the geneticist; little or no input is required from the decision maker in generating the numbers. Other uncertainties may be included in the problem definition, however, that can only be quantified by the decision maker. For example, if one of the options being considered is to rely on birth control to prevent conception, one needs to know the probability of the birth control method's being effective. While there are general guidelines available that give population-wide probabilities of failure, the probability of conception with some methods depends on individuating factors, such as how effectively they are used. The probability of failure can then only be specified after gathering relevant data from the patient.

Regardless of the source of the numerical probability, one faces the problem of having the patient understand the meaning of these numbers. Wertz, Sorenson, and Heeren (1985) discuss some of the factors that are involved in clients' perceptions of risks expressed as probabilities. The perception of risk is a major topic that I shall not discuss here (see paper by Vlek, this volume). It is necessary, however, to consider some of the problems as they apply to a decision analysis. The empirical meaning of a probability is a subject of dispute among philosophers and statisticians; it is not easy to convey the subtlety of some of the issues to someone who is unfamiliar with the use of numbers to describe beliefs. Murphy and Chase (1975) provide an interesting analysis of the use of Bayesian probabilities in genetics. They recognize some of the problems that arise when trying to explain what a Bayesian probability represents. If the concept is difficult to explain to an expert, it must be especially confusing to a patient.

Understanding new information consists of relating the information to schemata, which are representations of a person's knowledge about the world. When a person learns that there is a .4 probability of being a carrier for a genetic disorder, there may be no relevant knowledge schema within which the information can be understood. To solve this problem, a decision analysis provides its own method for helping a person develop a relevant scheme. This is the sensitivity analysis, which I discuss in the next section. The best way of interpreting any number that is used in a formal analysis is to show what effect that number has on the final outcome. This is the purpose of the sensitivity analysis. If the decision maker understands how the final outcome is affected by that .4 probability, how the desirability of an option changes if it drops to .3 or rises to .5, we can say that at a functional level she understands its meaning

A topic that arises when discussing probabilities is the effect that new information has in changing the probabilities. Bayesian approaches to probability were developed to show how probabilities should change; Bayes' theorem is a normative rule for revising one's opinions in the light of new information. It is clear from descriptive studies that the usual process of opinion revision is not a Bayesian one. Normative models such as Bayes' theorem, or other derivations from mathematical probability theory, are not successful as descriptive theories. Peterson and Pitz (1986) have outlined a descriptive theory of how people use information to express their confidence or uncertainty about future events. The theory is based on a distinction between using information to suggest new outcomes and using information to confirm old hypotheses. One of the implications of this theory is that people become increasingly confident in their prediction of future events, while at the same time becoming increasingly uncertain when asked to consider alternative outcomes. This apparently contradictory result occurs because different ways of phrasing a question lead people to adopt different strategies for processing the information. The finding has important implications for the quantification stage of a decision analysis, for it suggests possible sources of systematic inconsistencies in people's judgments.

Normative theories of judgment and decision making demand that judgments and decisions be mutually consistent. In practice, judgments and decisions are based on information processing strategies that seem to the decision maker be appropriate, but which can lead to major inconsistencies in judgments. It is the role of the formal analysis to help a decision maker recognize inconsistencies in his or her judgments. Before the analysis is complete, these inconsistencies must be resolved.

This discussion leads inevitably to the familiar concern with heuristics and biases. It has been suggested by some authors that people cannot make rational judgments of probability. How, then, can we justify using such judgments as part of a decision analysis? There are three points that ought to be made in this respect. First, as noted previously, such studies as those listed in Kahneman et al. (1982) are not universally taken to indicate the irrationality of human beings; Cohen (1981) has suggested that some of the published interpretations of the data show that it is the experimenters, not the subjects, who are wrong. Second, given that people make inconsistent judgments (and even Cohen admits that rational subjects can sometimes make errors because of performance limitations), one can make sure that the analysis includes procedures to identify and correct such inconsistencies. Finally, one wants to know what magnitude of error is likely to be involved. Relative to other sources of error that might occur (in defining the problem, for example), the distortions produced in the assigned probabilities may be unimportant. In the last resort, the sensitivity analysis can be used to assess the impact of such errors on the results.

Probability estimates are not the only numerical judgments required of a person during a decision analysis. An important part of the quantification process is assigning weights to the attributes and objectives. This too can be difficult for people who are unfamiliar with the process. They are forced to confront the often intolerable conflicts that lie at the heart of the decision problem.

Some authors have recommended using very simple approaches to weighting, which avoid many of the difficult judgments that a decision maker might otherwise have to make. For example, Janis and Mann (1977) propose a "balance sheet" approach to the solution of personal problems, which is a simplified form of MAUT. This approach has been used in genetic counseling by Schild (1981). Unfortunately, while they may be easy to use, simplified MAUT methods ignore one useful contribution of a formal decision analysis. This is a direct measurement of the trade-offs that a decision maker is willing to accept among the attributes. A multiattribute description of the decision maker's goals implies that there is conflict among the goals. Finding an optimal solution demands that the decision maker resolves the conflicts, which can only be done by defining acceptable trade-offs among the attributes that define these goals. Those forms of analysis that confront the decision maker with the conflicts and the trade-offs are likely to provide a better understanding and acceptance of the final decision.

Shapira (1981) has shown that trade-off functions are not always well behaved. Sometimes a decision maker finds it impossible to give up a quantity of attribute X, no matter how small, to obtain an improvement in attribute Y, no matter how large. If one attribute is truly incommensurate with another it is difficult to complete the formal analysis. The problem appears in extreme form when a decision maker finds all available options unacceptable because they lead to outcomes for which trade-offs are impossible. A woman may be unwilling under any conditions to accept the risk of a severely disabled infant, and be equally unwilling to undergo an abortion. In effect, such expressions of complete unacceptability lead to infinitely large weight on the relevant attributes, and the analysis cannot proceed. The difficult task faced by a counselor or a decision analyst is to find a way to permit the decision maker to resolve this extreme conflict. I suspect that one can only approach the problem by sensitizing the clients to the ubiquitousness of trade-offs in complex problems, and the impossibility of avoiding hard choices.

The third set of quantities needed for the analysis is the single attribute utilities. These are the evaluations of each scenario in terms of each attribute. This is the quantification process that is most controversial, for it is at this stage that the decision maker is asked to assign numerical values to emotionally charged outcomes. It is important to note that these numbers are nothing more than the expression of degrees of preference. It is possible, in fact, to hide the numbers from the decision maker by using graphic rating scales.

A key concern here is the time period over which the scenarios are evaluated. The value tree is likely to include attributes that represent both the short-term costs and benefits of an option (e.g., the immediate effect of the decision on other members of the family), and very long-term effects (the values and preferences associated with raising a sick child many years in the future). Beach et al. (1977), in describing a decision aid to help couples with birth planning, discuss the importance of distinguishing between short-term and long-term utilities. For many people the conflict between short-term and long-term concerns is at the heart of the decision problem. One of the major sources of difficulty that people encounter in dealing with this conflict is judging the desirability of a possible outcome a long time prior to its occurrence. In some cases the decision maker is asked to evaluate an outcome projected many years into the future. In the absence of direct experience with such outcomes a person will find this difficult to do. Christensen-Szalanski (1984) found that women making decisions about natural child birth expressed values many months prior to the delivery that changed as the delivery approached.

There have been a few attempts to deal theoretically with conflicts between short-term and long-term concerns, and with changing utilities over time. Christensen-Szalanski suggests that people incorporate a discounting of future outcomes into their judgments. Thaler and Shifrin (1981) have proposed that value judgments represent a balance between long-term planning and short-term gratification. These theories may have useful applications to genetic problems. A complete understanding of how people deal with decisions about genetic risk will require a more complete study of discounting effects and other ways of resolving conflicts between short-term and long-term outcomes.

Synthesis

The numerical judgments of probabilities, weights, and utilities are combined to generate aggregate measures of utility or expected utility for each option. While the process of aggregating the judgments is complex, it is readily automated and can be left to a computer or other mechanical aid. According to some textbook presentations of decision analysis, this is the final step, the solution of the problem. If it is the final step, then because it can be automated it creates no particular problems for the decision maker. In fact, arriving at the aggregate utilities for each option is not the end of the analysis, but only the beginning of a very useful exploration process.

A decision analysis, while it provides a numerical, aggregate utility for each option, does not offer a prescription for action. It is more helpful to think of it as helping the decision maker explore the dynamics of a problem. This exploration is achieved through a sensitivity analysis, which is the process by which the sensitivity of the results to changes in the analysis is examined. By systematically altering the numerical judgments one may determine the effects of each element on the final solution. One can explore the effects of changes in the problem description in the same way. The advantage to decision analysis using computers is that the decision maker can receive immediate feedback showing the effects of any changes on the final solution.

The sensitivity analysis offers a method by which the client acquires an understanding of the several factors involved in the analysis. To say that a person understands a probability, an attribute weight, or a utility, can mean many things. In some cases, "understanding" refers to the knowledge of how these quantities are defined and how they are related to the axiomatic foundations of the theory. To a client this kind of understanding is probably not important. Instead, I suggest that the most useful understanding for the client is one in which she recognizes how each quantity affects the final decision. This knowledge is acquired most readily when the decision maker can see how the aggregate utilities change as changes are made in the judgmental quantities.

Consider the role of attribute weights as an example. In principle, these weights describe the trade-offs that are acceptable to the decision maker. Making trade-off judgments between attributes is very difficult for most people; a decision maker may have to determine, for example, how much additional financial burden he or she is willing to accept in order to please her parents by providing them with grandchildren. No-one can make such a judgment without experiencing severe misgivings. However, the sensitivity analysis can demonstrate exactly how much of a trade-off is necessary in order to change the ordering of the aggregate utilities for each option. By finding the critical "swing weight", and discovering how sensitive the results are to changes in the trade-offs, the decision maker can better understand how the relative weight of the two attributes affects the results, and can be more comfortable in accepting the judgments that she makes.

This ability of the sensitivity analysis to provide clients with a better understanding of their problem is especially important when the counselor is reluctant to be directive. Many clients seeking genetic counseling would prefer that the counselor provide them with a recommended course of action, and most counselors are understandably reluctant to do this. A sensitivity analysis can provide an alternative to a more directive form of counseling. Any set of aggregate utilities is in a sense a recommendation for action, but it is a conditional recommendation. The results of the analysis can be interpreted in the following way : if you accept this model of the problem, and if the accompanying judgments are acceptable to you, then the option with maximum utility is the one that is most consistent with your judgments. Through the sensitivity analysis, the decision maker can see that if changes are made in the model or in the judgments, then the aggregate utilities change. It remains the responsibility of the client to select a complete representation of the problem that is acceptable. The representation includes the model of the problem, the judgments concerning the elements of the model, and the set of aggregate utilities that are derived as a result. If the complete analysis is a satisfactory description of the client's feelings, then the analysis is a "requisite" analysis of his or her problem.

Evaluating the effectiveness of decision aids

I have suggested ways in which a formal decision analysis might be helpful to clients who seek counseling about genetic risks. Most of the suggestions are speculative, however, and there is a need for empirical evidence that a decision analysis can provide assistance in the way I have suggested. Earlier I referred to evidence in support of the principle of decomposition, which indicated that judgments of simple events are more reliable and sensitive than are judgments of complex events. I noted also the finding by Sachs (1984) that personal decisions are often inconsistent with expressed preferences, and that such inconsistency is related to difficulty in accepting the decision. This evidence provides an a priori justification for using decision analysis, but it does not demonstrate that decisions made by means of a formal analysis are in any sense better than decisions made some other way.

What evidence is there that decision aiding technologies can be effective, especially in an area like genetic counseling? There is a small but growing literature concerned with the evaluation of decision aids (see Reidel, 1986, and Reidel and Pitz, 1986), but most of this literature deals with decision aids used in an organizational or military context. The difficulties faced by a person who is dealing with a highly emotional personal problem are likely to be different from those of the manager or the battalion commander. Do decision analyses overcome those difficulties?

Reidel and Pitz (1986) argue that evaluating decision aids can itself be approached as a problem in multiattribute utility analysis. The MAUT approach outlined above that is used to help a person make decisions about genetic risks can also be used to help some other person make decisions about a decision aid. There may be several goals or objectives to be achieved as a result of using the aid. A thorough discussion of relevant criteria is given by Rohrmann (1986). Measurable attributes can be defined that address these criteria, and weights can be assigned that reflect the importance of the attributes. Reidel and Pitz combine a MAUT approach to evaluation with a "life cycle" model. This model is based on the assumption that decision aiding procedures develop gradually, and that evaluation issues arise at every stage of development. They suggest how MAUT can be used at various stages to guide development and implementation of the aid.

Reidel and Pitz (1986) take the decision analytic approach to evaluation one step further, and point out that evaluation is a problem that involves multiple decision makers. The parties to the decision may include the user of the aid (the original decision maker), the agent of the organization responsible for purchasing or installing the aid, and the person or group of people who develop the aid. Reidel and Pitz suggest that a team approach to evaluation should be employed so that the interests of all of these parties are adequately represented.

An enduring problem in evaluating decision aids is finding a suitable criterion, or measure of effectiveness of the decision aids. In principle one would like to evaluate the outcome of the decision making process, and show that decisions reached through formal analysis lead to greater long term satisfaction for the decision maker than do decisions reached without such assistance. There are several reasons why it is difficult to do this. In most cases involving genetic risk, as well as other personal decisions, it is many years before the full impact of a decision can be known. A satisfactory study would take a long time, and few developers of decision aids are willing to make such an investment of time and effort. In addition, there are many uncertain, unpredictable factors that affect the final outcome. In effect, these factors introduce large amounts of error variance into any experimental comparison of outcomes.

Eventually a long-term study of the outcomes of alternative approaches to decision making is the only fully satisfactory approach, difficult as such a study will be. The MAUT approach to evaluation can overcome these difficulties to some extent. One partial solution is to use short-term measures of the decision maker's satisfaction with the decision procedure to evaluate its effectiveness. The suitability of these measures can be expressed through the attribute weights used in a MAUT analysis of the aid. There are obvious weaknesses with short-term measures; they provide no guarantee of long-term suitability of the decision. Nevertheless, a decision aiding procedure that does not generate a positive response by the decision maker is unlikely to prove effective in the long run. Short term measures can therefore be a useful part of a more complete evaluation.

A study related to issues of user satisfaction was carried out by Hartke (1986), who was interested in predictive judgments used in an organizational context. The methods he used were very similar to those employed in the quantification stage of a decision analysis. Hartke employed a factor analysis of various measures of user satisfaction, and found that a two factor solution was adequate for describing decision makers' reactions. One factor related to the ease or difficulty of the procedure, the other to the confidence that the decision maker had in his or her judgment. It is likely that these are the two factors that are of most concern to a decision maker who uses a formal decision analysis.

Reidel (1986) used these factors, along with a general index of satisfaction with the outcome, to measure user satisfaction with decision aids for helping people make career choices. She compared a decision analysis of the kind described in this paper with a pencil-and-paper version of a MAUT analysis (for which the sensitivity analysis could not be conducted) and the Strong-Campbell interest inventory, a test traditionally used to help people choose a career but which has none of the elements of a decision analysis. She found that general user satisfaction was greater for all three groups of subjects than for a control group that was left to its own devices. However, there were no differences among the three treatments. There were differences in terms of procedural difficulty; subjects who used either form of the decision analysis found the judgment procedures difficult to use. The result is sobering, although in retrospect not surprising. One might conclude that people find any formal procedure to be helpful, and that in the short-term at least they cannot differentiate between the effectiveness of an elaborate decision analysis and a simple inventory.

A second approach to the evaluation of decision aids is based on the assumption that a successful decision analysis should change the decision maker's understanding of the problem in some significant way. One might therefore seek cognitive changes that are associated with the analysis. It is unlikely that the time, effort and expense of a decision aiding procedure that does not produce any changes in the decision maker can be justified. In Reidel's study, this was where the decision analysis approach appeared to be most effective. She used a multidimensional scaling (MDS) to measure subjects' perceptions of career options. She found a greater change in the MDS structure for the decision analysis group than for the others. There was evidence, then, that by working through the decision analysis the decision makers changed their interpretation of the problem.

One other point needs to be made about evaluating decision aids. A complete decision analysis involves several stages (as outlined above), each of which leads the decision maker through many steps. A global evaluation of the decision aid may be necessary if decisions about the aid itself have to be made. Nevertheless, to develop an understanding of the strengths and weaknesses of the procedure, and to improve the procedure, it is important to evaluate the separate components of the aid. One might examine each part of each stage used in the decision analysis, and determine to what degree it provides useful support and assistance to the decision maker. The weakness of a study such as Reidel's is that it does not suggest which part of a decision analysis is responsible for any of the changes that are observed in the decision maker's understanding of the problem.

I have recently completed a couple of studies that address the effectiveness of parts of the decision analysis procedure. Neither study makes it possible to draw any strong conclusions, but they are illustrative of the kind of study that might be used for evaluation purposes. One experiment used as a criterion the changes that occurred in a decision maker's interpretation of the problem. The task for the decision maker was to make recommendations to a hypothetical government commission on prison reform. We examined the separate effects of the problem description, the quantification, and the sensitivity analysis components of the decision analysis. The results suggested that only the first stage, the problem definition, produced any significant changes in the decision maker's representation of the problem.

In a second study we used a hypothetical genetic risk problem. Subjects were couples who were either recently married, engaged, or at least good friends. They were asked to imagine that the woman was at risk of being a carrier for Duchenne Muscular Dystrophy, and told to work through the problem of whether or not to have children. While the problem was hypothetical, it was realistic enough to be involving for all the subjects. We were primarily concerned with the role of problem definition in helping the decision maker. Four groups of subjects were used. Two groups used a pre-defined problem structure; one structure was relatively complete, the other was considerably simplified. Two other groups built their own structure, using either the complete or the simplified definitions of the problem as starting points. We examined measures of user satisfaction; we also looked at the agreement between the partners (before and after the analysis) as a measure of change that might be informative. Unfortunately, we found no significant between-group differences. There were very large individual differences in subjects' ratings of the usefulness of a formal analysis for dealing with such a problem. These individual differences obscure any group differences that might be due to procedural variables. We have since replicated the study using a repeated-measures design, in which subjects were given experience with two or more methods for analyzing a problem. The effect of procedural variables are more apparent when subjects have experienced more than one problem solving procedure.

There is one other approach to evaluation that will occur regardless of the outcome of other approaches. Formal decision aids are available now; more will become available in the future. Some geneticists and counselors will use them; some will not. In the long run the "market place" will determine their success or failure. The efficiency of the market place is limited, however, if no information is available to the consumer. It is the responsibility of the psychologist, therefore, to provide information that might help a genetic counselor make a wise decision about the best way to assist patients.

Conclusion

The definitive study that shows that decision aids are effective in helping people make personal decisions has not yet been reported. There is every reason to believe that a formal analysis can be helpful if used carefully. In particular, two parts of the decision analysis procedure should help a person understand and cope with a problem. These are the problem definition and sensitivity analysis stages of the formal analysis. The former requires the decision maker to create a "requisite model" of the problem by decomposing it into its important elements. The sensitivity analysis permits the decision maker to explore the effects of changing judgments, and should provide him or her with a clearer understanding of the dynamics of the problem. The theoretical arguments for using these procedures are strong. One would feel more comfortable in recommending them, however, if there were some empirical demonstration of their effectiveness.

To anticipate the results of an extensive body of research that as yet does not exist, I predict some of its most important findings. These will consist of cautionary notes that must be considered before any decision analytic procedure is used to help a person deal with genetic risk. First, I expect that experience in using formal methods of analysis with simpler problems will be necessary before asking a person to deal in an analytic way with a really significant problem. Second, I expect that the issue of trade-offs will always be difficult to deal with. They are, after all, at the heart of every decision problem. Every option leads to both desirable and undesirable outcomes, and effecting a balance among these outcomes is not easy. I like to think, however, that the procedures I have described here will prove to be the most effective way of helping decision makers find solutions to their problems.

References

Adelman, L., Sticha, P.J. and Donnell, M.L.
An experimental investigation of the relative effectiveness of two techniques for structuring multiattributed hierarchies.
Organizational Behavior and Human Decision Processes 37, 188-196, 1986.

Beach, L.R., Townes, B.D., Campbell, F.L. and Keating, G.W.
Developing and testing a decision aid for birth planning decisions.
Organizational Behavior and Human Performance 15, 99-116, 1977.

Checkland, P.
Systems thinking, systems practice.
Chichester : Wiley, 1981.

Christensen-Szalanski, J.J.
Discount functions and the measurement of patients' values : Women's decisions during childbirth.
Medical Decision Making 4, 47-58, 1984.

Cohen, L.J. (1981).
Can human irrationality be experimentally demonstrated.
Behavioral and Brain Sciences 4, 317-331, 1981.

Connolly, T.
Hedge-clipping, tree-felling and the management of ambiguity.
In McCaskey, M.B, Pondy, L.R. and Thomas, H. (Eds.), Managing the challenge of ambiguity and change. New York : Wiley, 1986.

Edwards, W.
The theory of decision making.
Psychological Bulletin 51, 380-417, 1954.

Edwards, W. and Newman, J.R.
Multiattribute evaluation.
Beverly Hills : Sage, 1982.

Fischhoff, B.
Clinical decision analysis.
Operations Research 28, 28-43, 1980.

Fischhoff, B., Slovic, P. and Lichtenstein, S.
Fault trees : Sensitivity of estimated failure probabilities to problem representation.
J. Exp. Psychol. : Human Perception and Performance 4, 330-344, 1978.

Hartke, D.
Estimation of the standard deviation of employee job performance in dollars : The application of judgment theory to utility analysis.
Ph.D. Dissertation, Southern Illinois University, Carbondale, 1986.

Hogarth, R.M.
Beyond discrete biases : Functional and dysfunctional aspects of judgmental heuristics.
Psychological Bulletin 90, 197-217, 1981.

Humphreys, P. and Berkeley, D.
Handling uncertainty : Levels of analysis of decision problems.
In G. Wright (Ed.), Behavorial decision making. London : Plenum, 1985.

Humphreys, P. and McFadden, W.
Experiences with MAUT : Aiding decision structuring versus bootstrapping the decision maker.
Acta Psychol. 45, 51-69, 1980.

Janis, I.L. and Mann, L.
Decision Making.
New York : Free Press, 1977.

Jungermann, H.
Speculations about decision theoretic aids for personal decision making.
Acta Psychol. 45, 7-34, 1980.

Kahneman, D., Slovic, P. and Tversky, A.
Judgment under uncertainty : Heuristic and biases.
Cambridge, Cambridge University Press, 1982.

Keeney, R.L. and Raiffa, H.
Decisions with multiple objectives.
New York : Wiley, 1976.

Keeney, R.L.
Decision analysis : State of the field.
Operations Research 30, 803-838, 1982.

Murphy, E.A. and Chase, G. A.
Principles of genetic counseling.
Chicago : Year Book Medical Publishers, 1975.

Peterson, D.K. and Pitz, G.F.
Confidence, uncertainty, and the use of information.
Computer Information Systems Department, Southwest Missouri State

University, Springfield, 1986.

Phillips, L.D.
A theory of requisite decision modelling.
Acta Psychol. 55, 29-48, 1984.

Pitz, G.F. and McKillip, J.
Decision analysis for program evaluators.
Beverly Hills : Sage, 1984.

Pitz, G.F. and Reidel, S.
The content and structure of value tree representations.
Acta Psychol. 56, 59-70, 1984.

Pitz, G.F. and Sachs, N.J.
Judgment and decision : Theory and its application.
Ann. Rev. Psychol. 35, 139-163, 1984.

Pitz, G.F., Sachs, N.J. and Heerboth, J.
Procedures for eliciting choices in the analysis of individual decisions.
Organizational Behavior and Human Performance 26, 396-408, 1980.

Pitz, G.F., Sachs, N.J. and Brown, M.T.
Eliciting a formal problem structure for individual decision analysis.
Psychology Department, Southern Illinois University, Carbondale, 1980.

Reidel, S.
Model-based evaluation of decision aids.
Ph.D. Dissertation, Southern Illinois University, Carbondale, 1986.

Reidel, S. and Pitz, G.F.
Utilization oriented evaluation of decision support systems.
IEEE Transactions on Systems, Man, and Cybernetics, in press, 1986.

Rohrmann, B.
Evaluating the usefulness of decision aids : A methodological perspective.
In Brehmer, B., Jungermann, H., Lourens, P. and Sevón, G. (Eds.).
New Directions in research on decision making.
Elsevier, North-Holland, 1986.

Sachs, N.J.
The coherence hypothesis of birth control use : The relationship between preferences, chosen method, and the consistency of birth control use.
Ph.D. Dissertation, Southern Illinois University, Carbondale, 1984.

Sachs, N.J. and Pitz, G.F.

Choosing the best method of contraception. Application of decision analysis to contraceptive counseling and selection.
Psychology Department, Southern Illinois University, Carbondale, 1981.

Schild, S.
Social and psychological issues in genetic counseling.
In Applewhite, S.R., Busbee, D.L. and Borgaonkar, D.H., (Eds.), Genetic screening and counseling : A multidisciplinary perspective. Springfield, IL : Thomas, 1981.

Schild, S. and Black, R.B.
Social work and genetics : A guide for practice.
New York : Haworth, 1984.

Shapira, Z.
Making trade-offs between job attributes.
Organizational Behavior and Human Performance 28, 331-355, 1981.

Thaler, R. and Shifrin H.
An economic theory of self control.
J. Political Econ. 89, 392-406, 1981.

Von Neumann, J. and Morgenstern, O.
Theory of games and economic behavior.
Princeton, NJ : Princeton University Press, 1947.

Wertz, D.C., Sorenson, J.R. and Heeren, T.C.
Clients' interpretation of risks provided in genetic counseling.
School of Public Health, Boston University, 1985.

Wishuda, A.
Design of decision-aiding systems.
In Wright, G. (Ed.), Behavioral decision making. London : Plenum, 1985.

Wooler, S. and Wishuda, A.
An educational approach to designing computer-based career guidance systems.
Brit. J. Educat. Technol. 16 (2), 1985.

PRESCRIPTIVE MODELS TO SUPPORT DECISION MAKING IN GENETICS

Stephen G. PAUKER and Susan P. PAUKER

New England Medical Center, Tufts University School of Medicine
Harvard Community Health Plan, Massachusetts General Hospital, Harvard Medical School, Boston, Massachusetts, USA

SUMMARY

Formal prescriptive models can help patients and clinicians better understand the risks and uncertainties they face and better formulate well-reasoned decisions. Using Bayes rule, the clinician can interpret pedigrees, historical data, physical findings and laboratory data, providing individualized probabilities of various diagnoses and outcomes of pregnancy. With the advent of screening programs for genetic disease, it becomes increasingly important to consider the prior probabilities of disease when interpreting an abnormal screening test result. Decision trees provide a convenient formalism for structuring diagnostic, therapeutic and reproductive decisions; such trees can also enhance communication between clinicians and patients. Utility theory provides a mechanism for patients to understand the choices they face and to communicate their attitudes about potential reproductive outcomes in a manner which encourages the integration of those attitudes into appropriate decisions. Using a decision tree, the relevant probabilities and the patients' utilities, physicians can estimate the relative worth of various medical and reproductive options by calculating the expected utility of each. By performing relevant sensitivity analyses, clinicians and patients can understand the impact of various soft data, including the patients' attitudes toward various health outcomes, on the decision making process. Formal clinical decision analytic models can provide deeper understanding and improved decision making in clinical genetics.

INTRODUCTION

Uncertainty is to clinical genetics what DNA is to molecular genetics.

Birth Defects: Original Article Series, Volume 23, Number 2, pages 279–296

Perhaps to a greater extent than other medical specialists, geneticists have always recognized the central role of uncertainty in biology and have traditionally been quite comfortable using probability theory to describe that uncertainty. Indeed, one of the foci of genetic counseling has been to help communicate those uncertainties and their implications to prospective parents and individuals at risk. Over the past four decades, a formal mathematic approach to decision making in an uncertain world has been developed, initially in economics and management science (Luce and Raiffa, 1957; Raiffa, 1968; Von Neuman and Morgenstern, 1944). For the past two decades, these techniques have been applied in clinical medicine (Griner et al., 1981; Kassirer, 1976; Lusted, 1968; Vecchio, 1966; Weinstein et al., 1980). Not surprisingly, clinical genetics was one of the earliest medical domains for these applications, which initially focussed on the interpretation of laboratory data (Goldberg and Oakley, 1979) and pedigrees (Maag and Gold, 1975; Murphy and Chase, 1975; Murphy and Mutalik, 1969). A decade ago we developed a decision analytic model to augment routine genetic counseling about amniocentesis (Pauker and Pauker, 1977; 1979). In this paper, we summarize three general applications for decision analytic models in genetics : 1) interpreting data, 2) making choices, and 3) communicating and focussing values.

1. DATA INTERPRETATION

Bayes rule

One of the dominant tasks of the geneticists is data interpretation. Those data can arise from a variety of sources, for example, the family history, patients' symptoms, epidemiologic studies, the physical examination, imaging studies, and the laboratory. As these data become available in the evaluation of an individual patient or family, each new finding must be combined with other facts already revealed about the patient, forming an evolving sequence of diagnostic hypotheses or beliefs. Thus, as the workup proceeds, the likelihood of each diagnosis' being considered changes. Although the interpretation of the streams of data that constitute an individual case can be, and often is, made informally and implicitly, it is possible to perform this task quantitatively and to calculate the probability of each diagnostic possibility. One scheme for performing such calculations (Bayes rule) has been available for over two centuries and can be applied easily to clinical problem solving (Griner et al., 1981).

To understand Bayes rule, one must first define several terms. **Prior probability** is the likelihood of a diagnostic possibility **before** the new datum is known. The spectrum of diagnostic possibilities and their associated prior probabilities provides a convenient and useful summary of all available diagnostic information. **Posterior probability** is the likelihood of a diagnostic alternative **after** a new datum is known. The change from the spectrum of prior probabilities to the spectrum of posterior probabilities reflects the diagnostic information carried by the incremental finding. Thus, the terms prior and posterior probability refer to a particular finding. As clinical information becomes available, the posterior probability for $finding_i$ becomes the prior probability for $finding_{i+1}$.

The relevant probabilities that describe the performance of a diagnostic test are called its **conditional probabilities.** If there are n diagnoses being considered, then n conditional probabilities ($P_{finding/disease\ n}$) are required to interpret each finding. If i different test results are possible, then $i \times n$ conditional probabilities are required to characterize the test.

In the special situation that only one disease is being considered (i.e., if there are only two diagnostic hypotheses - "disease" and "no disease") and where the test being considered can have only two possible results (i.e., positive and negative), then the four relevant conditional probabilities are given special names :

$P_{positive/disease}$ is the test **sensitivity** or the true positive rate;

$P_{negative/no\ disease}$ is the test **specificity** or the true negative rate;

$P_{negative/disease}$ is the **false negative rate** and equals (1 - sensitivity);

and

$P_{positive/no\ disease}$ is the **false positive rate** and equals (1 - specificity).

In this case, Bayes rule states that $P_{disease/finding}$ equals

$$\frac{P_{disease} * P_{finding/disease}}{(P_{disease} * P_{finding/disease}) + ((1-P_{disease}) * P_{finding/no\ disease})}$$

where $P_{disease}$ is the prior probability, $P_{disease/finding}$ is the posterior probability, and $P_{finding/disease}$ and $P_{finding/no\ disease}$ are conditional probabilities of a particular finding.

The calculation can be automated by using a standard tabular formulation. The diagnoses are listed in column A, the prior probabilities in column B, and the conditional probabilities in column C. Column D is calculated as the product of columns B and C. The posterior probabilities (column E) are the ratio of each entry in column D to the sum of the entries in that column. Consider, for example, a woman who has a 50 % risk of being a carrier for Duchenne muscular dystrophy. Assume her creatine kinase level is determined after exercise and is found to be normal. Further assume that the sensitivity of the test is 66 % and that the specificity is 97 %. Table 1 demonstrates the calculations that reveal the posterior probability to be 26 %.

Table 1 : Bayes rule for interpreting a normal creatine kinase in a woman with a 50 % probability of being a carrier for Duchenne muscular dystrophy

Column A Diagnosis	**Column B** Prior Probability	**Column C** Conditional Probability	**Column D** Product	**Column E** Posterior Probability
Carrier	50	34	1700	0.259
Not carrier	50	97	4850	0.741
			6550	

On the other hand, consider the meaning of an elevated creatine kinase level in a woman (with a different pedigree) whose chance of being a carrier is only 1.5 %. As seen in Table 2, in that case the probability of the woman's being a carrier is increased. Thus, the posterior probabilities in these two situations are roughly equivalent even though one woman had a normal creatine kinase level while the other woman had an elevated level. Clearly, the prior probability must be considered in interpreting this test result.

Table 2 : Bayes rule for interpreting an elevated creatine kinase in a woman with a 1.5 % probability of being a carrier for Duchenne muscular dystrophy

Column A Diagnosis	**Column B** Prior Probability	**Column C** Conditional Probability	**Column D** Product	**Column E** Posterior Probability
Carrier	15	66	990	0.251
Not carrier	985	3	2955	0.749
			3945	

Pedigrees

In the two examples given above, the prior probability of the woman's being a carrier varied 32-fold. Presumably, in the first case, the woman had two affected brothers, whereas the second woman could have been the great-great-great-granddaughter of the first woman. However, the phenotypes in the pedigree can contain evidence that might not be used appropriately if Bayesian calculations are omitted (Murphy and Chase, 1975; Murphy and Mutalik, 1969). For example, if a woman who might be a carrier for a X-linked recessive disorder has an apparently unaffected son, the likelihood of her being a carrier should be diminished. The strength of the effect depends on the ratio of the likelihood of a carrier's having a son with a normal phenotype to the likelihood of a non-carrier's having a son with a normal phenotype. For example, consider a woman who has a brother and a maternal uncle with classical hemophilia. Traditional pedigree analysis would suggest that such a woman has a 50 % chance of being a carrier. Suppose that woman has two unaffected grown sons and a grown daughter who now presents for counseling. Clearly the daughter's chance of being a carrier is half the mother's chance, but is the mother's chance 50 %? Applying Bayes rule, we find that the probability of the woman's being a carrier is only 20 %. Thus, her daughter's chance of being a carrier is only 10 %, not 25 %. By replacing the exponents in column C of Table 3 with N, where N is the number of unaffected sons, one can show that the likelihood of being a carrier is $1/(2^N+1)$.

Table 3 : Bayes rule for interpreting the pedigree of a woman with a 50 % prior probability of being a carrier for classical hemophilia who has two unaffected sons

Column A Diagnosis	**Column B** Prior Probability	**Column C** Conditional Probability	**Column D** Product	**Column E** Posterior Probability
Carrier	50	50^2	125000	0.20
Not carrier	50	100^2	500000	0.80
			625000	

Physical findings

The same principles apply to the interpretation of the physical examination - the physical findings modify the prior probabilities, as a function of the conditional probabilities of each observed finding given each diagnosis. In the examples presented thus far only one diagnosis was being considered, i.e., carrier or not carrier. In practice any number of diagnoses can be considered in the Bayesian calculation.

Consider, for example, a tall, thin boy with ectopia lentis suspected of having either Marfan syndrome or homocystinuria who, on physical examination, is found not to display hyperextensibility. We have displayed estimated clinical prior probabilities (based on the pedigree and on disease prevalences) in column A. The Bayesian calculation reveals that homocystinuria has a higher posterior probability than Marfan syndrome despite the fact that its prevalence was lower.

Note two additional features of this example : 1) the application of Bayes rule is not restricted to settings in which only a single diagnosis is being considered; and 2) Bayes rule can be used to interpret positive as well as negative information. In fact, this is an example of the "normal finding phenomenon," in which normal findings occur with different frequencies in two different diagnoses being considered and such a finding thereby provides information useful in differential diagnosis (Gorry et al., 1978).

Table 4 : Bayes rule for interpreting the absence of hyperextensibility in a boy suspected of having either Marfan syndrome or homocystinuria

Column A Diagnosis	**Column B** Prior Probability	**Column C** Conditional Probability	**Column D** Product	**Column E** Posterior Probability
Marfan syndrome	40	20	800	0.12
Homocystinuria	10	90	900	0.14
Neither	50	99	4950	0.74
			6650	

Laboratory data

Although the principle applies to any finding, laboratory data are often continuous variables that are classified based on some **decision criterion** and are expressed as being either positive or negative. Clearly, if the laboratory changes the criterion (or even the way the test is performed), then the conditional probabilities (i.e., the sensitivity and specificity) will change and the interpretation of a test result should also change.

For example, consider a Tay-Sachs screening program that employs the determination of serum levels of hexosaminidase in prospective parents. Such programs typically report results as being normal or low, the latter suggesting the carrier state. Assume that a laboratory develops a problem with their assay and their criterion for an abnormal results such that 20 % of their results are abnormal and require follow-up evaluation with a leukocyte hexosaminidase test (a more time consuming and expensive procedure). Because the laboratory director knows that most of these results will eventually be shown to be "false positive", he or she labels all initially abnormal results as "inconclusive". Furthermore assume that test sensitivity remains very high, i.e., virtually all carriers have abnormal results on the initial screen.

Assuming these results apply to an Ashkenazi Jewish population with a carrier frequency of 1/30, we can see that for every 10,000 patients screened, there will be 2000 inconclusive results. Of these, only 333 will be carriers; thus, the posterior probability of a patient with an inconclusive result actually being a Tay-Sachs carrier is 16.7 %, a five-fold increase over the unscreened population.

Table 5 : Bayes rule for interpreting an inconclusive hexosaminidase level in a French Canadian being screened as a Tay-Sachs carrier

Column A Diagnosis	**Column B** Prior Probability	**Column C** Conditional Probability	**Column D** Product	**Column E** Posterior Probability
Carrier	1	100.0	100.0	0.106
Not carrier	49	17.2	842.8	0.894
			942.8	

Now suppose the same laboratory screens a man of French-Canadian descent, for whom the carrier frequency is only 1/50. What is the meaning of an initially inconclusive result? First, we must calculate the specificity of the inconclusive result. In the initial (Ashkenazi) population there would be 1667 inconclusive results among the 9667 non-carriers screened, providing a specificity of 17.2 %. Applying Bayes rule, we see that the chance of this man's being a carrier is only 10.6 %, compared to the 16.7 % appropriate for interpreting the same result in an Ashkenazi Jew.

Orthogonal data

When a laboratory test is performed to provide diagnostic information about the presence of one disease process, it may simultaneously provide information about other abnormalities. Thus, a finding that decreases the likelihood of the primary disease may actually increase the likelihood of another problem. A common example of this phenomenon is found when the maternal serum level of alpha-fetoprotein is used to screen for neural tube defects (Goldberg and Oakley, 1979; Pauker et al., 1981) but provides information about Down syndrome. For example, suppose a level below 0.5 multiples of the median were found in 30 % of pregnancies with Trisomy 21 but in only 5 % of unaffected pregnancies.

If a low maternal serum alpha-fetoprotein level were obtained when screening a 30 year-old woman (for whom the prevalence of Down syndrome at delivery would be 1/885), then Bayes rule would suggest that the risk is 0.0067 or 1/148, the risk that would be expected in a 39 year old woman at delivery.

On the other hand, if a level above the 0.5 multiples cutoff were found in a 40 year old woman (for whom the prevalence of a Down syndrome pregnancy would be 1/109), then the risk would still be 1/148, an almost insignificant decrease. Of course, the likelihood ratio for a normal maternal serum protein level (70/95 or 0.74) is based on all values above the 0.5 multiples of the median cutoff. If, rather than lumping all such values, one examined data for the specific level found, one could expect that levels falling toward the high end of the normal range would have far lower likelihood ratios and would imply far greater reduction in the risk of an affected pregnancy.

Table 6 : Bayes rule for interpreting low maternal serum alpha-fetoprotein level in a 30 year-old woman

Column A Diagnosis	**Column B** Prior Probability	**Column C** Conditional Probability	**Column D** Product	**Column E** Posterior Probability
Down syndrome	1	30	30	0.0067
Unaffected	884	5	4420	0.9933
			4450	

Table 7 : Bayes rule for interpreting normal maternal serum alpha fetoprotein level in a 40 year-old woman

Column A Diagnosis	**Column B** Prior Probability	**Column C** Conditional Probability	**Column D** Product	**Column E** Posterior Probability
Down syndrome	1	70	70	0.0068
Unaffected	108	95	10260	0.9932
			10330	

2. MAKING DECISIONS

Genetic counseling has traditionally been non-directive, providing patients with facts, trying to help them understand and retain those data, but providing them with little guidance in actually using that information to make decisions. Reproductive decision making, particularly with respect to genetic risk and the potential for diagnostic information, is a wonderful example of necessary decision making under the bounds of uncertainty. Based on our experience using the techniques of formal decision analysis in other medical settings, we developed a decision analytic model of the amniocentesis decision over a decade ago (Pauker and Pauker, 1977; 1979). We have applied that model extensively in genetic counseling over the past decade and review its basic structure here.

We present the amniocentesis model as a well-tested example of decision analysis in genetics. A similar approach can be used for a variety of reproductive decisions, varying from the use of ultrasound, through chorionic villous sampling, to fetoscopy, and even to intra-uterine shunting for hydrocephaly. In each case, the decision analytic method involves seven basic steps.

Principles of decision analysis

First, the question must be framed as an explicit choice among a limited set of alternatives. *Second,* the problem is structured as a **decision tree,** a formal diagram of the decision space constructed from three basic parts :

1) **decision nodes** which describe a complete and mutually exclusive set of choices that are under the control of the decision maker (such

nodes are depicted as squares);

2) **chances nodes** which describe a complete and mutually exclusive set of states of the world or potential future events which are not under the control of the decision maker but which rather are governed by the laws of chance (such nodes are depicted as circles); and

3) **terminal nodes** or outcomes scenarios that summarize the consequences of a given path of decisions and chances.

Third, each branch of each chance node is assigned a probability summarizing its likelihood. *Fourth,* each outcome state is associated with a relative value or **utility.** Such utilities are typically assigned by the decision maker and can be based on an arbitrary unit-free scale (corresponding to preferences) or can be based on some measurable units (e.g., monetary cost, years of life saved, affected children avoided, etc.). *Fifth,* the expected utility of each decision strategy is calculated. The decision maker is expected to select the option with the best utility. In most circumstances, the best strategy is the one associated with the highest utility, but if, as in the example below, greater utility values imply greater burden, then the best strategy is the one with the lowest (dis-)utility. There are two rules for calculating expected utility :

1) at a decision node, assign the utility of the best option because the decision maker can select that option;

2) at a chance node, the expected utility is the weighted average of the expected utility of its branches, where the weighting factor for each branch is the probability of its occurring.

Sixth, the model is used to perform sensitivity analyses, i.e., each of the relevant assumptions is varied to determine the affect of such variation on the apparently optimal decision. *Finally,* the results are interpreted so the decision maker has a better comprehension of the problem domain.

One of the central features of such directively-enhanced genetic counseling is the incorporation of the patients' attitudes toward alternative reproductive outcomes. Such attitudes (i.e., utilities) are typically assessed using the **lottery technique** in which the patient is presented with a set of alternative scenarios and is asked to make a choice between two such scenarios. The scenario descriptions are then altered systematically in a manner designed to help the patient understand his or her attitudes and expresss them quantitatively as a utility, which can then be incorporated into the decision model. Typically, the structured choice is between a certain outcome of intermediate value (e.g., therapeutic abortion) and a gamble between two outcomes, one better (e.g., an unaffected child) and one worse (e.g., an affected child). The odds of the gamble are then varied systematically until the patient is **indifferent** between the certain intermediate outcome and the gamble. The **principle of substitution** is then used to assign a utility to the intermediate outcome : if the patient is indifferent between that outcome and the gamble, then the utility of that outcome must equal the expected utility of the gamble, calculated using rule (2) described above.

The amniocentesis decision

For patients considering amniocentesis for prenatal diagnosis, as depicted by the decision tree in Figure 1, two options are available : no amniocentesis and amniocentesis. In either case, the pregnancy may end in a spontaneous abortion, although the likelihood of that event is somewhat higher (s versus $s+a$) after amniocentesis. In either case, the pregnancy may be affected (probability d) or unaffected. If amniocentesis is performed, the results may be positive (suggesting an affected fetus) or negative. If the pregnancy is unaffected, then the likelihood of a positive result (p) is the false positive rate, the complement of the test's specificity. If the pregnancy is affected, then the likelihood of a negative result (n) is the false negative rate, the complement of the test's sensitivity. We presume that a positive result will lead to a therapeutic abortion. Although it might be possible for a couple to select amniocentesis if they were unwilling to have an elective abortion for a positive result, our model is not appropriate for counseling such couples because they are presumably seeking something from the procedure which our decision model does not adequately include.

The next step is to assign utilities to each of the seven potential outcomes. Note that we do not distinguish between a true positive result and a false positive result because they would not be prospectively distinguished and either would result in a therapeutic abortion. Furthermore, if a chromosomal analysis is successful on the fetus and shared with the couple, then an additional outcome must be considered. The couple must then assign a relative disutility to it. We assign a disutility of zero to the best outcome (an unaffected child without amniocentesis) and a disutility of 100 to the worst outcome (an affected child despite amniocentesis). Table 8 summarizes the symbols used to depict the five remaining intermediate outcomes.

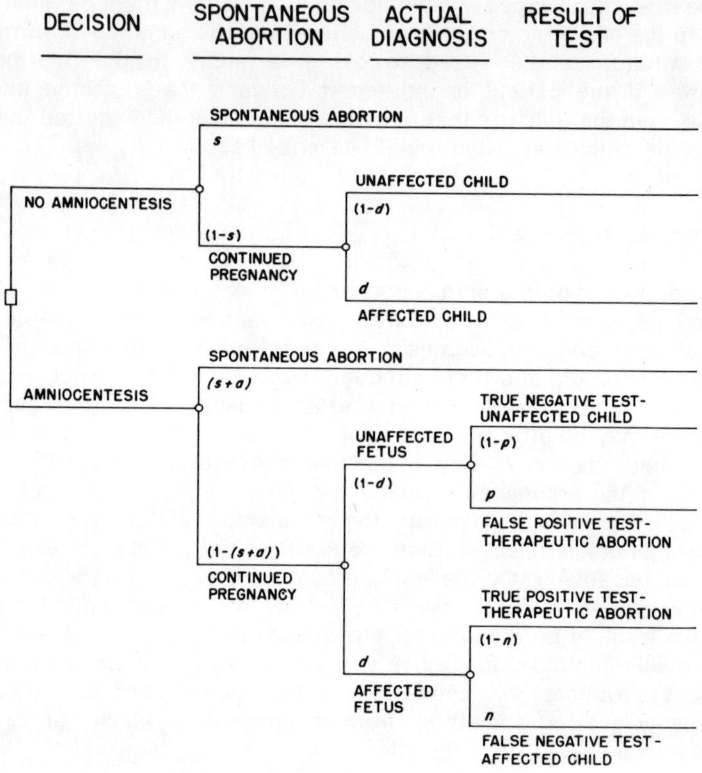

Figure 1 : Decision Model of the Amniocentesis Decision.

The square node at the left denotes the main decision point. Each circular node denotes a chance event. The letter in italics represent the probability of each chance outcome. Note that this decision tree has been "flipped", i.e., the state of the pregnancy proceeds the results of the amniocentesis, to avoid the algebraic complexities of Bayes rule. Reproduced from (Pauker and Pauker, 1977).

In most circumstances, an affected child would be almost as bad an outcome without amniocentesis as with and an unaffected child would be almost as good an outcome after amniocentesis as without the test. Thus U_{uc} approximates zero and U_{as} approximates 100. Applying the above rules about weighted averages, we find that the **expected disutility of no amniocentesis** is

$$100 - s(100d - U_{sas})$$

and the **expected utility of amniocentesis is**

$$(pU_{ta} + d((1-p)U_{ta} + n(100-U_{ta}))(1-(s+a)) + (s+a)U_{sac}$$

These two expressions can be determined for each prospective parent. If the expected disutility of amniocentesis is less than the expected disutility of no amniocentesis, then amniocentesis should be encouraged, and vice versa.

Table 8. Symbols for Utilities in Amniocentesis Model

Outcome	Symbol
Unaffected Child After Amniocentesis	U_{uc}
Spontaneous Abortion	
Without Amniocentesis	U_{sas}
After Amniocentesis	U_{sac}
Therapeutic Abortion	U_{ta}
Affected Child Without Amniocentesis	U_{as}

In most circumstances, the variables that change the most from patient to patient are the utilities (i.e., the patients' attitudes toward reproductive outcomes) and the risk of an affected pregnancy (Pauker et al., 1981; 1982; Pauker and Pauker, this symposium). In such circumstances, it is useful to calculate the **threshold risk of an affected pregnancy,** based on the patient's attitudes : if the actual risk exceeds the threshold risk, then amniocentesis should be recommended; if the actual risk is less than the threshold risk, then amniocentesis should not be recommended. If we define r to be the relative risk of amniocentesis (i.e., $a/(1-s)$) and S to be the odds of spontaneous abortion without amniocentesis (i.e., $s/(1-s)$), then the threshold risk equals

$$Threshold = \frac{(1-r)pU_{ta} + (r+S)U_{sac} - (S)U_{sas}}{(1-r)((p-(1-n))U_{ta} - 100n) + 100}$$

In particular circumstances, the risk of amniocentesis and the false positive and false negative rates are fixed, so the equation can be reduced to a nomogram that depends on the three utilities, U_{ta}, U_{sac}, and U_{sas}.

The difference between the disutility of spontaneous mid-trimester abortion after amniocentesis (U_{sac}) and the same result without amniocentesis (U_{sas}) can be viewed as a measure of the guilt or regret associated with making a choice that results in a poor outcome. Of course, the vast majority of spontaneous abortions after amniocentesis (3.1 % of 3.5 %) would occur even without the procedure; thus, it might be inappropriate for patients to attach the burden of regret to all 3.5 %. This problem can be modelled by considering the two disutilities associated with spontaneous abortion to be equal (U_{sa}). In that case, the threshold risk equals approximately

$$Threshold = \frac{(1-r)pU_{ta} + rU_{sa}}{(1-r)((p-(1-n))U_{ta} - 100n) + 100}$$

In the case of Down syndrome, if one takes the risk of amniocentesis to be approximately 1/250 (above a baseline risk of spontaneous miscarriage of 1/30 for apparently healthy second trimester pregnancies) and the false positive and false negative rates to be approximately 0.5 % each, then the threshold risk of an affected child equals approximately

$$Threshold = \frac{U_{ta} + 7U_{sac} - 6U_{sas}}{250(100 - U_{ta})}$$

Again, if the burdens of spontaneous abortion with and without amniocentesis are equal, then the threshold risk is approximately

$$Threshold = \frac{U_{ta} + U_{sa}}{250(100 - U_{ta})}$$

Clearly, if a prospective parent will experience substantially more regret if spontaneous abortion occurs after amniocentesis compared to the same result in the absence of amniocentesis, then such a couple should have a substantially higher threshold risk of having an affected child. For example, in the extreme, and perhaps limiting, case in which spontaneous abortion without amniocentesis might be completely discounted (i.e., have a disutility of zero) and a spontaneous abortion after amniocentesis might have a disutility equal to that of an elective abortion, then the simpler equation would underestimate the threshold risk by a factor of eight.

Cost-Benefit and Cost-Effectiveness analysis

Sometimes it is not appropriate to consider only the attitudes of the prospective parent in making recommendations about reproductive options. When making policy choices in a world of limited resources, be it for society as a whole or for a particular insurance carrier or other health provider, it may be important to consider potential alternative uses for each health care dollar. In such circumstances, a very similar analysis can be used. The major differences would occur in assigned utilities : rather than being based on the attitudes of a single patient, they might be based on the conglomerate views of society and might reflect the financial costs of testing and of an affected child. If all outcomes can be reduced to a single monetary equivalent, then one performs a **cost-benefit analysis** by which one can select the best policy for society or for the insurance carrier. If one keeps financial costs and health outcomes separate, then one performs a **cost-effectiveness analysis.** Although such analyses allow one to calculate the additional cost per unit of health benefit achieved, they rarely allow one to conclude in any absolute sense whether a given program is justified or not. Rather, cost-effectiveness analyses are used to compare programs and allow the policy maker to make a rational choice as to whether resources should be allocated to one program or another.

3. COMMUNICATION AND VALUES

One of the major benefits of formal explicit prescriptive decision models is that such models enhance communication, in this case between the clinical geneticist and the patient, and encourage both partners in the decision to understand their attitudes and their values better.

Decision structures as language

Significant efforts have been made by the genetics community to understand the nature of the counseling relationship and to enhance communication and patient retention in that setting. In that context, we believe that a formal decision model, such as the ones presented here, can be shown to patients and enchance communication and understanding. The decision model can be viewed as a very specialized language for describing potential events and decisions in an uncertain world. These models help the patient understand what choices he or she can make and what the consequences of those choices may be. The models also emphasize to the patient what events are governed by chance, what outcomes will be conditioned on those chance events, and what the array of potential outcomes is.

Confronting choices

The use of formal decision models, particularly if patients are asked to make choices in the hypothetical lotteries needed for utility assessment, requires that each patient confront his own values in an explicit and very real way. It is insufficient for the patient to say merely that he or she desires an amniocentesis. Rather, he or she must consider explicitly an entire spectrum of scenarios and state under what circumstances elective therapeutic abortion or spontaneous abortion would be acceptable and under what circumstances those outcomes would be unacceptable.

This process of explicitly confronting one's values is far from simple and sometimes is not benign. Both patients and physicians can be stressed in such circumstances. The task is neither simple nor is it appropriate for all patients and all counsellors. Rather it is a tool that might be offered in appropriate circumstances.

CONCLUSIONS

Clinical genetics is concerned with making diagnoses, describing outcomes, and making choices in an uncertain world. Much of that world can be described in probabilistic terms. Formal prescriptive models can enhance the performance of those tasks.

REFERENCES

Goldberg, M.F. and Oakley, G.P. Jr
Interpreting elevated amniotic fluid alpha-fetoprotein levels in clinical practice : Use of predictive value positive concept.
Am. J. Obstet. Gynecol. 133, 126-132, 1979.

Gorry, G.A., Pauker, S.G. and Schwartz, W.B.
The diagnostic importance of the normal finding.
New Engl. J. Med. 298, 486-489, 1978.

Griner, P.F., Mayewski, R.J., Mushlin, A.I. et al.
Selection and interpretation of diagnostic tests and procedures.
Ann. Internal Med. 94, 553-600, 1981.

Kassirer, J.P.
The principles of clinical decision making : An introduction to decision analysis.
Yale J. Biol. Med. 49, 149-164, 1976.

Luce, R.D. and Raiffa, H.
Games and Decisions.
Wiley (New York), 1957.

Lusted, L.B.
Introduction to medical decision making.
Charles C. Thomas (Springfield), 1968.

Maag, U.R. and Gold, R.J.M.
A simple combinatorial method for calculating genetic risks.
Clin. Genet. 7, 361-367, 1975.

Murphy, E.A. and Chase, G.A.
Principles of genetic counseling.
Yearbook (Chicago), 1975.

Murphy, E.A. and Mutalik, G.S.
The application of Bayesian methods in genetic counseling.
Human Heredity 19, 126-151, 1969.

Pauker, S.P. and Pauker, S.G.
Prenatal diagnosis : a directive approach to genetic counseling using decision analysis.
Yale J. Biol. Med. 50, 275-289, 1977.

Pauker, S.P. and Pauker, S.G.
The amniocentesis decision : an explicit guide for parents.
in : Risk, Communication, and Decision Making in Genetic Counseling (Epstein C.J., Curry C.J.R., Packman S., Sherman S., Hall B.D., eds), Part C of Ann Review of Birth Defects, 1978. National Foundation-March of Dimes. Birth Defects Original Article Series XV:5C, Alan R. Liss (New York), pp 289-324, 1979.

Pauker, S.G., Pauker, S.P. and McNeil, B.J.
Implications of prospective parents' attitudes on alternative policies regarding prenatal diagnosis.
in : Critical Issues in Medical Technology (McNeil, B.J., Cravalho, E.G., eds), Auburn House (Cambridge, Mass), pp 343-357,1982.

Pauker, S.G., Pauker, S.P. and McNeil, B.J.
The effect of private attitudes on public policy : prenatal screening for neural tube defects as prototype.
Medical Decision Making 1, 103-114, 1981.

Raiffa, H.
Decision Analysis : Introductory Lectures on Choices under Uncertainty.
Addison-Wesley (Reading, Mass), 1968.

Vecchio, T.J.
Predictive value of a single diagnostic test in unselected populations.

New Engl. J. Med. 274, 1171-1173, 1966.

VonNeuman, J. and Morgenstern, O.
Theory of Games and Economic Behavior.
Princeton University Press (Princeton), 1944.

Weinstein, M.C., Fineberg, H.V., Elstein, A.S. et al.
Clinical Decision Analysis.
WB Saunders (Philadelphia), 1980.

GENERAL DISCUSSION

The second day of the symposium ended with a general discussion under the chairmanship of J.J. Cassiman and G. d'Ydewalle. Any participant could make a statement or could ask questions to the speakers or the audience . The two hours discussion was typed and transcribed as faithfully as possible. The editors have only made minor abbreviations or comments for the sake of clarity. The rest is as it was voiced by the different intervenants.
As the reader will notice, the discussion starts off with a certain antagonism between counselors and psychologists, but ends with a public declaration of mutual respect and interest. Nevertheless, much more discussion and actual field work will be needed to find complete harmony between the two fields.

F. Hecht : We have two groups of people here : one group doing genetic counseling and another group looking at how it should be done. My question therefore is : those of us who are doing genetic counseling are they using models?

Editorial note : *a minority of the genetic counselors present used models.*

St. Pauker : Dr. Hecht made a point that the models that were built and presented by a variety of people here are not being used. I would like to know why this is so? Is it that the models are inappropriate? Is it that they are wrong? Is it that they don't work? Is it that we are not

Birth Defects: Original Article Series, Volume 23, Number 2, pages 297–313 communicating? Is it that the modelers don't really understand genetics? What's the problem? It is clear that the models are not being used by many people and the real issue is why.

F. Hecht : Well let me ask the contrary question : How many of the people who have a strong interest in models are going in and doing genetic counseling on a regular basis to determine whether the models work with patients? I would suggest that one of the problems right now is the failure for the model-builders to go in and really see whether their models work well in genetic counseling. People doing genetic counseling like myself obviously should get much more experience with the models.

C. Vlek : It would appear to me that we are just at the beginning of what could be a serious attempt to bring two fields together. The preliminary questions pertain to the existing demands for genetic counseling and to the conditions that should be fulfilled in order to bring modelers, decision theorists and geneticists fruitfully together. There are certain barriers on the road to that sort of cooperation and there are also certain critical questions about the demand and the extent to which the demand could be dealt with by the modelers and the decision theorists. These should be answered first, before one embarks into a major project, trying out several types of models for their success in genetic counseling.

G. Pitz : I didn't take a careful count of the answers to Dr. Hecht's original question, but I think it was about a 10 % response rate to his question "How many are using models?". I find that response rate about right. If it were much higher than that, I would feel that I was waisting my time being here. If it were lower than that, I would worry that I was waisting my time speaking to people who are not interested in listening to me.

St. Pauker : I think that genetics is no longer unique. Genetics is a very interesting application but people who work in the area don't need it. We are happy to work in that area. If the genetics community feels that they have the answers, that they know how to do counseling and that they feel that modeling is not appropriate, then it makes it more difficult. I think that this has not been the case. Genetics is an area where much can be done, but it really depends on communication and conferences such as this one between both sets of people. People now need to come and listen, but people should also begin to work in their own countries : there are geneticists here, there are decision makers here, everywhere, and if those people begin to talk together about practical cases, it will grow. If they don't talk at an individual level, it will not.

P. Humphreys : I think one of the problems is how the question was just framed : why are people not working with models, is in the word "model" itself. Surely, it is a model when we present it at a conference. But what

are we modeling? First, we are not necessarily modeling the problem, we are certainly not modeling the solution : we are trying to help the decision making process. Second, decision analytic models have been around for a long time as have other ones. We have analyzed questionnaires in the same way. When it comes to the more interactive processes, as decision analytic models are, when they are used in practice, you find that if you analyze the success of the model, sometimes it works, sometimes it doesn't. What tells us that it is going to work? Look at who is using it. People who like decision analytic models, and are skilled at building them and who often have a history building and developing the ideas behind them, do very well with them. They are the people who have gone out into the consultancy in the field. These people really do rather well, not with their "model", but with their "tool".
Today we see models being used as tools and we have to ask, what are we trying to do : although we have a model or a problem representation, we are not trying to say that by representing the problem we will have the solution. In practice we are going to help in "supporting the decision making process" by making use of this tool. The real decision process probably isn't modeled. Should you need to model the real decision process and say, well we need more cognitive psychology? I think that is wrong. I think the question is to discover how to use models as tools appropriately : this means sensitivity of the user or the counselor about when models are going to be appropriate and how they are going to provide support. I think this is the beginning, which Charles Vlek mentioned, and which we are beginning to work at.

G. d'Ydewalle : Actually, the core issue of some papers of this morning and definitely of many interventions during the two days is rather critical to models. Psychologists in general are slightly afraid to apply directly models to one particular setting : I don't think the message was just to use the models as they are.

F. Hecht : In the U.S., people who are in medical genetics have generally gone through some years of training. They then go out and go to work and if they are pediatric geneticists, they tend to see dysmorphologic problems, which lend themselves often very poorly to quantitation. Most medical geneticists also get immured in prenatal diagnosis and are spending most of their time talking to 35 year old women and so on. I think that anything that is to be developed, has to be an ongoing interaction between the model builders and the clinical geneticists. It cannot be a one-time process. It must be an ongoing interaction in order for it to be useful.

J. Edwards : I was privileged to be with various bosses in medicine who were very distinguished. I thought they seemed to reach very good diagnosis and they gave very good advice. When I asked them "how" they did it, they gave the most absurd answers. This of course goes back to Socrates and the poets and this is well known in all fields of critical endeavor. But it does seem a fact of life that people, who are able to make very good judgements, often do it by methods which do not stand up to very good analysis.

Now, I feel a bit guilty by haven't held my hand up saying I do genetic counseling which in fact I do because the Oxford region has 2,5 million people and Dr. Lindman and myself have to share out the various problems, which include over 1300 amniocenteses a year and a very large Duchenne and Huntington interest : so, we do have a lot of blood on our hands and I can speak, I think with some knowledge. I was also running the chromosome laboratories. So the question is what use have these models? Well, I personally found them extremely useful. Hearing the models this morning from the model group, I thought that was a very interesting use of terms and use of descriptions and it was very valuable. I thought it was really in the same sort of situation as chess and warfare. Chess is obviously a very difficult and structured game and it introduces a lot of problems in analysis and difficulties. I'm not quite sure how good the algorithm that you discussed this morning is on the chess board. The qualitative models and the concept of model is extremely valuable and anybody who produced a model has obviously got very clear ideas and it has been a great pleasure to hear the Boston model expanded so lucidly, but models are not actually transportable. One can learn a lot by a model : it is a great discipline for the modelers and it is an education for the spectators, but on the whole, these models lack exportability and this is a problem.

The problem with a numerical model is that you got to feed it with numerical data. To put a numerical or cost value on human life, and then put that into a machine, puts you in exactly the same position as arbitrary saying "do this and do that". But basically whatever happens, there are two rates : there is a failure rate, that is the birth of people with some defect, and there is a casualty rate which in your analysis was 82 % at the age of 30; that is the termination of normal foetuses. Whatever one does, one has to have some sort of trading, some sort of agreement as to the relative costs or distress. On your flow diagram (Dr. Pauker) there was no branch for a termination of a normal foetus and I personally find this a very distressing event and it certainly happens. We try to keep it as rare as possible except in Duchenne where by plan it has to be 50 % at present, in many of our cases. This cannot be dissociated from any sort of procedure and this is why I do not like a numerical input model because it's impossible to devise numerical values to put into the model.

St. Pauker : I agree fully. If any outcome is relevant to the decision maker, it needs to be included in a model. If termination of an affected or normal foetus is different that needs to be specified explicitly. The view of putting quantitation on what appears to be things that are difficult to quantitate really misses the point of that quantitation. All that quantitation represents is a set of preferences. Let us consider the quantitation of the termination of a non-affected foetus. If I gave you two choices, having a Down's child or terminating a non-affected foetus, and those are the only two choices, you can always say one of three things : I rather terminate a Down's child or I rather terminate a normal foetus or I am indifferent between the two. Whichever of those three responses you give, you are in essence quantitating those on a single scale. Whether you like it or not, making a choice, I can turn that choice via decision theory into a scale. The scale only represents, if you will, a summary of the choices that you or the decision maker would make under those environments. The only way you can say that something cannot be quantitated is, if you say that you aren't willing to make that decision. If you aren't willing to make that decision, than you shouldn't be coming to see a counselor.

P. Humphreys : I just like to add a little bit more to that last point. There are some studies in medical decision making on the value of a life and the results are perhaps a little bit embarrassing if you look at them without realizing what they mean and that is if you go across different diseases and say what's the value of keeping you alive. This is for existing people, not for unborn children. The answer also depends "where" you are ill. How much are you worth if you've got let's say, a cardiac problem? How do they calculate this? Which amount of medical resources are put into prolonging life for particular amounts of time? The other problem is the value of the life to whom. When you come to the questions of the value of the life of an unborn child, again you can say, well the value to whom and in this case, general models, even culturely based analyses, are not adequate. You have to look at the various stakeholders involved. Of course one of the trickiest questions is the ethical question. We have to face this at an individual level. I think this is one of the biggest problems with people who are used to models of stable processes including genetic processes. The process, which we model in trying to support counseling, is never stable. It is very hard to generalize the model from one person to another, particularly the model with values in it. Often, even the structure of the model cannot be generalized across and this means that what the modeler, if you call us modelers, can offer really, is not pre-structured models with all values in it, except for one, and you just plug the patient in and get the answer. We have to say all we can offer are the techniques out of which you can generate models, but this is going to be a skill. You have to master how to generate the solution for the person. Isn't this what good counselors always claim they want to do anyway? Isn't this what they have moaned about models not letting them do before by forcing them into a particular framework? I think the way forward then, is how can we start the dialog, how to teach people how they can generate things in the language they want to use, how they can work with the client, how to use the insights, not of the models but the processes by which modelers can generate models in this area.

G. Pitz : I like to come back to the quantification issue because I think this may be the point at which the most interesting arguments begin. The accusation that, when using the decision analytic techniques, I'm quantifying things that should not be quantified, is one that I have to face almost every day. I want to make very clear that what I mean by quantification is simply that you, the decision maker, prefer a to b and you can tell me something about the degree to which you prefer a to b. You could for example tell me that your preference for a over b exceeds the magnitude of your preference for c over d. If you are willing to make that kind of statement about your preferences that's what I mean by quantification and I mean nothing more than that. Nevertheless, the objection is raised frequently by those with whom one tries to go through this kind of formalized decision analytic process. There are two things that need to be kept separate in the discussion of these models : one is their theoretical foundation which in many ways is strongly mathematical, the other is the way in which they are used in practice, which can only be effective in the hands of a skilled individual who is capable of guiding a person through the judgements that they need to make in order to arrive at a decision. You can evaluate those two components of the analysis separately. You can look at its formal basis and say "Is this indeed a requisite model for this kind of problem?" The argument is then going to be very abstract, theoretical and often mathematical. If the answer is positive, you can then ask : "is the individual using this approach, doing so in a skilled way exhibiting the kinds of talents that we would expect in any other counselor?". If the answer to that is yes, it has always been the case in my experience, that even the most reluctant individual finds the process illuminating rather than discouraging.

L. Thomassen : I would like to make a general remark. Perhaps the question should not be "what model and how to use it" but we should turn for a moment to another point : "Why do we need this model and isn't it a basic problem, a problem of communication and of understanding between physician and counselor?". I personally would find it a pity if the input of psychological expertise would only be a model. I would very much prefer if the basic understanding of human beings, the psychological aspect, would be given more attention in the education of genetic counselors. I would like to make this general remark. Models are only tools : we should never forget that the basic goal is to have a good communication and understanding of each other.

J.J. Cassiman : Dr. Humphreys, I think the remark Mrs Thomassen just made comes back to one of the points you made in your talk. But I am sorry to say that many of us did not quite get the point you were making in your talk because we are not used to the terminology you used; it may surprise you but we are "simple minds". When you were talking about first level, I think everybody got the message what the first level was, but about second and especially the third level (you wanted counselors to get to the second and the third level, I think), could you rephrase this in one minute so that people clearly get the message you want them to get.

Editorial note : *The reader is referred to the contribution of P. Humphreys at this symposium.*

P. Humphreys : In the dialog of counseling, the second level is very typically the way in which most counselors will work, when they find themselves in an information-providing situation, where they do not particularly want to get involved in depth and psychodynamic models of the patient. And this is the way of negotiating effectively let's say with the patient. We are trying to work at the second level. The sort of things that is happening is that there is a frame, a structure within which that it is agreed, "this defines the problem". It may be like the decision analytic model which the Paukers showed, actually as agreed between the patient and the doctor. They might understand what it means in different ways but they say somehow "This is the problem" and they would like the doctor or the counselor to help them explore the pathways themselves, to say "What if this would happen? You give me some information about what might be important here but I would like to explore it with you. Don't just tell me what to do; I like to think about the what-ifs". The easy way to think about it is what are the "what-ifs", but they do not want to be given the need in the type of frame J. Pitz was talking about, the multi-attribute frame, and to have to think up for themselves which criteria really matter. They like a list of criteria which they can work from and explore on those criteria and get some idea about how important those criteria are, working out with the analysts themselves. The next level up is when in fact you say : *"well let's see how you want to think about the problem; you've got a value-problem; you want to see which criteria really matter; let us consider the probability of having a child with Down Syndrome; let's assume whatever reason you've got, that you need to think about what would be the key criteria that should matter in distinguishing your life in those conditions, to say "I have a normal child" or say "I remain without child". If you are working the next level up, then you are left very much in working at which criteria really matter to you".* This is quite often meant to say in more psychodynamically oriented counselors where they have a patient who doesn't like any of the alternatives : they are desperate because everything is awful and somehow they want to find the criterium on which they can find the silver lining. They just want to get a criterium introduced so that this person can make this important. But the person takes response, waiting to find the criteria or in the Pauker' model the person would actually take the responsibility for building the decision tree. It's a personal decision tree about things they can do, like move to another country or find a new life. Above that level, you get into someone who wants to really deal with the whole way of coping with the problem in all its aspects for themselves. That isn't seen so often in practice.

G. d'Ydewalle : You are assuming a kind of total flexibility of the counselor and the client. However, in the genetic counseling situation, there are many immediate reactions to some questions; it's a very dynamic situation and also with a lot of emotional aspects involved. So, I am surprised that the whole problem of the overloading of the short-term memory, due to all what is going on, has been neglected and it's almost impossible for a rational being to cope with that. Moreover, as it is a really emotionally loaded situation, I'm pretty sure that very often you get a kind of, what we call in psychology, "functional fixedness" to one or another particular aspect of the problem space. How could you break that down, because that is one of the tasks of the counselor?

P. Humphreys : The first issue about short-term memory is that, if you ever trust that you're exploring within a structure, which in some way is coherent, this means if you ask a what-if question in one corner, in a decision tree you look at the impacts, all the way through the tree. The same in changing the importance of a criterium. This means you have the freedom, to work on one part of the problem and not loose sight of the rest because you know you haven't got to keep all in mind and make all the compensations. Let's say you don't have to handle too much at once. This is one of the reasons why we try to build coherent structures. Whenever you decompose, people might say "Why decompose, why look at values on lots of attitudes instead of one, when you know the information increases exponentially as we introduce these?" The answer is, it's o.k. if you have a coherent structure, it is like you explore one thing and come round to the rest later on and you only get the real freedom of commitments. This is a point which you don't see in academic presentations of the model. I like to stress again, it is "exploration through" which is so important. And what is most important is when in the end people think "Now if we change this, I think I know what would happen". They begin to feel the model so personally because they can anticipate. They don't know how because that would be more than what is in their short-term memory but they then feel they have got it in a sense. They may not be happy but at least now they have got their problem, they can explore it, and they feel somehow, with all the memory limitations, they found something. Now, "functional fixedness" is partly to do that, but also a little bit more complicated because in my presentation, I concentrated on the cognitive aspects and left out many of the emotional aspects. It is not always that either we can just think about this part of the problem or that part of the problem. That is why we have a frame, a sensitivity training really for consultants and counselors, as you look at different parts of the cognitive side of the problem. I just answer the question cognitively because otherwise we get into a very interesting but a very long discussion. Just sticking on the cognitive side, if you look at how people focus within a frame, if you can look at how people focus at the second level, you find that they explore some pathways and not others. In counseling, you let them explore through the whole frame, so they understand it. Another type of functional fixedness is where you just concentrate on at the next level up, on one frame above another. You spend all your time exploring the probabilities and forget about values. This is often a problem when you are talking with a probability inclined counselor. At the next level up, you may find people only exploring one part of the small world and not others. They forget about relationships with their partner for example and the impact of that. So, we can use this framework I was talking about, to see how people get into functional fixedness for reasons that go outside of the frame because they are motivational and not purely cognitive. We can at least see the results of that and we can see at what level the problem is. Then you have to work hard. The reason may not be just not having thought about it but there may be another one that has to be handled motivationally but you can find where it is in the representation : whether it is very fine grained in one corner or very global about which part of the world they are looking at. You can do this just by thinking of the levels. These levels are not a model, they are just simple sensitivity training levels.

J.J. Cassiman : Let's go back to the geneticists now and ask a question to the people who presented models and decision making processes today. Would you agree that the genetic counseling sessions, as they are done at the present time, are done fairly well, and are using some of the information you have given us today ? The second part of my question would be : would you agree that one of the reasons of the fairly strong reaction from genetic counselors to what you proposed or some of it, would be the fact that they don't like to be analyzed in the way they approach the situation?

C. Vlek : There are several reasons to explain the resistance that seems to exist among clinical geneticists against the use of formal tools for judgement and decision making. Let me just enumerate four of them. One is that of course, there is a lack of data on mistakes, errors and failures that are being made under the current procedures. If we have more complaints filed against what happens under current procedures, we could get an idea about the demand for better procedures. Second, that there is of course also a lack of demonstrations of how better procedures work or that formal procedures can work better and please both the client and the counselor more than current procedures do. I think a meeting like this could lead to an explication of alternative formal tools for improved clinical counseling, genetic counseling. Of course these should be evaluated for their practicality. The third rather important reason seems to me to be a traditional overestimation of the value of intuitive judgement, which seems to be especially strong in medical circles. That may have something to do with the fourth point which isn't quite negligible : I sometimes get the impression that some medical clinicians are in need of defending their traditional power positions. Of course, the use of formal tools is an attempt to break through these traditional power positions, some of which I think have to be shared with the clients or other people. So what I think we should try to do in order to be constructive and positive, is to establish some agreement about the possible advantages of using formal methods and techniques for judgement and decision making under uncertainty. One set of advantages has to be with the structuring and the consciousness raising of these methods. You have to explicate yourself, you have to get to some dialog with the counselor and you have to do that in a particular language. That, of course, will increase communicability which may do away with a lot of misunderstandings that currently seem to occur between counselors and clients. Increasing communicability gives you a potential for conflict resolution as we have heard demonstrated this morning. Finally, I think that the sort of traditional resistance that I heard mirrored in some remarks of Dr. Edwards makes us totally unfit for answering some of the questions raised by Prof. Van den Berghe in his opening address. If advances in genetic research push us, push society towards facing more and more specific ethical questions, being more explicit about particular societal preferences on our genetic inheritance, we have to become more explicit, we have to have a conceptual language, we have to be willing to use formal tools and methods. Otherwise, we'll just let things come over us.

F. Hecht : I just want to make sure I understand one of your points correctly : by approaching things more formally, you think we can be potentially more effective ? Why not do it all by computer then? I don't see why we need a future generation of clinicians like myself who are going to make intuitive mistakes. What has being left out here is that there is an art that is hard to define, and this is not to defend the genetic counseling that goes on with no rational basis, but there is an art to genetic counseling and part of that defies model building.

St. Pauker : First of all, there are many arts : practicing medicine is an art and practicing decision making is an art. Being a practitioner of one art does not preclude being a practitioner of the other : they all help. I have to be in the relatively unique position that I do more than one art and I think I did it reasonably well. I detect an antagonism between decision makers and physicians. I am fogged at that antagonism, because I have both sides of my brain who are fighting with each other because I belong at both ends of that spectrum. I think we need to step back and say basically that we are both on the same side of the same problem. The problem is that we picked the wrong word to start. The word "modeling" and "modeler" creates anxiety and antagonism. It makes people paranoid even though we barely mentioned computers here. They make physicians believe that the computers will take over their practice. I think the appropriate thing to talk about is what you're doing as geneticists or as genetic counselors. What I do as a cardiologist and what I do as a decision analyst, is what I call "decision support" and we all do that. We all work on how to take a decision that needs to be made and to help people make that decision better. If a particular tool or particular model helps, that's great. I think we have to look at ways, that we are working on the same side to cover the same task.

G. Pitz : One of the topics that has come up a number of times over the last two days has been the fact that when patients receive information from a counselor concerning genetic disease, they interpret that information in the light of their own expectations, their own scripts and schemas. They hear not what the counselor says but what fits with their conceptions of the problem. The difficulty is that that is a universal mode of processing information. When I stand up here and talk about formal models of decision analysis, what people hear is not what I say. What people hear is what fits with their conceptions of what a person, talking about formal models of decision analysis, is likely to talk about. I hear in Dr. Hecht's comments no resemblance to what I was talking about.

C. Vlek : I sympathize with the question of Dr. Hecht because even Dr. Pauker has to admit that there is a potential in the work he is doing for developing computer programs - and they already exist - which dispense of Dr. Pauker's efforts and lead the client through an interactive interview of the type you have developed over the last ten years, where the client is just giving yes or no answers while the computer program, according to a specific model, develops a specified model of the situation, asks for probability assessments (perhaps from some knowledge representation bases, which experts have made available), asks for the clients preferences, which the client has to provide on the spot, using certain utility scaling procedures which also could be automated because they are algorithmic. The ethical question that rises here of course is "Would you like that? Where remains the art of clinical decision making?" As decision theorists, we have to admit that that is a potential future that we should have to guard, but at the same time we might wish to stimulate, because it can bring some relief. But, let us please not exaggerate these beautiful tools. "The balance lies somewhere in the middle. I like neither totally intuitive decision making when I have a vexing problem to consider, nor do I like an endless infinite analysis. For, some tools may be useful but I don't want to be automated myself.

F. Hecht : Along that line, for prenatal diagnosis, a most common situation involving advanced maternal age and other indications, one can utilize an interaction between the patient and the computer to deal with a good bit of the transaction. Then one can have the patient meet with the counselor to discuss additional issues and weigh some of those things and get a bit of a more human aspect in order to get some sort of hybridization between a formal approach, which is computer based and incidentally collects data which you can analyze later, and the aspect that is more artful.

J. Edwards : We shouldn't be critical of these decision models : they seem to be very valuable and helpful as models and they can direct ones views. However, there is a big difference in the word "counselor" as it's being used. I think I will agree with Dr. Hecht that some of us who were trained in medicine require medicine as a decision making activity of some difficulty, which like all professions, has its problems and its beliefs, hierarchies, structures and its bad habits. Nevertheless, to some extent, it's trying its best to accommodate these things. Certainly in Great Britain, we just do not have counselors in the sense that the word exists in some other communities : we only let medically qualified people with postgraduate experience in pediatrics or something relevant, obstetrics or similar, loose in this situation. This may be a bad thing but this is how it works, we do not have counseling divorced from medicine and try not to integrate it.

J. Kere : We have a medical problem here, which is the counseling situation, and then we have the conservative cure with the old kind of counseling but we now also have a radical cure for that, that is using the model. In medicine, we usually make a clinical trial between these two cures and then we evaluate the results and decide if it's useful to use the new radical cure. I would like to hear some comments of both groups here about how to evaluate the outcome of these two methods.

S. Pauker : I like to kickoff that discussion with a case. This is one of the cases that I presented in my paper in this symposium from a data base of 850; it is particularly significant for what we have been talking about the outcome (see case 8 p. 164). It relates to what we talked about earlier, whether you judge the decision by the outcome, which in this case is extremely negative, the worst outcome, or whether you discuss it by how she felt in terms of her comfort, whatever that is, with the decision process. I think this is a good kickoff for a discussion about outcome.

J.J. Cassiman : I would like to have somebody, who comes from a completely different field, the ethical and moral field, give his impressions on what has been said thusfar.

G. Van Steendam : The subject of this symposium was "decision making". I've got the idea that there are at least two levels in decision making and I think all or nearly all the papers, were related to the first level. I mean, all the papers were trying to help people to make the right decision about what to do with their own values. The problem is that there is a second level of decision, the decisions about the values themselves. We assume people have their values but don't find them, don't know them, don't communicate them and we didn't treat the problem, we didn't speak about the problem of people not knowing their values, or not even knowing how to shape a value, when they are willing to change their values for example. I'm just asking myself if there is any model or any way to help these people in their decision making about the values themselves?

J. Porter : It was mentioned that there were two groups here, the theorists on the one side that really don't or have very little contact with the actual patient and the doctors on the other hand who have all the contact with the patients. I just like to mention that there is a very important middlegroup which is the psychologists here and they happen to be the quietest group. I know some psychologists who are in the middle between the theorists and the genetic counselors : they are the ones who are actually doing research and trying to bring the two fields together. I just would like to know if there's anyone here who is actually working in that kind of area, trying to bring the two fields together and actually trying to please the two camps. It's a great shame that we have not yet had the nerve to actually stand up and say "Let's change the area and let's have some input from those people who have looked analytically at the counseling process itself".

G. Evers-Kiebooms : I think you have raised a very important question since it was the main purpose of this meeting to bridge the gap between two groups : first the researchers working in the field of risk perception and decision making and secondly people working as genetic counselors and psychologists involved in research or more clinical psychological activities in genetic centers.

C. Vlek : I hate not to be a woman for the moment, but it may please the lady to hear that by far the majority of the speakers of the second session of the symposium are psychologists. Let me also try to answer part of your question. First of all, you asked for ongoing research. I know of some very active people in the Department of Medical Sociology at Groningen University, who are doing research on attitudes of women vis-à-vis amniocentesis, judgement and decision processes in genetic counseling, the sort of work I think that you are asking questions about. You complained about the fact that we seemed to address only "the middle part" of what is going on in genetic counseling, the middle part being the risk judgement and decision making part (the prior part being that you have to receive and deal with a client who comes in in a hectic emotional state, severely under stress; and the later part being that you send away the client with some sort of advice, with some clarification of his or her problems and the client has to cope with his or her situation at home). Regarding the first part, my functional view would be that it is the task of genetic counselors to attempt to transform the emotional state of the client into something workable, which means that you may try to point at the deleterious effects of stress on judgement and decision making. For example, Janis and Mann have some beautiful research on that. You may attempt to get the patient gradually think and talk in terms of possible courses of action, possible ways of dealing with negative consequences instead of raising hell about all the bad things she or he expects, that is just expressive behavior and not functional. You have to try to turn expressive behavior into functional behavior, not disrespecting the expression of emotions, of course. If they come to you, they pay money for your assistance. The least you can do is to try to help them to turn from expressive behavior into functional behavior. Concerning the later part, once you've gone through some sort of decision procedure or counseling procedure, I think perhaps more attention should be paid to an assessment of the demands that a situation at home will put upon the client and an assessment of the abilities and possible indication of tricks and strategies for the client to cope with that situation. So the whole idea of stress, appraising task demands and assessing coping abilities, is somewhat underrated and should be incorporated into the whole genetic counseling procedure, but I must confess that I have too little experience with genetic counseling to be able to appraise whether I tell anything new.

J. Edwards : We haven't actually heard from the consumer. We have heard from the intermediaries and when the market place was mentioned during the symposium, it was actually the "marketer" rather than the market "place" and there has been a remarkable lack of informed consumers discussing it. There has been almost no literature written by patients about what they demand, although in Oxford we have a large number of patients, who are very knowledgeable and psychologists. When the time comes they seem extraordinarily disinterested in trying to make use of their experience to undertake surveys of what people want and what their values are. There is very little data on what I might call normal expectations to pregnancy : whether the people want to be messed around by counselors, whether they want to talk about it, what they want to have done, what are their risks? Apart from a study in Birmingham by Sarah Bundey, which resulted in a very good article on the attitudes of 40-years-old college graduates towards amniocentesis, I really know very little of what the informed consumer expects from well-meaning males and other technocrats and people.

J.J. Cassiman : I don't know Dr. Edwards if you are aware that you are sitting next to a consumer and I would like to ask Dr. Evers-Kiebooms to phrase the question that consumers have put to her.

G. Evers-Kiebooms : In Leuven, we have very close collaboration between the genetic centre and some associations of concerned patients and families. All the research we were doing about cystic fibrosis was in collaboration with the Belgian Cystic Fibrosis Association, and the same was true for the Huntington Disease Association. For other studies we were working with other associations too. This is a very good means to get feedback, and to know the real problems and the real reactions of the families concerned. One of the reactions of the President of the Huntington Disease Association in Belgium is that we were talking all the time about amniocentesis and pregnancy interruption in the case of a positive result. When there will be presymptomatic diagnosis of the Huntington disease, detection will be done on adolescents or on adult asymptomatic persons. So, we must be aware of the fact that all those persons will have to live and to cope with the positive result.

J. Edwards : Sorry, I was misunderstood. I was meaning, if I might use the term without offence "normal women", women without the terrible problems of already having had a child with some disorder or having had a family of Huntingtons. I was meaning a random section of women. I know you did a beautiful work and this fills a very big gap but there is still a gap of what one might call the normal potential consumer.

St. Pauker : I'm not quite sure how things go in Britain but I'm confused by the use of the restriction of consumer to the woman. In the States, it takes two people to make a pregnancy and in most circumstances I would think that the potential father is as much an important consumer of counseling and provider of decision making as the mother. I am somewhat bothered by what might be going on in Britain.

J.J. Cassiman : Let's try to round up the discussion.

S. Pauker : I just want to say that this conference has served a very important liaison because for us it's the first time we become familiar with the psychology literature. It certainly has existed, as long as ours and perhaps longer. This conference has served that function of bridging. The points, made in the paper of Humphreys and Berkeley, and other points mentioned here, bring up aspects of decision making that we now need to incorporate into what we do and model the concept of the levels which is another way of looking at how one approaches the decision making. They are very exciting and bring up all kinds of new ideas for how to look at this. I'm just as you say bringing in the societies for helping people to look at the consumer. For us, in a sense, we are the consumer of how to do this thinking about decision making and we will go forth with this information and have new networks for talking to people about it. So this conference is the first time that, as far as I know, it hasn't just been my husband and I talking to each other, bringing two fields together, where we are really trying to move forward. In the New England Journal where there will be a review article very soon about decision making, in which genetics and the psychological aspects of the counseling will show to be prominent. In the decision society that my husband helped to start, we start to see people talking more and more about counseling as it applies in other fields, particularly genetics. I think you will see more and more of this : that is what I was meaning about taking the time to percolate. But this conference has served that function more than anything I have seen in the whole time we have been at this.

J.J. Cassiman : We will try to formulate some conclusions if that's any way possible. Would you agree that if geneticists are somewhat reticent to use decision making tools in genetic counseling, that there may be a role for clinical psychologists, accepted on the one hand by the genetic counselors and understanding on the other hand the people who are working in decision making? Would you agree that there may be an important role for them as "go-between" between the two fields?

E. Meulepas : I am afraid of the phenomenon traduttore traditore. If you have the go-between psychologists who have to translate mathematics in words in order that the clinicians should understand them, I rather prefer that the model makers themselves as Mohammed would go to the mountain and translate it themselves into words. I rather prefer the mathematician to translate in ordinary language and not to use a go-between psychologist who maybe has chosen the study of psychology because he didn't know enough mathematics.

J. Porter : As stated previously from the other side of the room (= the model builders), and they are psychologists as well, there are different aspects of psychology. The psychologists here that do the practical research have the theoretical know-how of how to do those mathematical formulations and they can interpret the results very well

J.J. Cassiman : Any other comments from the two fields, the genetic counselors and the people from the psychology field?

P. Humphreys : Perhaps I should say this, I can wear several hats sometimes because I do spend about a quarter of my time in organization of decision making, working directly with clients who pay me. So, we have to see how our tools work that way. I'm also a psychologist. I'm also involved in building software responsable for a unit where a lot of software is built, that's where I was doing consultancy. Maybe I can wear more than one hat but unfortunately I can not wear the hat of a genetic counselor or even a psychologist working with genetic counselors and that's why we didn't bring any of that in. In terms of go-between, I think it is probably the wrong word. People need to bring the skills they really have. Clinical psychologists have different skills from modelers, have different skills from people who have a full understanding of the genetic side of genetic counseling and these skills need to be brought together. My feeling is that this needs to be a joint effort, but to make it a joint effort it also means each of us has to learn if not everybody's language, at least one other person's language to get the communication and to think about not how our tools are good for us, but how we can redevelop what matters in this joint context we are all trying to work in.

J. Dumon : I only want to make a comment as a clinical geneticist. Ten or twenty years ago, what we could do for patients with a genetic problem was only "Mendelian counseling", giving them some risk figures. Now, more and more medical technology enables us to offer them a lot of possibilities, like chorion biopsy, amniocentesis, DNA-analysis etc. I feel that we need some backup with or without models. We need to know exactly what we are doing for the patient, for the family. Not only what we are doing for ourselves scientifically, medically etc., but what we are doing for the real patient, the person in flesh and blood. I think that as Mrs. Porter and Dr. G. Evers-Kiebooms said, we need clinical psychologists to question the patients on : "What did the guy tell you? how did you understand what he told you, how did you cope emotionally with what he or she told you?" So, I think there is room for clinical psychologists in genetic departments.

J.J. Cassiman : We'll stop the discussion here. I thank those who participated and those who listened. It's a discussion that could go on for many more hours and days and maybe this is a good reason to plan something for the near future.

LIST OF PARTICIPANTS

S. AGHAMOHAMMADI, The University of Sussex, Biology Building, Centre for Medical Research, Falmer, BRIGHTON SUSSEX BN1 9QG, U.K.

Montserrat BAIGET, Hospital de la Santa Creu I Sant Pau, Servei d'Hematologia, Avgda. S. Antoni, M.ª Claret 167, 08025 BARCELONA, SPAIN

Marie Françoise BERTHEAS, Labo Hématologie Cytogénétique, CHRU St-Etienne, Hôpital Nord, Av. Albert Raimond, 42277 ST.PRIEST-EN-JAREZ Cedex, FRANCE

Anne BILLEN, Tiensestraat 102, B-3000 LEUVEN, BELGIUM

Anne Marie BLOCK, Department of Genetics and Endocrinology, Cancer Cell Center, Roswell Park Memorial Institute, 666 Elm Street, BUFFALO NY 14263, U.S.A.

Andrea BOOGAERTS, Boogaardstraat 9, B-2800 MECHELEN, BELGIUM

Aldar Slavic BOURINBAIAR, King's College Hospital, Haematology Department, Denmark Hill, LONDON SE5 9RS, ENGLAND

Sabine BROCATUS, Kerkhovensesteenweg 425, B-3900 LOMMEL, BELGIUM

Stefaan CEUPPENS, Steendreef 11, B-2959 ELEWIJT, BELGIUM

Trees CLOOSTERMANS, Losbergenlaan 18, B-3200 KESSEL-LO, BELGIUM

Paola Silvia DAL CIN, Roswell Park Memorial Institute, Department of Genetics and Endocrinology, 666 Elm Street, BUFFALO NY 14263, U.S.A.

Roger DE MEYER, Université Catholique de Louvain, Cliniques Universitaires Saint-Luc, Département de Pédiatrie, Avenue Hippocrate 10, B-1200 BRUXELLES, BELGIUM

Lieve DENAYER, K.U. Leuven, Centrum voor Menselijke Erfelijkheid, Campus Gasthuisberg, Herestraat, B-3000 LEUVEN, BELGIUM

Jan P. DUMANSKI, Department of Clinical Genetics, Karolinska Sjukhuset, P.O. Box 60500, 104 01 STOCKHOLM 60, SWEDEN

Jan DUMON, Medische Genetica - U.I.A., Universiteitsplein 1, B-2610 WILRIJK, BELGIUM

Bernd DWORNICZAK, Zentrum Für Molekulare Biologie, Universität Heidelberg, Im Neuenheimer Feld 282, 6900 HEIDELBERG 1, GERMANY

María Teresa FERRO, Servicio de Genetica Medica, Ministerio de Sanidad y Seguridad Social, MADRID-34, SPAIN

P.G. FRETS, Erasmus Universiteit Rotterdam, Afdeling Klinische Genetica, Postbus 1738, 3000 DR ROTTERDAM, NEDERLAND

M. FREUND, U.C.L., Service de Pédiatrie, Avenue Hippocrate 10, B-1200 BRUXELLES, BELGIUM

Irène GARCIA, Département de Pédiatrie et Génétique, Institut Universitaire de Génétique Médicale, CMU - 9 av. de Champel, 1211 GENEVE, SUISSE

Dorotea GARGANO, Via Enrico Fermi 23, 50047 PRATO, FIRENZE, ITALY

Francesca GHIONE, Dipartimento di pediatria "Cesare Cocchi", Ospedale Meyer, Via Luca Giordano 13, 50132 FIRENZE, ITALY

Hit Kishori GOSWAMI, Department of Genetics, Bhopal University, BHOPAL 462 026, INDIA

L.C.P. GOVAERTS, Afdeling Erfelijkheidsvoorlichting, Anthropogenetisch Instituut, Ant. Deusinglaan 4, 9713 AW GRONINGEN, NEDERLAND

Marcel GULICKX, De Dries 6, B-2130 BRASSCHAAT, BELGIUM

Wolfram HENN, Institut für Humangenetik, Universität, Bau 68, 6650 HOMBURG/SAAR, GERMANY

Luc HENS, Vrije Universiteit Brussel, Laarbeeklaan 103, B-1090 BRUSSEL, BELGIUM

Jo HUYS, Standonckstraat 3, B-3000 LEUVEN, BELGIUM

Elly IPPEL, Stichting Klinisch Genetisch Centrum, Postbus 18009, 3501 CA UTRECHT, NEDERLAND

Juha KERE, University of Helsinki, Department of Medical Genetics, Haartmaninkatu 3, 00290 HELSINKI 29, FINLAND

Irene LARRIPA, Academia Nacional de Medicina de Buenos Aires, Instituto de Investigaciones Hematologicas, Section Citogenetica, PACHECO DE MELO 3081 (1425), BUENOS AIRES

Dominique LEROUX, Laboratoire de Cytogénétique, Centre Hospitalier Régional et Universitaire de Grenoble, B.P. 217 X, 38043 GRENOBLE CEDEX, FRANCE

I. LIEBAERS, Medische Genetika, V.U.B., Laarbeeklaan 103/E, B-1090 BRUSSEL, BELGIUM

Jeanne-Marie LIBOUTON, Cliniques Universitaires Saint-Luc, Service de Pédiatrie, Avenue Hippocrate 10, B-1200 BRUXELLES, BELGIUM

Valerie LINDGREN, National Institutes of Health, Building 41, Room D201, BETHESDA, MARYLAND 20892, U.S.A.

Antonio MARTINO, p.za B. Zumbini 72, 87100 COSENZA, ITALY

H. MEIJER, Rijksuniversiteit Limburg, Capaciteitsgroep Genetica/ Celbiologie, Postbus 616, 6200 MD MAASTRICHT, NEDERLAND

Thomas MEITINGER, Genetics Laboratory, Department of Biochemistry, South Parks Road, OXFORD OX1 3QU, ENGLAND

Nicole MICHIELS, Lismortel 27, B-3900 LOMMEL, BELGIUM

Agnès MOINE, Centre Départemental de Transfusion Sanguine de la Savoie, Faubourg Maché, B.P. 1125, 73011 CHAMBERY CEDEX, FRANCE

Hans MORREAU, Afdeling Celbiologie & Genetica, Erasmus Universiteit Rotterdam, Postbus 1738, 3000 DR ROTTERDAM, NEDERLAND

Ulrich MUELLER, Adolf Martars Strasse 10, 1000 BERLIN 31, WEST GERMANY

Pat NESS, 704 Symphony Place, 1117 Marquette Avenue South, MINNEAPOLIS, MINNESOTA 55403, U.S.A.

Giuseppe NOVELLI, Cattedra di Genetica, Università degli Studi, Via saffi 2, 61029 URBINO (PS), ITALY

Virginia NUNES, Hospital de la Santa Creu I Sant Pau, Servei d'Hematologia, Avgda. S. Antoni M.[a] Claret 167, 08025 BARCELONA, SPAIN

Stefan OEYEN, Kerkhovensesteenweg 425, B-3900 LOMMEL, BELGIUM

Huguette PISON, Laboratoire de Cytogénétique, Centre Hosp. Régional et Univ. de Grenoble, B.P. 217 X, 38043 GRENOBLE CEDEX, FRANCE

Berardino PORFIRIO, II Università degli Studi di Roma, Dipartimento di sanita' publica e biologia cellulare, Via Orazio Raimondo, 00173 ROMA, ITALY

Janice Adele PORTER, Clinical Genetics, Birmingham Maternity Hospital, Edgbaston, BIRMINGHAM B15 2TG, ENGLAND

Robert RANYARD, Psychology Department, Higher Education, Deane Rd., BOLTON BL3 5AB, GREAT BRITAIN

Alvaro RINGRESSI, V.L. Bardelli 7, 50 139 FIRENZE, ITALY

Antonella ROSETTI, Università di Perugia, Instituto Di Clinica Medica Generale e Terapia Medica I, Policlinico Monteluce, 06100 PERUGIA, ITALY

B. ROZENDAL, Katholieke Universiteit Nijmegen, Sint Radboudziekenhuis, Geert Grooteplein Zuid 20, Postbus 9101, 6500 HB NIJMEGEN, NEDERLAND

SAI-MEI HE, Department of Clinical Genetics, Karolinska Hospital, P.O. Box 60500, 104 01 STOCKHOLM, SWEDEN

Sheila N.J. SAIT, Roswell Park Memorial Institute, Department of Genetics and Endocrinology, 666 Elm Street, BUFFALO NY 14263, U.S.A.

Detlev SCHINDLER, Universität Würzburg, Humangenetik, Koellikerstrasse 2, 8700 WURZBURG, GERMANY

Peter SCHMID, Universität Ulm, Abteilung Klinische Genetik, Oberer Eselsberg, M 25, 7900 ULM, GERMANY

Constance SCHRANDER-STUMPEL, Lenculenstraat 19B, 6211 KP MAASTRICHT, NEDERLAND

Cathérine SERCK-DEROM, Kwadenplasstraat 20, B-3740 DESTELBERGEN (HEUSDEN), BELGIUM

Françoise SERVILLE, Résidence Dauphine, 120, Avenue Louis Barthou,

33200 BORDEAUX, FRANCE

Luca SINEO, Università degli Studi di Firenze, Instituto di Antropologia, Via del Proconsolo 12, 50122 FIRENZE, ITALY

Christine SMULDERS, M. van Coehoornstraat 11A, 6217 LR MAASTRICHT, NEDERLAND

Mirja SOMER, Department of Medical Genetics, Kalevankatu 16, SF-00100 HELSINKI 10, FINLAND

Jean Raymond TEYSSIER, Centre Hospitalier Régional et Universitaire de Reims, Hôpital Maison Blanche, Cytogénétique, 45, Rue Cognacq-Jay, 51092 REIMS Cedex, FRANCE

Ulrike THIES, Institut für Humangenetik, Universitätskliniken Göttingen, Gosslerstrasse 12d, 3400 GOTTINGEN, GERMANY

Iongvah THINGNGANING, Department of Chemistry, Science College, KOHIMA 797 001, NAGALAND

Loes THOMASSEN-BREPOLS, Bovenover 10, 3062 CC ROTTERDAM, NEDERLAND

Christine VAN BROECKHOVEN, Universitaire Instelling Antwerpen, Departement Biochemie, Universiteitsplein 1, B-2610 ANTWERPEN-WILRIJK, BELGIUM

Henny VAN DEN BOSSCHE, Dienst Medische Genetica, Academisch Ziekenhuis, Blok A, De Pintelaan 185, B-9000 GENT, BELGIUM

Annick VAN DEN BRUL, Hoogstraat 7, B-1870 WOLVERTEM, BELGIUM

August VAN ELSEN, Labo voor Genetica, Universitaire Instelling Antwerpen, Universiteitsplein 1, B-2610 ANTWERPEN-WILRIJK, BELGIUM

A.J. VAN ESSEN, Afdeling Erfelijkheidsvoorlichting, Anthropogenetisch Instituut, Ant. Deusinglaan 4, 9713 AW GRONINGEN, NEDERLAND

Hugo VAN HEUVERSWIJN, Innogenetics, Industriepark Zwijnaarde 7, box 4, B-9710 GENT, BELGIUM

Luc VAN HOVE, Dienst Hematologie, U.Z. Gasthuisberg, Herestraat, B-3000 LEUVEN, BELGIUM

Bernard A. VAN OOST, p/a Prof. Dr. H.H. Ropers, Faculteit der

Geneeskunde en Tandheelkunde, Anthropogenetisch Instituut, Postbus 9101, 6500 HB NIJMEGEN, NEDERLAND

Guido VAN STEENDAM, Craenendonck 15, B-3000 LEUVEN, BELGIUM

Lars O. VEJERSLEV, The John F. Kennedy Institute, Department of Medical Genetics, 7 Gl. Landevej, DK 2600 GLOSTRUP, DENMARK

C. VERELLEN-DUMOULIN, Université Catholique de Louvain, Cliniques Universitaires Saint-Luc, Département de Pédiatrie, Avenue Hippocrate 10, B-1200 BRUXELLES, BELGIQUE

A. VERHEST, Département Cytogénétique, Institut Jules Bordet, 1 rue Heger Bordet, B-1000 BRUXELLES, BELGIQUE

Martin WERNER, Institut für Humangenetik, Universität, Bau 68, 6650 HOMBURG/SAAR, GERMANY

Bernhard ZABEL, Klinikum der Johannes Gutenberg-Universität, Kinderklinik und Kinder-Poliklinik, Postfach 3960, Langenbeckstrasse 1, 6500 MAINZ, GERMANY

Index